TABLE OF CONTENTS

Welcome to the
PHYSICAL
EDUCATION
PROGRAM

MISSION STATEMENT

Physical Education is an integral part of the total education process. Our educators believe in a sound mind and a sound body at any ability level. Schools are responsible for teaching students to use skills in real-world settings. Our mission in Physical Education is to help students reach their maximum potential in order to ensure a healthy, productive life. Physical Education explains how and why the body moves, promoting students' mental and social development through performing physical activities. The course also provides students with the knowledge and skills to become healthy and active individuals. By participating regularly in a broad spectrum of activities, students—regardless of ability level—are able to meet physical challenges; develop essential motor skills; assess their individual abilities; appreciate the joy of human movement; and develop strategies for physical improvement.

PHYSICAL EDUCATION REQUIREMENTS

REQUIREMENTS FOR PHYSICAL EDUCATION

- Students in grades 7-12 should complete **72 hours** of Physical Education activities for a passing grade. In other words, you should average three hours of activity per week for 24 weeks.

- Your school will notify you if they require more or less than 72 hours.

- You may begin documenting your hours from the first day of your school year until your completion date.

- Each week, record your hours and activities in the electronic Physical Education Log. Save the Physical Education Log in your user file on your computer.

- Record your activities by the day. Do not group activities by the week or month.

- Record no more than three activity hours per day in your log. If you record more than three hours per day, your instructor will give you a chance to fix your log to fit this criterion.

- The Physical Education department understands that when you play a sport, your competitions and practices may last longer than three hours. That is acceptable and is why we ask that you fill out the Organized or Team Sports Verification Log instead of the Physical Education Log.

- You can find the Organized or Team Sports Verification Log online in your Physical Education course or on page 7 of this workbook.

- The Physical Education Log and the Organized or Team Sports Verification Log are the **only** forms accepted for Physical Education credit. We do not accept handwritten forms.

- Submit your Physical Education Log or Organized or Sports Team Sports Verification log through your Physical Education course.

- It is recommended that you record **50 percent** of your Physical Education activities from this workbook.

You may choose to participate in any of the activities shown in the chart below; be sure to record these in your Physical Education Log or Organized or Team Sports Verification Log. Work is not an acceptable Physical Education activity. Examples of work include occupations, yard work, household chores, etc. Any activity not listed below must be pre-approved by your Physical Education instructor.

Sports	Lifetime/Leisure	Fitness
Archery	Biking/Scooter/	Aerobics
Baseball	Skateboarding	Calisthenics
Basketball	Bowling	Cardio Videos
Football	Canoe/Kayak	Fitness Videos
Golf	Dance	Gymnastics
Hockey	Frisbee/Bocce/Target Games	Jump Rope
Lacrosse	Horseback Riding	Martial Arts
Racket Sports	Kickball/Four Square	Stationary Exercise
Soccer	Playground Activities	Equipment
Swimming	Skiing/Skating/Snowboarding	Yoga
Volleyball	Tag/Active Games	Zumba®
Water Sports	Walking/Running	
Wrestling	Wall Climbing	

PHYSICAL EDUCATION FORMS

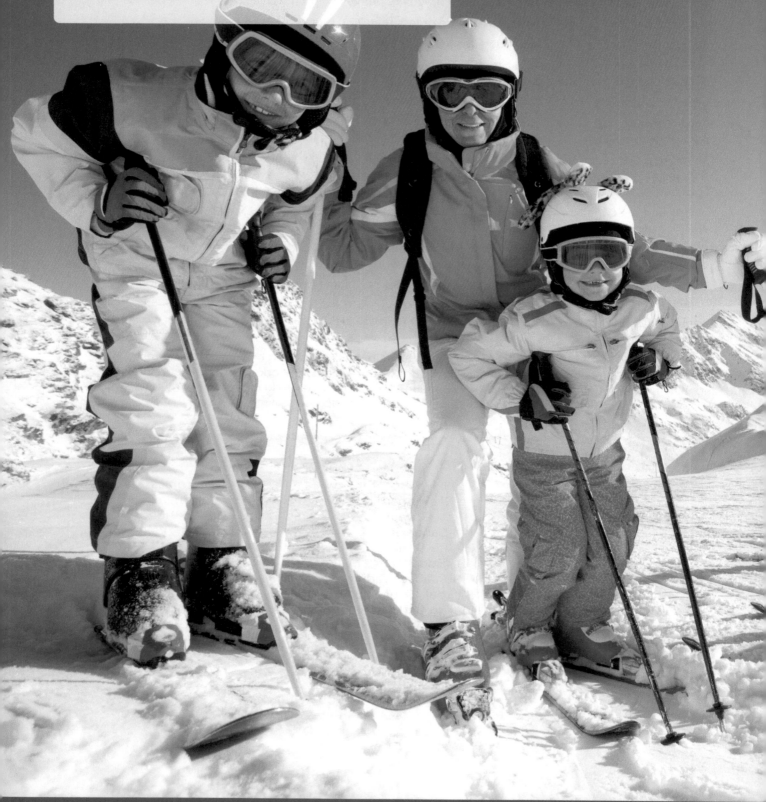

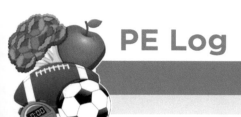

PE Log

The PE Log (Physical Education Log) will track the various activities that you complete as part of the requirements for this course. It is recommended that you complete no more than three activity hours per day.

To complete the PE Log, enter your information in the open fields below. Then, in the table, enter the date you completed the activity, the name of the activity, the amount of time you participated (in hours), and the kit item (if applicable). **Note:** Farm work, part time jobs, and household chores do not count as valid activities.

You must complete all areas of this form in order to receive credit.

Remember to save this document to your computer. You will be instructed to submit the log periodically throughout the course; therefore, you should always be adding your hours to the log. When prompted to submit the log, turn in your completed PE Log to your instructor through your Physical Education course.

Student Name and ID:

_____

Telephone Number:

_____

Instructor and Course Name:

_____

Email Address:

_____

Parent/Guardian:

_____

Total Activity Hours **(72 Hours Required):**

_____

You may choose to **add** any of the following **unorganized** activities to the Physical Education Log: swimming, basketball, archery, Ultimate Frisbee, walking, running, hiking, biking, wall climbing, golf, bowling, weight lifting, aerobics, cardio, football, snowboarding, volleyball, tumbling/gymnastics, calisthenics, stretching, skiing, canoeing, kayaking, martial arts, horseback riding, Wii Fit, yoga, Zumba, dance, fencing, racket sports, softball, or baseball.

PE Log

Date	Physical Activity	Participation Time (in hours)	Physical Education Kit Item
09-01	Running	.25	electronic movement band

ORGANIZED OR TEAM SPORTS VERIFICATION LOG

- This form can be submitted in place of or in conjunction with the Physical Education Log.
- The fields on this document should not be altered.
- Remember to save this document to your computer.
- Submit completed electronic sports verification log through your physical education course.
- The sports verification log is for organized or team sports only.
- Please remember to complete the rest of your Physical Education course upon submitting this form.
- Please only list the HOURS, not minutes, of your activities. If you want to list minutes, use decimals such as 0.25 for 15 minutes.

Student Name: _____

Student ID#: _____ Student Grade Level: _____

Physical Education Instructor: _____

Coach's Name: _____ Home School District:_____

Telephone Number: ( ) - _____ Email Address: _____

Total Activity Hours:_____ **(72 hours are required)** Parent/Guardian: _____

Students may include organized or team sports from the fall, winter, or spring seasons. Sports may include, but are not limited to: football, golf, soccer, volleyball, tennis, cross country, field hockey, baseball, softball, track, lacrosse, basketball, wrestling, rifling, gymnastics, swimming and diving.

Date	Sport Played	HOURS ONLY	Game or Practice
09-01	Football	1.5 hours	Game

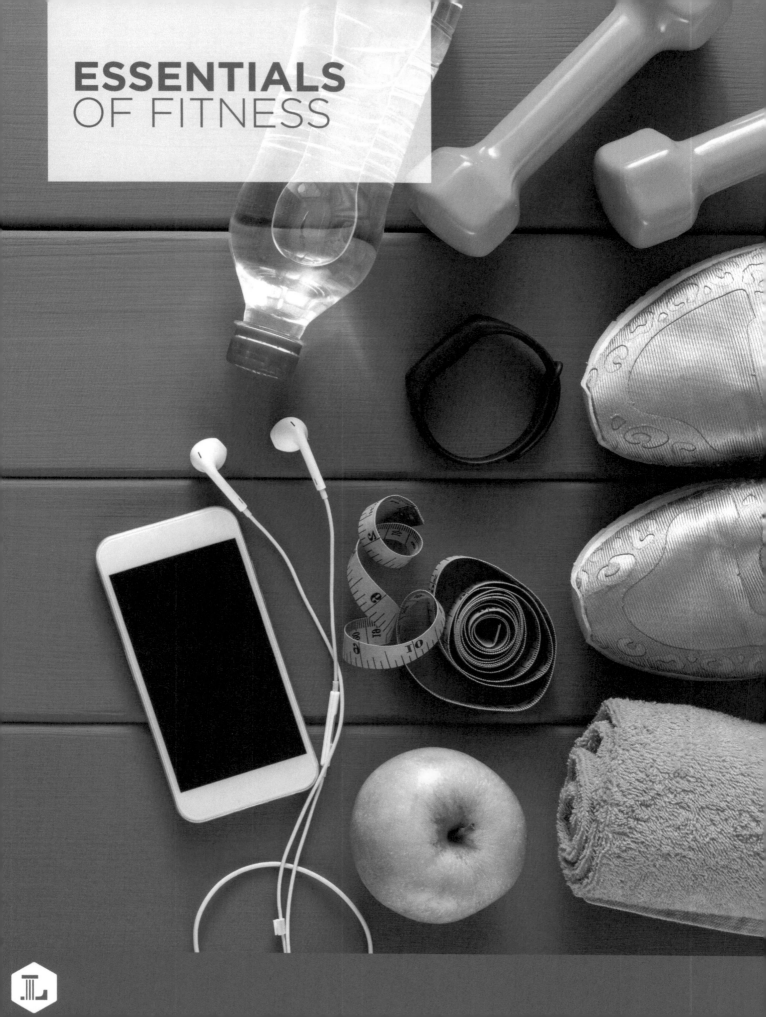

ESSENTIALS
OF FITNESS

HEALTH-RELATED FITNESS COMPONENTS

Health-related fitness components are the areas that make up total fitness. It is important to be balanced in all categories and to stay active in order to ensure good physical health. Staying active has many benefits, such as decreasing the risk of illness and chronic disease; increasing metabolic rate, which allows for food to be converted into energy more easily; building muscular strength and endurance; burning more calories; increasing heart and lung function; and so on. The 5 health-related fitness components provide a guideline on which to base your fitness levels and set goals for your workouts and exercise routines.

BODY COMPOSITION
the ratio of fat to muscle

CARDIOVASCULAR ENDURANCE
the ability of your heart and lungs to supply oxygen to your body

FLEXIBILITY
the ability of your muscles and joints to move through a full range of motion

MUSCULAR ENDURANCE
the ability of your muscles to exert force for an extended period of time

MUSCULAR STRENGTH
the ability of your muscles to exert maximum force in a single effort

SKILL-RELATED COMPONENTS

Skill-related components are the different areas of physical functioning. The 6 skill-related components are not as important for overall health and wellness as the health-related fitness components, but they are vital parts of basic, everyday movements. These components are associated not only with sports and activities but also with daily functions, such as climbing stairs or crossing the street. Being skillful in these areas can also allow you to perform better during athletics.

AGILITY
the ability to change the position of your body quickly but with control

BALANCE
The ability to maintain stabilization while moving and staying still

COORDINATION
the ability to use your senses together with moving body parts

POWER
the ability to use speed and force in movement and actions

REACTION TIME
the ability to move quickly when responding to stimuli

SPEED
the ability to cover a distance within a short period of time

WELLNESS-RELATED COMPONENTS

Wellness-related components are the other aspects of a good quality of life. It takes more than physical fitness to have overall wellness. To live a balanced life, you need to take care of all areas of your mind, body, and spirit. Practicing good habits in the 5 areas of health and wellness can allow you to grow as a person and develop confidence and purpose. This can lead to a joyful, productive life.

EMOTIONAL HEALTH
the ability to control and express your emotions appropriately

ENVIRONMENTAL HEALTH
the ability to maintain a clean and safe area around you

MENTAL HEALTH
the ability to recognize reality and cope with the demands of life

SOCIAL HEALTH
the ability to interact with people and have appropriate relationships

SPIRITUAL HEALTH
the ability to have direction and purpose

Discuss the health-related, skill-related, and wellness-related components with a trusted friend or an adult. List the components that are most important to you and the exercises that you can do to improve and maintain your overall physical and emotional health.

Question	Answer
What components do I want to improve upon or maintain?	
What can I do to reach my goal?	

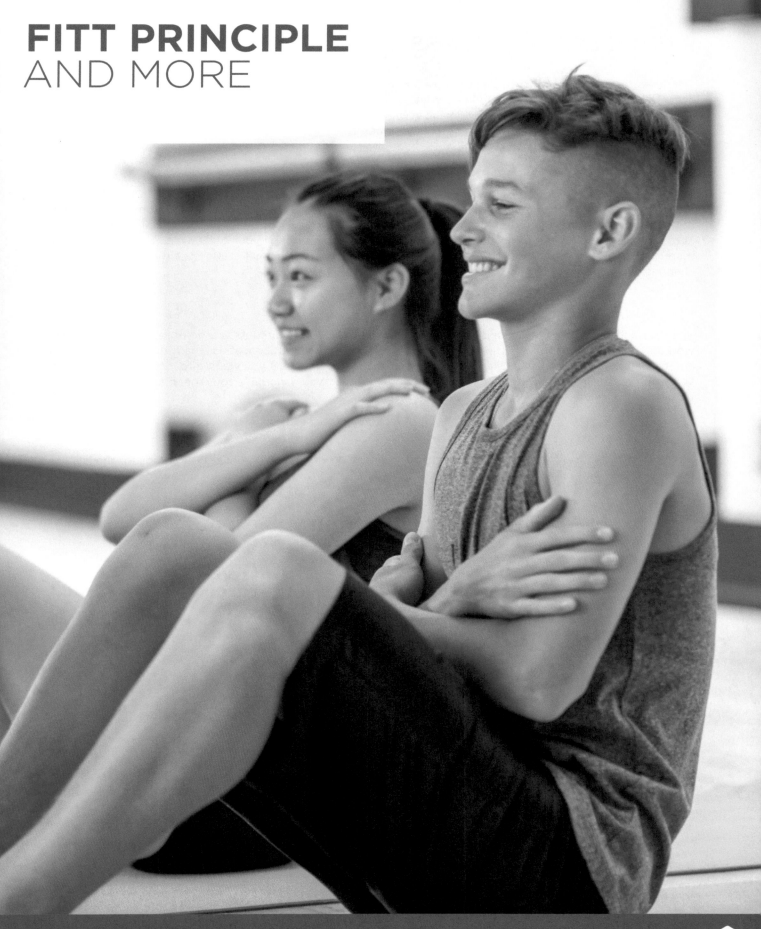

FITT PRINCIPLE
AND MORE

PRINCIPLES OF FITNESS

The fitness principles below provide structure for creating your own workout plan. Each of the principles has its own classifications, but they all work in coordination with each other to ensure a quality program that will lead to maximum results. After you have a specific goal written, make sure that you review each of the principles thoroughly to create a suitable plan that meets your needs.

THE OVERLOAD PRINCIPLE

The overload principle describes how your body reacts to the workload that is placed upon it. Your body responds to the amount of exercise and training that you make it do and adapts to it. It becomes accustomed to the exercise and the amount of effort that is needed. At this point, you no longer have to work as hard to perform, so change no longer occurs. You consistently want to challenge your body by increasing its workload, therefore increasing your fitness level. You can increase its workload in small stages, but these will lead to big changes over time.

THE SPECIFICITY PRINCIPLE

The specificity principle corresponds to your goals and the types of workouts you do or muscles you use. Your workouts should correspond to the goal at hand. You want to be intentional about the exercises you perform and the muscles you use to focus on reaching your goal. For example, if you wanted to increase your mile time, you would want to concentrate on exercises or workouts that would increase your speed and improve your cardiovascular endurance.

THE FITT PRINCIPLE

The FITT principle is a formula for designing your exercise program. The acronym *FITT* stands for the key components of a good workout.

Frequency: how often you exercise
example: 3 times per week

Intensity: how hard you exercise
example: 80 percent of your maximum heart rate

Time: how long you exercise
example: 60 minutes

Type: what kind of exercise
example: cardiovascular endurance workout, such as running on a treadmill

THE REST AND RECOVERY PRINCIPLE

The rest and recovery principle is very important for reaching your goals and preventing injury. While it is vital to work out consistently to maximize your potential, it is also just as important to rest the muscles that were used to allow growth and development. It is suggested that you push your muscles past the point of exhaustion, as explained in the overload principle, but you do not want to overstrain your muscles and cause injury. For example, when you are strength training, you never want to work the same muscles 2 days in a row because your body needs time to rest and recover.

THE USE OR LOSE PRINCIPLE

The use or lose principle simply stated is the principle that if you do not use it, you will lose it. When you work out or otherwise move your body, you build up your muscles and increase your strength, which is hypertrophy; however, if you do not stay active, you will lose your strength and your muscles will atrophy. Finding a balance of activity and exercise is important to your overall health and wellness. Staying active keeps your body physically healthy and your brain mentally healthy. Possible alternatives are lack of muscle tone, lack of strength, illness, becoming overweight, lower energy levels, and so on.

Limit sitting at computers, playing video games, and watching TV.

Every day, walk or stay active for at least **60 minutes.**

Activity Recommendations

3 to 5 times per week, give your heart and lungs an aerobic workout.

3 or more times per week, strengthen and stretch your muscles.

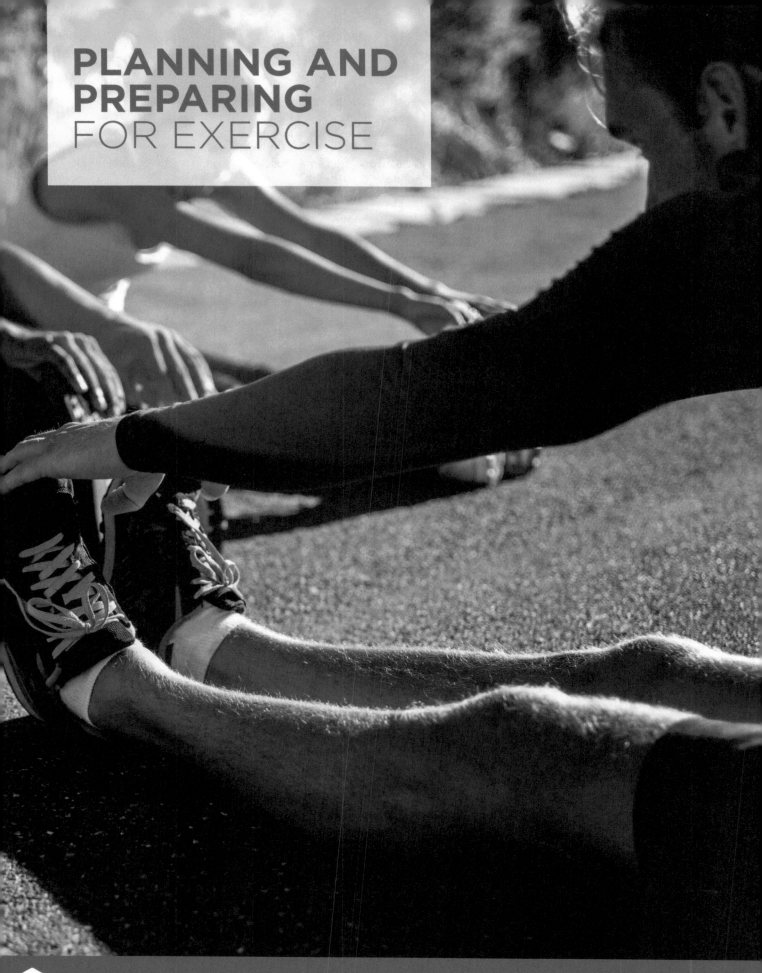

PLANNING AND PREPARING
FOR EXERCISE

WARM-UP AND COOL-DOWN

Before beginning a workout or exercise program or performing moderate to vigorous activity, you need to be sure that you are physically and mentally prepared. There are steps to take prior to participating in physical activity to ensure safety, success, and results. Having a set plan to follow when you are exercising allows you to maximize your time and allows you to reach your goals more efficiently. Knowing how to properly prepare your body for physical activity helps you prevent injury and keeps you safe. The following warm-up, cool-down, and weather precaution information will provide tools and tips for you to design a workout routine or activity session suited for your needs.

The importance of a warm-up is that it prepares your body for exercise. A good warm-up should increase your heart rate, breathing rate, and body temperature. You can do traditional warm-up activities like jumping jacks or jumping rope, or you can perform other warm-up activities like using cardiovascular endurance equipment, dancing, or walking. Once you have completed your warm-up, you are ready to begin your exercise. Reversely, when you have finished your exercise, you should do a cool-down. Your body needs to return to baseline—your heart rate, breathing rate, and body temperature must all decrease back to a resting level. Some examples of cool-down activities include stretching, walking, and relaxation practices such as deep breathing and guided imagery. Warming up and cooling down are essential to the physical activity process.

WARM-UP SUGGESTIONS:

1. Complete 3 sets of 10 to 15 repetitions of each of the exercises below.

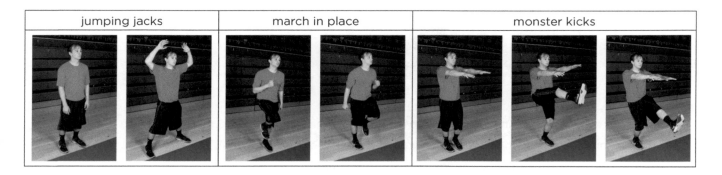

jumping jacks	march in place	monster kicks

2. Use a piece of cardiovascular equipment such as a treadmill, stationary bike, or elliptical for 5 to 10 minutes. Your heart rate, breathing rate, and body temperature should all increase during this time.

COOL-DOWN SUGGESTIONS:

1. Gradually slow your exercise or activity until you are at a walking pace. Continue walking for 5 to 10 minutes or until your heart rate and breathing rate are at a resting rate or slightly above. Finish your cool-down with the static stretches found in the Stretching section of this manual, or create your own stretching routine. This will increase your flexibility and decrease muscle soreness and tightness.

2. Follow the deep breathing sequence of in through your nose and out through your mouth until your breathing is back to normal. While you are breathing, close your eyes and focus on a place that is relaxing to you, such as a beach. Think about the way you feel when you are at this place, physically and mentally. When you are fully relaxed, slowly open your eyes and "awaken" your body.

WEATHER PRECAUTIONS RELATED TO EXERCISE

COLD TEMPERATURES
Cold-weather sports can be fun, but you need to be safe!

Tips for a Safe Workout
- Let someone know where and when you are exercising, or have someone accompany you.
- Layer your clothes. If you get warm, you can take a layer off, but do not take off your coat!
- Wear hats, gloves or mittens, and waterproof boots.
- Go inside if your teeth are chattering or if you are shivering.
- Hydrate! You need water in cold weather as well as in hot weather. Warm drinks and soups can also help warm you up.
- Watch out for slippery surfaces.
- Exercise in safe areas only.

Dangers: Frostbite and Hypothermia
Frostbite: If you are not wearing enough protective clothing, any exposed skin tissue can freeze. This most commonly happens to noses, ears, fingers, and toes.
Hypothermia: This is what occurs when your core body temperature drops. It can result from exposure to cold weather or being in cold water. Symptoms include shivering, a lack of energy, mental confusion, and even more severe symptoms. Do not allow your body to get to this point. When you start shivering, go inside!

HOT TEMPERATURES
Exercising in hot temperatures can be dangerous. Pay attention to your body's signals: Stop exercising and cool down immediately if you are feeling fatigued and are not feeling well.

Tips for a Safe Workout
- Let someone know where and when you are exercising, or have someone accompany you.
- Know the temperature of your exercise environment. Avoid exercising in high temperatures.
- Take it easy in hot temperatures. Take breaks, shorten your workout time, or go indoors to an air-conditioned facility.
- Drink water before you are thirsty, and keep hydrated.
- Wear sunscreen and a sun hat.
- Dress in cool, loose, light-colored clothing.

Dangers: Heat Cramps, Fainting, Heat Exhaustion, and Heatstroke
Heat cramps: Abrupt muscle pain that is caused by heat is heat cramps.
Fainting: You can experience light-headedness or collapsing as a result of exercising, especially in hot conditions.
Heat exhaustion: Heat exhaustion occurs when your core body temperature increases. Sweaty, cold, clammy skin in addition to heat cramps and fainting are symptoms of heat exhaustion. Untreated heat exhaustion leads to heatstroke. Get medical help and cool down your body temperature immediately.
Heatstroke: This occurs when your core body temperature rises above 104 degrees Fahrenheit (40 degrees Celsius). At this stage, the body does not sweat. This is a life-threatening situation that requires medical attention.

Other Precautions to Take
Special note: Pay attention to the humidity level as well as the temperature. Exercising in a high-humidity condition contributes to elevated body temperature and excessive sweating.
For more information, research the signs and symptoms of weather-related health conditions in addition to prevention methods and first aid. Get advice from your doctor about exercising in cold and hot temperatures.

FITNESS TESTS

Fitness tests allow you to assess your current fitness levels. The tests measure the main fitness components: cardiovascular endurance, flexibility, muscular strength, muscular endurance, and the subcomponents speed and agility. The results of the tests will allow you to evaluate your fitness levels and decide which areas you would like to work on in order to increase your overall health and wellness. It is recommended that you take the fitness tests 3 times during the school year (pre, mid, and post).

CARDIOVASCULAR ENDURANCE
ENDURANCE WALK/RUN

The endurance walk/run measures heart and lung endurance. Map out a safe 1-mile route to complete the test. You will need a stopwatch to time your run. It is recommended that you run at a steady pace for the entire mile. Walking may be combined with running, but you are encouraged to complete the test in the shortest amount of time possible.

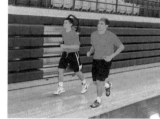

FLEXIBILITY
V-SIT AND REACH

The V-sit and reach measures the flexibility of your lower back and hamstrings. Mark a straight 2-foot line with a piece of tape, rope, or tape measure on the floor to use as a baseline. Use a tape measure or yardstick to draw a 4-foot measuring line perpendicular to the midpoint of the baseline, extending 2 feet on either side and marked in half inches. The point where the lines intersect is the 0 point. Take off your shoes and sit on the floor with the measuring line between your legs. Place your heels directly behind the baseline, with your feet 8 to 12 inches apart. With your palms facing down, place your hands on top of each other and on the measuring line. Have a partner hold your legs flat while you slowly reach forward as far as possible, keeping your fingers on the line and your feet flexed. You may practice up to 3 times. Then, complete the exercise a final time, holding the distance for 3 seconds. Record your score.

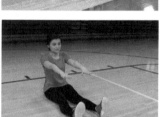

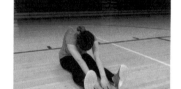

- Keep your legs straight and flex your feet.

- Do not bounce.

- Slowly reach forward. Hold for 3 seconds.

MUSCULAR ENDURANCE
BENT-KNEE SIT-UP

This activity measures your abdominal strength and endurance. Set a stopwatch for 1 minute. Lying down on your back, flex your knees and place your feet flat on the floor about 12 inches from your buttocks. Cross your arms in front of your chest. Keeping your arms in the same position, use your trunk to sit up and touch your elbows to your thighs. Return to the starting position so that your shoulder blades touch the ground. Do not let your head or neck touch the ground. A partner should hold your feet and count how many curl-ups you complete in 1 minute.

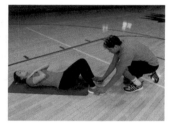

- Do not count curl-ups if you are bouncing off the floor, if your arms are not crossed in front of your chest, or if your elbows do not touch your thighs when you are sitting up.

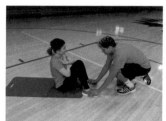

MUSCULAR STRENGTH
FLEXED-ARM HANG, RIGHT-ANGLE PUSH-UPS, AND PULL-UPS

These activities measure upper-body strength and endurance. You only have to complete 1 of these 3 tests.

FLEXED-ARM HANG

Using either an overhand grip (your palms facing away from your body) or an underhand grip (your palms facing toward your body), assume the flexed-arm hang position by bending your elbows and clearing the bar with your chin (place your chin above the bar, but do not rest it on the bar). Keep your chest close to the bar. Try to keep your body as still as possible and to not swing your legs or place your feet on surrounding objects or walls. Time yourself in this position until your chin touches or drops below the bar.

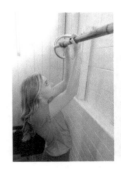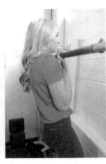

- This is a good skill to practice before attempting pull-ups.

- You may use a chair or have someone lift you to the position.

- When you are finished, let go of the bar slowly and carefully to avoid injury.

RIGHT-ANGLE PUSH-UPS

Situate your body on a mat in a push-up position. Place your hands under your shoulders and point your fingers forward. Keep your legs straight, parallel, and slightly apart, supporting your feet with your toes. Straighten your arms, keeping your back and knees straight. Then, lower your body and bend your elbows 90 degrees. Keep your chest 4 to 5 inches from the floor. Return to the up position. The push-ups should be done to a metronome pace of 1 complete push-up every 3 seconds. Do as many consecutive push-ups as possible until you cannot complete 1 within the set pace.

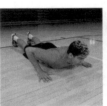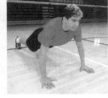
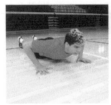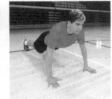

- Record only the push-ups that you do with proper form.

- Record only the push-ups that you do to the metronome pace.

- Your stomach and legs should not touch the ground. Keep your back straight.

PULL-UPS OR CHIN-UPS

Hang from a horizontal bar at a height where your arms are fully extended and your feet are not touching the ground. You may do a pull-up using an overhand grip (your palms facing away from your body) or a chin-up using an underhand grip (your palms facing toward your body). Pull yourself up until your chin is above the bar; then, return to the full hanging position. Perform as many correct pull-ups or chin-ups as you can.

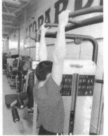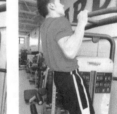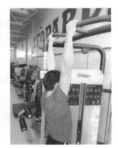

- Pull-ups should be done slowly and safely by controlling your body back to the starting position.

- Kicking or bending your legs or swinging is prohibited during the test.

SPEED AND AGILITY
SHUTTLE RUN

This sprinting activity measures the subcomponents speed and agility. Mark 2 lines 30 feet apart. Place 2 small items from your Physical Education Kit on 1 of the lines. Start on the opposite line. Use a stopwatch to time yourself in seconds. On a "ready, go" signal, start the stopwatch. Run to pick up 1 item and run back to the starting line, placing the item behind the starting line. Then, run back to pick up the second item and return to the starting line, but hold on to the object and run through the line.

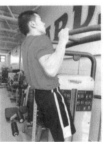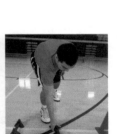
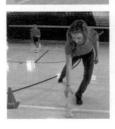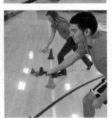

- Do not throw the items.

- It is important that you run through the starting line to achieve a better time.

FITNESS PERFORMANCE SCORECARD

Student Name: _____ Gender: _____

Fitness Challenge	Date: Age: Grade: Height: Weight: Test #1	Date: Age: Grade: Height: Weight: Test #2	Date: Age: Grade: Height: Weight: Test #3
Endurance Walk/Run			
V-Sit and Reach			
Bent-Knee Sit-Up			
Flexed-Arm Hang			
Right-Angle Push-Ups			
Pull-Ups or Chin-Ups			
Shuttle Run			

PHYSICAL EDUCATION PERFORMANCE CHART

Fitness performance charts are tools that you can use to identify your fitness levels based on national averages. The results can show your strengths and weaknesses in relation to your physical fitness and help you set attainable fitness goals.

Compare your scores to the fitness performance chart to see if you have attained your fitness levels. Find your age at the top of the chart and go down the column to see the average and outstanding scores for your fitness levels. Pick an event from the left-hand column and go across the row until you reach your age group. There are 2 groups of scores on the chart: attainment and outstanding achievement. The attainment standard is an average score that represents the 50th percentile based on the current fitness survey. The outstanding achievement is a score at the 85th percentile based on the current fitness survey.

GIRLS' FITNESS PERFORMANCE CHART

EVENTS	LEVEL OF PERFORMANCE	AGE LEVELS												
		6	7	8	9	10	11	12	13	14	15	16	17	18
ENDURANCE WALK/RUN (Minutes & Seconds)	ATTAINMENT STANDARDS	¼ mile 2:30	¼ mile 2:24	¼ mile 5:02	¼ mile 4:57	¾ mile 7:30	¾ mile 7:25	1 mile 9:54	1 mile 9:50	1 mile 9:50	1 mile 9:50	1 mile 9:52	1 mile 9:54	1 mile 9:50
	OUTSTANDING ACHIEVEMENT	2:05	1:55	3:58	3:53	6:10	6:06	8:15	8:04	8:08	8:00	8:07	8:16	8:16
V-SIT & REACH (inches)	ATTAINMENT STANDARDS	2.5	2	2	2	3	3	3.5	3.5	4.5	5	5.5	4.5	4.5
	OUTSTANDING ACHIEVEMENT	5.5	5	4.5	5.5	6	6.5	7	7	8	8	9	9	8
BENT-KNEE SIT-UPS (One-Minute Time Limit)	ATTAINMENT STANDARDS	22	25	29	31	32	33	35	25	36	35	35	35	36
	OUTSTANDING ACHIEVEMENT	31	34	38	30	40	42	43	45	45	44	44	44	44
FLEXED-ARM HANG* (Seconds & Tenths)	ATTAINMENT STANDARDS	6	7	8	8.5	10	12.4	15	15.9	14	13	12	11	10
	OUTSTANDING ACHIEVEMENT	14.7	19	19.5	22	24	25	32	35	35	29	30	30	28
RIGHT-ANGLE PUSH-UPS (#)	ATTAINMENT STANDARDS	6	8	9	12	13	11	10	11	10	15	12	16	16
	OUTSTANDING ACHIEVEMENT	9	14	17	18	20	20	20	21	20	21	24	25	25
PULL-UPS/CHIN-UPS (#)	ATTAINMENT STANDARDS	1	1	1	1	1	1	1	1	1	1	1	1	1
	OUTSTANDING ACHIEVEMENT	2	2	2	2	2	2	2	2	2	2	2	2	2
SHUTTLE RUN (Seconds)	ATTAINMENT STANDARDS	14.2	13.5	13.1	12.2	12.2	11.8	11.6	11.2	11.2	11.2	11.2	11.2	11.1
	OUTSTANDING ACHIEVEMENT	12.9	12.5	12	11.5	11.3	10.9	10.5	10.3	10.4	10.4	10.4	10.2	10.2

* Modified Fitness Test ▪ Attainment Standards (Represents the 50th percentile) ▪ Outstanding Standards (Represents the 85th percentile)

BOYS' FITNESS PERFORMANCE CHART

EVENTS	LEVEL OF PERFORMANCE	AGE LEVELS												
		6	7	8	9	10	11	12	13	14	15	16	17	18
ENDURANCE WALK/RUN (Minutes & Seconds)	ATTAINMENT STANDARDS	¼ mile 2:21	¼ mile 2:10	¼ mile 4:22	¼ mile 4:14	¾ mile 6:30	¾ mile 6:30	1 mile 8:34	1 mile 7:54	1 mile 7:33	1 mile 7:27	1 mile 7:21	1 mile 7:08	1 mile 7:08
	OUTSTANDING ACHIEVEMENT	1:55	1:48	3:30	3:30	5:30	5:19	7:10	6:45	6:28	6:18	6:14	6:12	6:12
V-SIT & REACH (inches)	ATTAINMENT STANDARDS	1	1	0.5	1	1	1	1	0.5	1	2	3	3	3
	OUTSTANDING ACHIEVEMENT	3.5	3.5	3	3	4	4	4	3.5	4.5	5	6	7	7
BENT-KNEE SIT-UPS (One-Minute Time Limit)	ATTAINMENT STANDARDS	22	28	31	32	35	37	40	42	45	45	45	45	45
	OUTSTANDING ACHIEVEMENT	31	36	39	43	45	48	49	51	53	53	53	55	55
FLEXED-ARM HANG* (Seconds & Tenths)	ATTAINMENT STANDARDS	8	12	18	22	25	29	35	40	42	45	48	50	55
	OUTSTANDING ACHIEVEMENT	17	22	27	31	35	37	40	45	48	52	60	68	70
RIGHT-ANGLE PUSH-UPS (#)	ATTAINMENT STANDARDS	7	8	9	12	14	15	18	24	24	30	30	37	38
	OUTSTANDING ACHIEVEMENT	9	14	17	18	22	27	31	39	40	42	44	53	55
PULL-UPS/CHIN-UPS (#)	ATTAINMENT STANDARDS	1	1	1	2	2	2	2	3	5	6	7	8	9
	OUTSTANDING ACHIEVEMENT	2	4	5	5	6	6	7	7	10	11	11	13	14
SHUTTLE RUN (Seconds)	ATTAINMENT STANDARDS	13.3	12.8	12.2	11.9	11.5	11.1	10.6	10.2	9.9	9.7	9.4	9.4	9.3
	OUTSTANDING ACHIEVEMENT	12.1	11.5	11.1	10.9	10.3	10	9.8	9.5	9.1	9	8.7	8.7	8.6

* Modified Fitness Test ▪ Attainment Standards (Represents the 50th percentile) ▪ Outstanding Standards (Represents the 85th percentile)

WORKING WITH A PURPOSE: GOAL SETTING

Evaluate and discuss your fitness test results with a trusted adult, and then use the following SMART goal plan to design an exercise program for yourself. Do not compare your results to the results of others. Everyone's body is different.

Have you heard the saying "failing to plan is planning to fail"? This is true of beginning a workout regimen. Starting a workout may be intimidating and confusing, but setting goals and plans for how to achieve those goals will set you up for success and put you on the right track. After performing your fitness tests and reviewing your results, you will have a better understanding of what areas you may need to improve in. Decide which area or areas you would like to work on and why. Knowing why you should be proficient in an area will allow you to have a better understanding of its importance and will keep you working toward improvement. Write a SMART goal and a plan based on the fitness principles and components.

Specific   Measurable   Attainable   Realistic   Timely

Short-Term Goal(s):

_____

_____

_____

_____

_____

_____

_____

_____

Plan(s):

_____

_____

_____

_____

_____

_____

_____

_____

HEALTH-RELATED FITNESS COMPONENTS

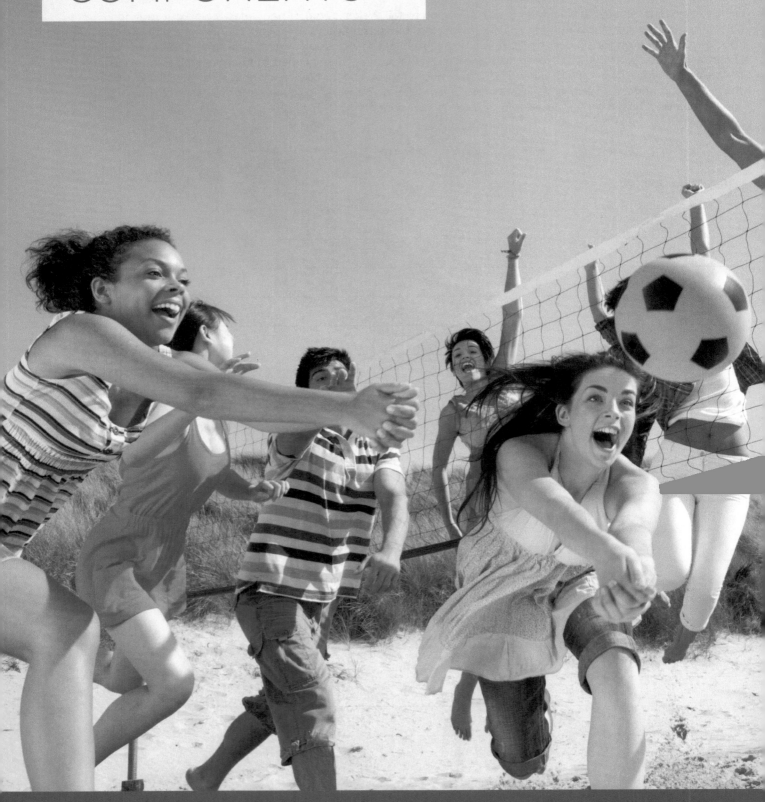

5 COMPONENTS OF HEALTH-RELATED PHYSICAL FITNESS

Total fitness is defined by how well your body performs in different categories. There are 5 specific categories that you must focus on in order to allow your body to work the way it was intended to. These health-related fitness components act as a guideline for planning your workout regimen based on your goals.

1. **BODY COMPOSITION:** the ratio of fat to muscle
2. **CARDIOVASCULAR ENDURANCE:** the ability of your heart and lungs to supply oxygen to your body
3. **FLEXIBILITY:** the ability of your muscles and joints to move through a full range of motion
4. **MUSCULAR ENDURANCE:** the ability of your muscles to exert force for an extended period of time
5. **MUSCULAR STRENGTH:** the ability of your muscles to exert maximum force in a single effort

Your goal should be to do a combination of physical and mental activities that allow you to perform tasks and meet the demands of everyday life. Life can be physically and mentally straining; but, if you continually work on your health and wellness daily, you will have a better chance at maintaining an overall good quality of life. Find activities and exercises that you enjoy so that you stay active for a lifetime. Activities in this manual will provide ideas of physical movement and exercises that you can do with or without equipment.

Cardiovascular Endurance
The body's ability to deliver oxygen and nutrients and to remove waste products.

Recommended Exercise: Running

Body Composition
The way in which your body is made up in terms of lean and fat mass.

Recommended Exercise: Swimming

Muscular Strength
The degree to which a muscle can exert force by contracting against resistance.

Recommended Exercise: Weight Training

Flexibility
The ability to move joints and muscles through their full range of movements.

Recommended Exercise: Yoga

Muscular Endurance
The ability of a muscle or group of muscles to continually generate a force over a sustained period of time.

Recommended Exercise: Rowing

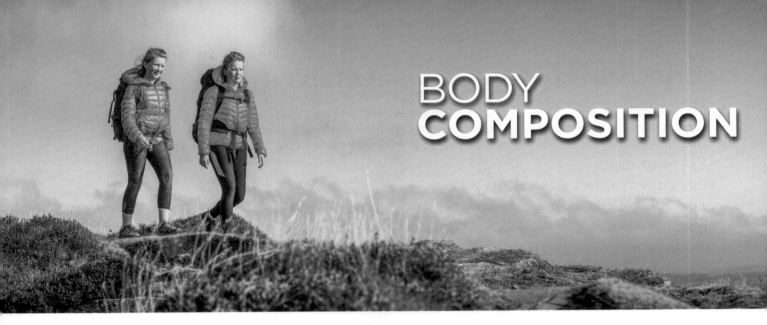

BODY COMPOSITION

Body composition describes the percentages of fat, bone, muscle, and water in your body. Your body is made up of fat mass and fat-free mass. Most commonly, body composition refers to the percentage of fat that makes up body mass and how that relates to fitness. Body composition and weight determine leanness, or the amount of fat in your body. Lean muscle burns more calories than fat and helps your body be more efficient.

WHY BODY COMPOSITION MATTERS

A person who has more muscle and less fat has a body that is more efficient at burning calories than the body of a person who has less muscle and more fat. Muscles burn more calories than fat; so, a lean, strong body will burn more calories and have a better metabolism than a less lean, weaker body. A body is also more efficient when it is exercising if it has lean muscle. Lean muscle makes you more capable of completing high-intensity exercises that burn more calories and create greater improvements. Paying attention to and attending to your body composition is important for your overall health.

HOW TO CHANGE BODY COMPOSITION

It is possible to change your body composition; however, this can be difficult. Some people may lack motivation or may just not have a lot of available time, but it is important to try to control your body composition. There are some things that you can do in order to help change your body composition and increase your metabolism.

- Eat healthy meals and snacks.
- Eat small, frequent meals.
- Do not skip breakfast. A healthy breakfast kickstarts your metabolism.
- It takes 20 minutes for your body to feel full, so it should take you about 20 minutes to eat a meal. Do not have a second helping of food until after 20 minutes have passed.
- Exercise often, incorporating the 5 components of fitness.
- Set goals for yourself.

HOW TO MEASURE BODY COMPOSITION

Many people do not often think about measuring body composition or even think that it is important; it is not a common practice to be measured, but there are several methods of measuring body composition, such as hydrostatic weighing, bioelectrical impedance, and skinfold calipers. Using skinfold calipers is the most common method of measuring body composition because skinfold calipers can be found in many health clubs. Skinfold calipers are used to measure folds of fat on your body. A personal trainer will measure from 3 different locations on your body to estimate an overall body fat percentage.

BODY MASS INDEX (BMI)

Body mass index is a weight-to-height ratio. It measures body weight, not body fat. Doctors use your body mass index to determine if your weight is healthy. Below is a BMI chart for you to use.

BODY MASS INDEX CHART FOR YOUNG ADULTS

weight in pounds

height in inches	80	90	100	110	120	130	140	150	160	170	180	190	200	210	220	230	240	250
48	24.4	27.5	30.5	33.6	36.6	39.7	42.7	45.8	48.8	51.9	54.9	58	61	64.1	67.1	70.2	73.2	76.3
50	22.5	25.3	28.1	30.9	33.7	36.6	39.4	42.2	45	47.8	50.6	53.4	56.2	59.1	61.9	64.7	67.5	70.3
52	20.8	23.4	26	28.6	31.2	33.8	36.4	39	41.6	44.2	46.8	49.4	52	54.6	57.2	59.8	62.4	65
54	19.3	21.7	24.1	26.5	28.9	31.3	33.8	36.2	38.6	41	43.4	45.8	48.2	50.6	53	55.4	57.9	60.3
56	17.9	20.2	22.4	24.7	26.9	29.1	31.4	33.6	35.9	38.1	40.4	42.6	44.8	47.1	49.3	51.6	53.8	56
58	16.7	18.8	20.9	23	25.1	27.2	29.3	31.3	33.4	35.5	37.6	39.7	41.8	43.9	46	48.1	50.2	52.2
60	15.6	17.6	19.5	21.5	23.4	25.4	27.3	29.3	31.2	33.2	35.2	37.1	39.1	41	43	44.9	46.9	48.8
62	14.6	16.5	18.3	20.1	21.9	23.8	25.6	27.4	29.3	31.1	32.9	34.7	36.6	38.4	40.2	42.1	43.9	45.7
64	13.7	15.4	17.2	18.9	20.6	22.3	24	25.7	27.5	29.2	30.9	32.6	34.3	36	37.8	39.5	41.2	42.9
66	12.9	14.5	16.1	17.8	19.4	21	22.6	24.2	25.8	27.4	29	30.7	32.3	33.9	35.5	37.1	38.7	40.3
68	12.2	13.7	15.2	16.7	18.2	19.8	21.3	22.8	24.3	25.8	27.4	28.9	30.4	31.9	33.4	35	36.5	38
70	11.5	12.9	14.3	15.8	17.2	18.7	20.1	21.5	23	24.4	25.8	27.3	28.7	30.1	31.6	33	34.4	35.9
72	10.8	12.2	13.6	14.9	16.3	17.6	19	20.3	21.7	23.1	24.4	25.8	27.1	28.5	29.8	31.2	32.5	33.9
74	10.3	11.6	12.8	14.1	15.4	16.7	18	19.3	20.5	21.8	23.1	24.4	25.7	27	28.2	29.5	30.8	32.1
76	9.74	11	12.2	13.4	14.6	15.8	17	18.3	19.5	20.7	21.9	23.1	24.3	25.6	26.8	28	29.2	30.4
78	9.24	10.4	11.6	12.7	13.9	15	16.2	17.3	18.5	19.6	20.8	22	23.1	24.3	25.4	26.6	27.7	28.9
80	8.79	9.89	11	12.1	13.2	14.3	15.4	16.5	17.6	18.7	19.8	20.9	22	23.1	24.2	25.3	26.4	27.5
82	8.36	9.41	10.5	11.5	12.5	13.6	14.6	15.7	16.7	17.8	18.8	19.9	20.9	22	23	24	25.1	26.1
84	7.97	8.97	9.96	11	12	13	13.9	14.9	15.9	16.9	17.9	18.9	19.9	20.9	21.9	22.9	23.9	24.9
86	7.6	8.55	9.51	10.5	11.4	12.4	13.3	14.3	15.2	16.2	17.1	18.1	19	20	20.9	21.9	22.8	23.8

Optimal: 18.5 - 25

Overweight: 25.1 - 30

Obese: 30.1 - 40

Severely Obese: Greater than 40.1

Underweight: 17.5 - 18.4

Severely Underweight: Less than 17.5

A way to determine body fat is to measure with skinfold calipers. This method measures the thicknesses of folds of skin from different locations on your body to calculate a percentage of body fat. A weightlifter may have a higher body weight due to muscles weighing more than fat, which would show a high BMI; however, the same weightlifter measuring with skinfold calipers would get a more accurate measure of body fat.

Being overweight or underweight can be a health risk. Be smart about unrealistic media or social portrayals of idealized body images. Common sense is important to weight control. Eating healthy and exercising moderately are important components of maintaining a healthy body weight.

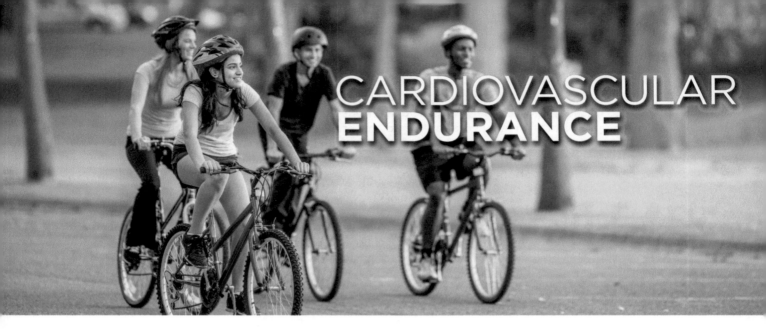

CARDIOVASCULAR ENDURANCE

Cardiovascular endurance is the ability of your heart to provide oxygen to your muscles during physical activity for a prolonged period of time. This is one of the most important components of physical fitness. Cardiovascular exercise—also called cardio or aerobic exercise—strengthens your heart and lungs and involves large muscle groups such as your leg muscles. Cardiovascular endurance helps your heart transport oxygen in the blood to all your working muscles. It also helps with how well your muscles use that oxygen. To give your heart a proper workout, make sure you do your cardio exercise within your target heart rate zone.

Having a healthy heart is extremely important to your overall wellness. There are different ways to strengthen your heart. In addition to using traditional equipment in a gym, you can exercise at home or in your community. For example, you can do a high-intensity circuit workout. You can also do outdoor activities such as hiking, biking, kayaking, and so on. It is important to find activities that you enjoy so that you are eager to stay active throughout your life.

PULSE

Your pulse is your heart rate, or the number of times your heart beats in a minute. Your pulse is the result of your heart pumping blood through your arteries. When your heart contracts, or pumps, blood moves through blood vessels in your body called arteries. The arteries pulsate as blood rushes through them. You can feel this pulsation in different locations on your body. During exercise, your heart pumps harder to move oxygenated blood to your muscles. Knowing how to check your pulse can help you evaluate your exercise program.

HOW TO CHECK YOUR PULSE

The most common areas to find your pulse are your wrist and your neck.

Wrist (radial artery): Place the tips of your index and middle fingers just below the base of your wrist on the same side as your thumb. Press lightly until you feel a steady pulse.

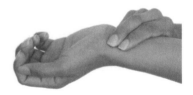

Neck (carotid artery): Find the center of your neck with your index and middle fingers. Then, place your fingers on either side of your windpipe. Press lightly until you feel a steady pulse.

- Be sure to use your same hand as the side of the neck you are taking your pulse on; for example, you would use your right hand to feel your pulse on the right side of your neck.

- Do not use your thumb. Your thumb has a pulse and could interfere with calculating a proper pulse rate.

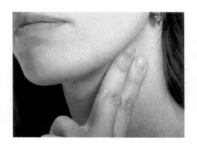

Once you have found your pulse, use a watch with a second hand and count your pulse for 15 seconds. Multiply that number by 4 to find your resting heart rate, or how many times your heart beats per minute while your body is at rest. A healthy resting heart rate for someone between the ages of 14 and 21 is between 60 and 100 beats per minute. The better your fitness levels, the lower your heart rate will be.

Use the formula below to calculate your resting heart rate.

pulse after 15 seconds × 4 = resting heart rate

HEART RATE

Being fit means exercising enough to make physical changes to your body. Cardiovascular exercise improves your aerobic capacity and heart rate and helps you maintain your body weight. It is important to keep your heart rate between 60 percent and 80 percent of your maximum heart rate when you are working out. If your exercise is too light, you will not benefit from the workout. If it is too intense, the workout could potentially be hazardous to your body. The table below shows the most favorable pulse rate levels by age and goal.

Use the formula below to calculate your maximum heart rate.

220 - your age = predicted maximum heart rate

TARGET HEART RATE

You experience the most benefits when you exercise in your target heart rate zone. Usually, this is when your exercising heart rate is 60 percent to 80 percent of your maximum heart rate. Do not exercise above 85 percent of your maximum heart rate as this may increase cardiovascular and orthopedic risks. When you are beginning an exercise program, you may need to gradually build up to a level that is within your target heart rate zone. If the exercise feels too hard, slow down. Do not push your body too hard, especially in the beginning.

HOW TO FIND YOUR TARGET HEART RATE ZONE

Maximum Heart Beats per Minute

220 – your age = _____

Multiply the number that you found by 0.6 (60 percent) and 0.8 (80 percent).

Example:

220 – 15 (age) = 205

205 x 0.6 (60% intensity) = 123 (target heart rate)

205 x 0.8 (80% intensity) = 164 (target heart rate)

HEART RATE ZONES FOR CHILDREN AND ADOLESCENTS

HEART RATE ZONE	FEELS LIKE	EXAMPLE ACTIVITIES	BENEFITS
Performance — 100-90%	**VIGOROUS TO VIGOROUS+** • very exhausting • fast breathing • muscles may feel tired	• short sprints • soccer • basketball	Develops maximum performance and speed.
Healthy Heart — 90-70%	**MODERATE TO VIGOROUS** • easy to heavy breathing • light muscular strain • average sweating	• games • jogging • cycling • dancing	Improves aerobic fitness and performance capacity.
Active — 70-60%	**EASY TO MODERATE** • easy, comfortable breathing • low muscle load • light sweating	• warm-up and cool-down • brisk walking • playing catch • volleyball	Improves basic endurance and muscle tone.

EXERCISE INCREASES BRAIN POWER AND MUSCULAR STRENGTH!

What was your heart rate during your previous workout? _____

Were you in your target heart rate zone? _____

Another way to measure the intensity of your workout is to use the *Borg Rating of Perceived Exertion (RPE) Scale. The RPE scale uses numerical values to determine how hard you are exercising. Number 6 represents no physical exertion. Number 20 represents maximum exertion. The exertion level increases with the value of the number from 6 to 20. Review the chart below.

Scale Range	Level of Exertion
6	No Exertion
7	Extremely Light
8	
9	Very Light
10	
11	Light
12	
13	Somewhat Hard
14	
15	Hard
16	
17	Very Hard
18	
19	Extremely Hard
20	Maximum Exertion

- Numbers 6–11 represent how you should feel using little or no effort, such as when you are lying in bed or sitting in a chair. You can talk in complete sentences and breathing is restful.

- Numbers 12–16 represent how you should feel while you are exercising. This is your target heart rate zone for exercise. Talking while exercising becomes harder, and breathing is deeper.

- Numbers 17–20 represent working too hard. You cannot talk, and breathing is labored or you are breathless. Never push yourself to maximum exertion.

What was your RPE number during your previous workout? _____

Was your intensity level between numbers 12 and 16? _____

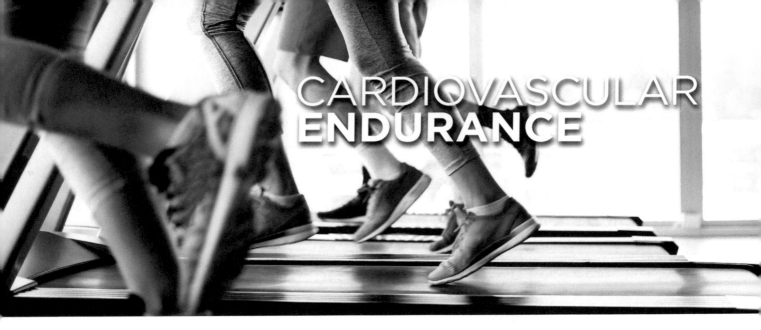

CARDIOVASCULAR ENDURANCE ACTIVITIES

AT THE GYM Always have a certified trainer instruct you on the use of an exercise machine.	OUTSIDE THE GYM Always alert someone to where you are going. Never swim alone.
circuit training	aerobics
elliptical trainer	biking
stair-climbing machine	hiking
stationary bike	swimming
treadmill	walking or running

BENEFITS OF CARDIOVASCULAR ENDURANCE

IMPROVE CARDIORESPIRATORY FUNCTION

- Cardio helps strengthen your heart and lungs. If you work out for at least 30 minutes 3 to 5 times per week, you can lower your risk of heart disease, cancer, diabetes, and many other chronic health problems.

- Cardio increases your heart rate, your breathing rate, and your endurance. At a moderately brisk level, your heart rate increases but you can still carry on a conversation.

- You can divide your 30-minute workout into 10-minute increments throughout the day and still receive effective health benefits. Performing a cardio activity at a moderately-brisk pace will decrease your risk of developing diabetes, obesity, high blood pressure, high blood cholesterol, heart disease, and some forms of cancer.

DECREASE RISK OF HEART DISEASE

- According to the Center for Disease Control and Prevention, heart disease causes approximately 1 in 4 deaths in the United States every year. The most common type of heart disease is coronary artery disease which is a buildup of plaque in the arteries.

ACHIEVE WEIGHT-LOSS GOALS

- If you work out at the right intensity, you will burn calories and will move toward your weight-loss goals.

IMPROVE JOINT RANGE OF MOTION

- If you are recovering from back, hip, knee, or ankle injuries, you may have some stiffness in your joints. Doing a gentle walking program can help loosen your joints and help them regain flexibility.

LOWER CHOLESTEROL

- Another major health issue that cardiovascular exercise can prevent is high cholesterol. High cholesterol is a result of eating fatty foods and not exercising. It can cause the arteries within the body to harden, which can limit the blood flow to the heart. Because blood carries oxygen to the heart, any lack of blood can result in chest pain, blockage, and even a heart attack. People who have higher cholesterol levels have an increased risk of heart attack and stroke. By consistently performing cardiovascular exercise, cholesterol levels can often be lowered and controlled, as needed.

PREVENT OSTEOPOROSIS

- Exercises, especially leg exercises, are very beneficial in the prevention of osteoporosis. This condition occurs when bones lose mass, which leads to a decrease in the stability of the bone tissue, thus making the bones more fragile.
- Other than getting the proper amount of calcium, the main methods of prevention of fragile bones are resistance training and cardiovascular exercise, which are achieved simultaneously by performing certain cardiovascular exercises.

MANAGE STRESS

- Working out can be a strategy for stress management that helps to combat depression and insomnia as well as improve brain function.

CALORIE AND FAT BURNING

When you do a cardiovascular endurance exercise, choose an exercise that you are interested in, such as riding a bike, walking or running on a treadmill or outside, using a stair-climbing machine, or even swimming. It is good to change your cardio workout from time to time. There are 2 groups of cardiovascular training.

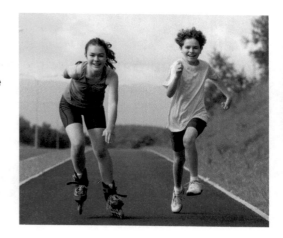

1. **Low Intensity (60-Percent Intensity)**
   - When you are doing low-intensity cardiovascular training, you want to be in the intensity range of 50 to 60 percent. You can perform this type of exercise longer, which will in turn burn more fat. Low-intensity training also helps prevent your joints from being overworked.

2. **High Intensity (80-Percent Intensity)**
   - When you are doing high-intensity cardiovascular training, you want to be in the intensity range of 70 to 80 percent.

   This type of exercise burns a lot of calories and helps increase your metabolism. A good way to perform a high-intensity workout is to incorporate interval training. Interval training is moving from an initial intensity of exercise to another intensity of exercise in different set-time intervals.

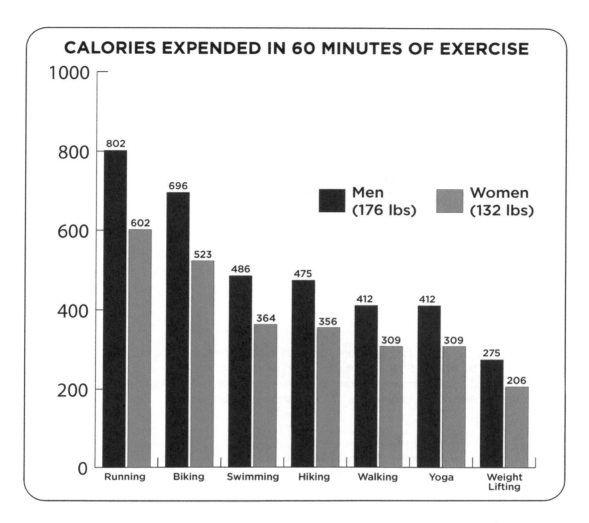

CALORIES EXPENDED IN 60 MINUTES OF EXERCISE

Legend: Men (176 lbs), Women (132 lbs)

Exercise	Men (176 lbs)	Women (132 lbs)
Running	802	602
Biking	696	523
Swimming	486	364
Hiking	475	356
Walking	412	309
Yoga	412	309
Weight Lifting	275	206

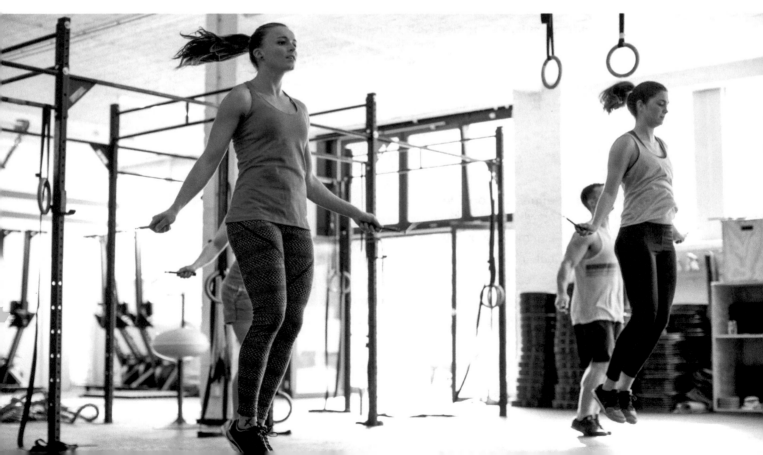

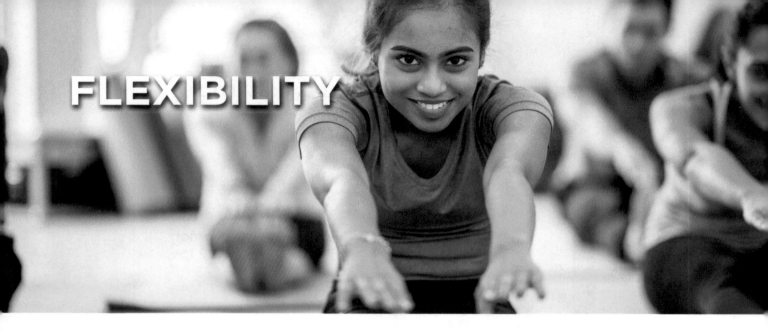

FLEXIBILITY

Flexibility is the ability of your joints to move through a full range of motion. You can achieve flexibility by stretching. It is important to include flexibility in your everyday workout. As you get older, you tend to lose your flexibility. Increasing your flexibility improves how well your body can perform during physical activity, reducing your risk of injury. Having good flexibility allows you to do things such as tie your shoes and pick objects up off the ground.

Flexibility increases your performance in cardiovascular endurance, muscular strength, and muscular endurance. Stretching each joint area before exercising helps prepare your body to exercise. Stretching each joint area after exercising helps you maintain overall flexibility. There are 2 types of stretches: static and dynamic. **Static stretches** are positions that you hold for a desired amount of time. These types of stretches focus on your flexibility. **Dynamic stretches** are movements that you do in order to loosen up your joints. These types of stretches are commonly done before completing a vigorous workout or activity.

Proprioceptive Neuromuscular Facilitation (PNF) stretching is a stretching technique that requires 2 people. It combines static stretching with isometric contracting of a muscle group in the pattern stretch, isometric contraction, and then stretch again. Isometric contracting is contracting a muscle against a fixed resistance without visibly moving the muscle. This is an advanced stretching method that is used by physical therapists for rehabilitation and by more advanced athletes, usually at the college level or higher, for deeper stretching. Consult and work with an athletic trainer or physical therapist for PNF stretching. PNF stretching that is done incorrectly and without a trained professional can result in serious injury.

This manual includes a variety of static and dynamic stretches for each major body part that will help you increase your flexibility.

Below are some guidelines to consider.
- Move your muscles slowly and gently.
- Keep your body in alignment, supporting your limbs and trunk.
- Never force movement. Instead, work with your body and its structure.
- Stretching is okay, but feeling pain is not. If you feel pain, numbness, or tingling, stop immediately.
- Rest between stretches to avoid overexerting your muscles.
- Breathe during your stretches to avoid muscle tension.

Below are some terms to know.

- **extension:** movement of a joint to lengthen the muscle

- **flexion:** movement of a joint to shorten the muscle

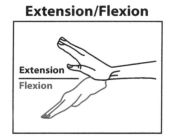

Extension/Flexion

- **abduction:** movement of a joint so that the limb is turned away from the middle of the body

- **adduction:** movement of a joint so that the limb is turned toward the middle of the body

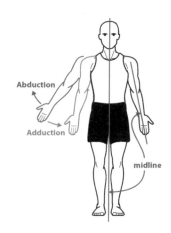

STRETCHING EXERCISES

Tips for Proper Static Stretching

- Stretch slowly and steadily. Relax and hold stretches without bouncing.
- Hold each stretch for 20 to 30 seconds.
- Repeat each stretch 2 to 3 times. Remember to do both the right side and the left side.
- Stretch before and after physical activity.

STATIC STRETCHES

NECK STRETCH

muscle focus: sternocleidomastoids and upper trapezii

- Either standing or sitting, look straight ahead so that your head is in a neutral position.
- Tilt your head slowly to the right so that your ear almost touches your shoulder.
- Hold this position for 20 to 30 seconds.
- Bring your head back up to the neutral position.
- Repeat this on the left side.
- Repeat the stretch 2 to 3 times on each side.

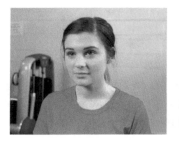
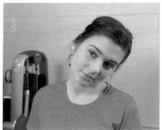

SIDE STRETCH

muscle focus: latissimi dorsi and abdominal muscles

- Stand with your feet hip-width apart.
- Place your right hand on your right hip.
- Tilt your body to the right while bringing your left hand and arm up over your head.
- Hold this position for 20 to 30 seconds.
- Stand back up to the starting position.
- Repeat this on the left side.
- Repeat the stretch 2 to 3 times on each side.

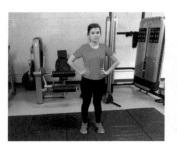
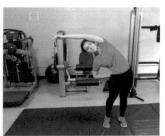

SHOULDER AND TRICEP STRETCH

muscle focus: triceps and deltoids

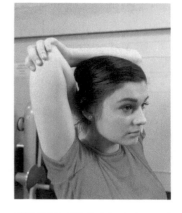

- Raise your right arm to the ceiling.
- Bend your right elbow so that your hand is reaching down your back.
- Bring your left hand up to your right elbow.
- Pull your right elbow with your left hand to stretch your triceps and shoulder.
- Hold this for 20 to 30 seconds.
- Repeat this on the left side.
- Repeat the stretch 2 to 3 times on each side.

LOWER BACK AND HIP STRETCH

muscle focus: glutei maximi, iliotibial tracts (IT bands), sartorii, quadrati lumborum, and sacrospinali

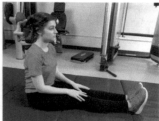

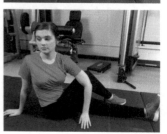

- Start in a seated position with your legs straight out in front of you.
- Bend your right knee and bring it up over your left leg so that your right foot is on the ground next to your left thigh.
- Twist your body to the right, placing your left elbow on the outside of your right thigh.
- Push with your left elbow on your right thigh for a deeper stretch.
- Hold this for 20 to 30 seconds.
- Repeat this on the left side.
- Repeat the stretch 2 to 3 times on each side.

HAMSTRING STRETCH

muscle focus: hamstrings

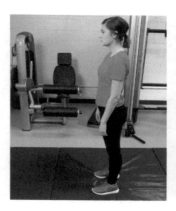

- Stand with your feet hip-width apart.
- Stepping forward with your right foot, point your toes up and place your heel on the ground.
- Bending forward, bend your left knee and keep your right leg straight.
- Place both hands on your right upper thigh and push down slightly.
- Hold this for 20 to 30 seconds.
- Repeat this on the left side.
- Repeat the stretch 2 to 3 times on each side.

QUADRICEP STRETCH

muscle focus: quadriceps

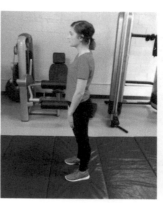

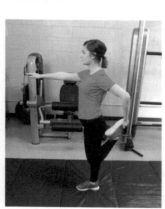

- Stand with your feet together.
- Focus on a single spot or hold onto something for balance.
- Bending your right knee, bring your right foot up to your buttocks.
- Grab your right ankle with your right hand.

- Pull your foot to your buttocks. Push your hips forward.
- Hold this for 20 to 30 seconds.
- Repeat this with your left foot.
- Repeat the stretch 2 to 3 times on each side.

GROIN STRETCH

muscle focus: adductor muscles

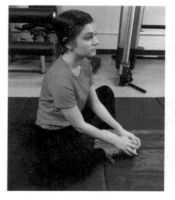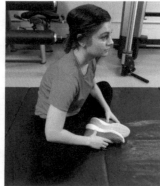

- Sit on the floor with your knees bent to your sides and the bottoms of your feet together.
- Place your elbows on your knees.
- Push down on your knees with your elbows.
- Pull your feet and legs closer to your body to intensify the stretch.
- Hold this for 20 to 30 seconds.
- Repeat the stretch 2 to 3 times on each side.

DYNAMIC STRETCHES:

MONSTER KICKS

muscle focus: hamstrings, glutei maximi, and abdominal muscles

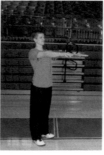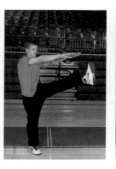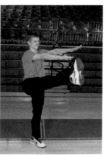

- Start on a solid surface and designate a specific distance to travel.
- Start with your feet together and your arms straight out in front of you.
- Take a step forward and kick with your opposite leg to try to touch your hands. Keep your kicking leg as straight as you can with your foot flexed.
- Continue this kicking pattern, alternating legs for the entire distance. Then, continue this back to the starting position.
- Repeat this cycle 2 to 3 more times.

HIGH KNEES

muscle focus: quadriceps, hamstrings, calves, glutei maximi, and abdominal muscles

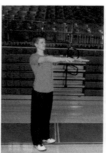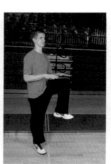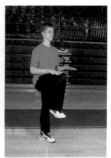

- Start on a solid surface and designate a specific distance to travel.
- Take small, quick steps, raising your knees toward your chest. Travel in a straight line to the designated area.
- Move at your own pace. Note that the faster you move your feet and the faster you travel, the more intense the exercise will be.
- Continue this back to the starting position.
- Repeat this cycle 2 to 3 more times.

LUNGE TWISTS

muscle focus: quadriceps, hamstrings, glutei maximi, and abdominal muscles

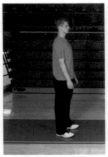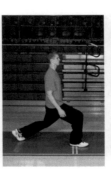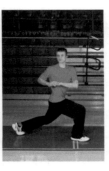

- Start on a solid surface and designate a specific distance to travel.

- Take a large step forward.

- Bend your front knee and create a 90-degree angle with each of your legs.

- Place your elbows on your stomach and keep your back straight. Turn your torso to the side of your front foot.

- Pick your back leg up to return to the starting position.

- Continue this pattern, alternating legs for the entire distance. Then, continue this back to the starting position.

- Repeat this cycle 2 to 3 more times.

REAR KICKS

muscle focus: quadriceps and hamstrings

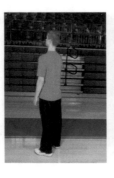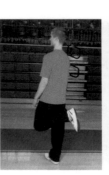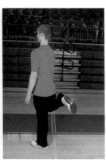

- Start on a solid surface and designate a specific distance to travel.

- Stand with your feet together.

- Flexing your foot, bend your right knee to swing your heel toward your buttocks, but do not allow your foot to touch your body.

- Alternate your feet each time.

- Move at your own pace to the designated spot. Then, continue this back to the starting position. Note that the faster you move your feet, the more intense the exercise will be.

- Repeat this cycle 2 to 3 more times.

ARM CIRCLES

muscle focus: deltoids

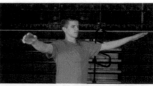

- Stand with your feet shoulder-width apart and your arms out to your sides so that they are parallel to the ground.

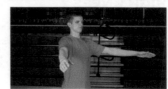

- Keeping your arms straight, move them in a forward circular motion.

- Perform 10 small circles and 10 big circles; then, switch directions and move your arms in a backward circular motion.

- Repeat this cycle 2 to 3 more times.

CARIOCA

muscle focus: abductors, adductors, quadriceps, hamstrings, and abdominal muscles

- Stand with your back straight and your feet together.

- Step to the side with your left foot; then, cross your right foot in front of your left foot.

- Step again to the side with your left foot; then, cross your right foot behind your left foot.

- Repeat this 5 times to the left; then, continue this 5 times to the right.

- Repeat this cycle 2 to 3 more times.

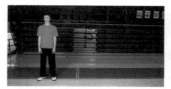 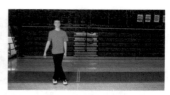
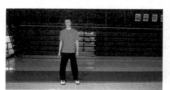 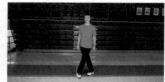

INCHWORMS

muscle focus: hamstrings and abdominal muscles

- Stand with your back straight and your feet slightly apart.

- Try to keep your legs straight while bending at your waist to put your hands on the ground.

- Walk your hands out until your body is in a plank (push-up) position.

- Hold the plank for 1 second; then, walk your feet toward your hands.

- Complete 2 to 3 sets of 10 repetitions.

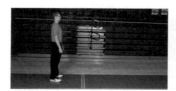 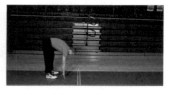
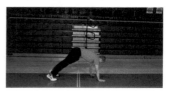

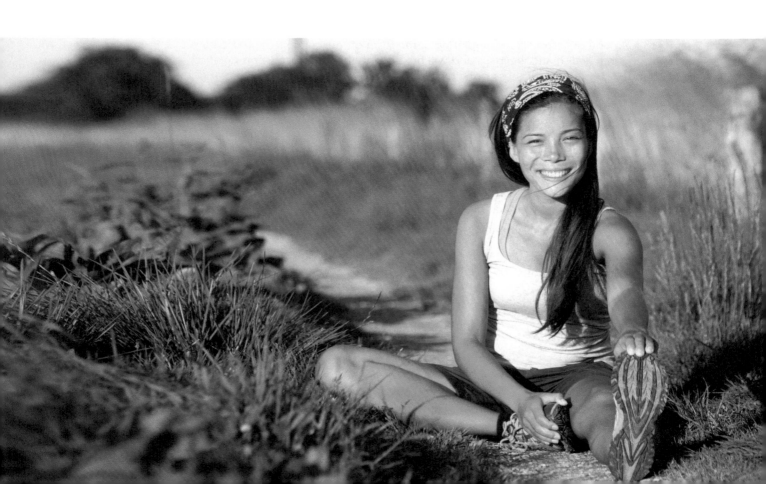

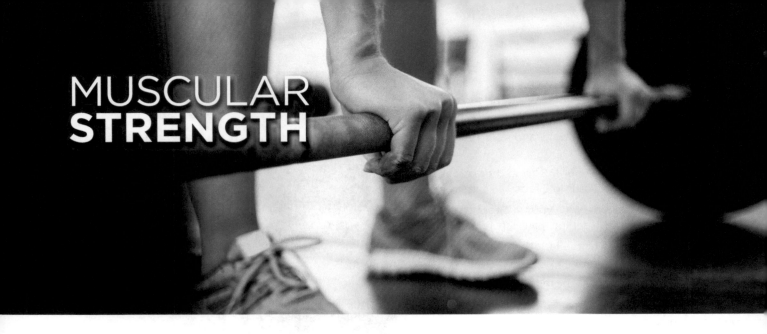

MUSCULAR STRENGTH

MUSCULAR STRENGTH

Muscular strength refers to the amount of force a muscle can produce. Muscular strength is a vital part of a balanced exercise routine, which includes anaerobic activity and flexibility. Without muscular strength, your body would be weak and unable to perform daily activities.

Having poor muscular strength increases your chance of getting hurt during activities. Some of the benefits of muscular strength training are that it builds muscle, burns fat, and increases your overall health.

Muscular strength exercises denote lifting more weight for fewer repetitions. Your muscles will start to get stronger when they are worked past the point of fatigue, or the point where they have very little or no energy left. Note that you should only lift only what you can handle; you should not lift weights that are too heavy for you.

Muscular strength training includes resistance methods like using free weights, weight machines, and resistance bands to help you build muscle. Completing some form of muscular strength training 3 to 5 times per week will help your overall health and wellness and will help maintain your muscle composition.
Be sure to review the basic fitness principles before beginning a workout regimen to build muscular strength.

Basic Rules for Muscular Strength Training

- Lift weights at least 3 times per week, every other day.
- Do not lift the same muscle group 2 days in a row.
- Warm up before lifting. **Never begin lifting on cold muscles.**
- Generally, to improve muscular strength, complete 3 to 5 sets of 8 to 12 repetitions.
- Use a spotter for safety when necessary.
- Complete any heavy-resistance exercises with low repetitions. Do not lift weights that are too heavy for you.
- A supervisor or coach should help you set up your program based on your needs.
- Cool down at the end of your workout, stretching the muscles that you used.

DUMBBELL CHEST PRESSES

muscle focus: chest muscles, pectoralis majors, deltoids, and triceps

- Lie with your back flat on a weight bench and your feet flat on the floor.
- Grip a dumbbell firmly with each of your hands.

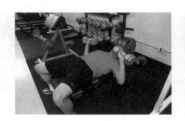 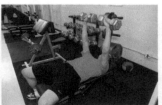

- Start with the dumbbells level with your chest and your arms bent at 90-degree angles.
- Raise the dumbbells straight up above your chest. Do not lock your elbows.
- Lower the dumbbells back to your chest and press them back up again.
- Complete 3 to 5 sets of 8 to 12 repetitions.

DUMBBELL INCLINE CHEST PRESSES

muscle focus: chest muscles, pectoralis majors, and deltoids

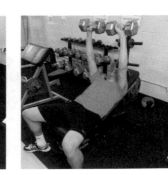

- Adjust a weight bench so that it is at a 45-degree angle with the floor.
- Sit with your back flat on the bench and your feet flat on the floor.
- Grip a dumbbell firmly with each of your hands.
- Start with the dumbbells level with your chest and your arms bent at 90-degree angles.
- Raise the dumbbells straight up above your chest. Do not lock your elbows.
- Lower the dumbbells back to your chest and press them back up again.
- Complete 3 to 5 sets of 8 to 12 repetitions.

SHOULDER PRESSES

muscle focus: deltoids

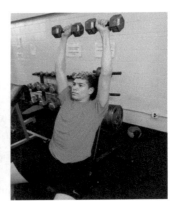

- Sit straight up either on a weight bench or in a chair.
- Hold a pair of dumbbells by your ears and keep them in line with your shoulders. Bend both elbows to 90-degree angles.
- Lift the dumbbells straight up above your head and straighten your elbows. Do not lock your elbows.
- Lower the dumbbells back to your ears and bend both elbows back to 90 degrees.
- Complete 3 to 5 sets of 8 to 12 repetitions.

OVERHEAD TRICEP EXTENSIONS

muscle focus: triceps

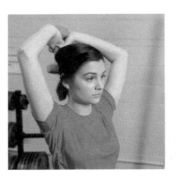

- Stand with your feet hip-width apart.
- Hold a dumbbell behind your head with both hands. Bend both elbows 90 degrees.
- Straighten your elbows while lifting the dumbbell above your head toward the ceiling.
- Bring the dumbbell back to the starting position.
- Complete 3 to 5 sets of 8 to 12 repetitions.

BARBELL BICEP CURLS

muscle focus: biceps and abdominal muscles

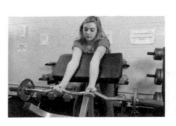
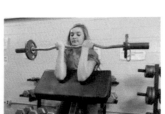

- Sitting straight up, place your arms flat on a padded surface.

- Keeping your arms straight, hold the barbell with both hands in front of your stomach. Do not lock your elbows.
- Curl the barbell slowly up to your chin.
- Bring the barbell slowly back to the starting position. Remember to not lock your elbows and to not use your back when you are exerting force.
- Complete 3 to 5 sets of 8 to 12 repetitions.

ALTERNATING BICEP CURLS (DUMBBELL OR MACHINE)

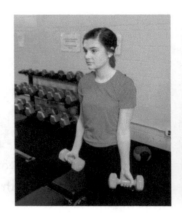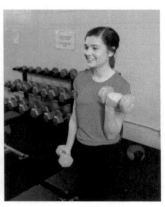

muscle focus: biceps and abdominal muscles

Dumbbells
- Hold a dumbbell in each hand, with your arms down to your sides and your palms facing away from you.
- Keep your arms straight and your elbows close to your sides.
- Bending your right elbow, lift the dumbbell up toward your right shoulder.
- Straightening your elbow, bring the dumbbell slowly back to the starting position. Remember to not lock your elbow or use your back to exert force.
- Repeat this on the left side.
- Complete 3 to 5 sets of 8 to 12 repetitions.

Machine (Not Alternating)

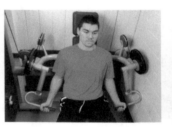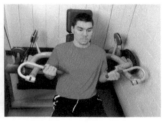

- Sit in the seat on the machine.
- Adjust the weight to a weight that you can handle. Do not attempt a weight that is too heavy for you.
- Grab a handle in each hand. Your arms should be extended at your sides.
- Bending your elbows, lift the handles up toward your shoulders.
- Straightening your elbows, bring the handles slowly back to the starting position. Remember to not lock your elbows.
- Complete 3 to 5 sets of 8 to 12 repetitions.

1-ARM DUMBBELL ROW

muscle focus: latissimi dorsi, rhomboids, lower trapezii, and erector spinae

- Hold a dumbbell with your right hand.
- Place your left knee and left hand on a sturdy bench.
- Extend your right arm toward the floor.
- Bending your right elbow, pull the dumbbell up toward your right side. Your elbow should be pointing up toward the ceiling.
- Lower the dumbbell slowly back to the starting position.
- Repeat this on the left side.
- Complete 3 to 5 sets of 8 to 12 repetitions.

PULL-UPS

muscle focus: latissimi dorsi and biceps

- Find a bar that is secure enough to hold your body weight.
- Hold onto the bar with both hands. Your hands should be placed wider than your shoulders, or outside of your shoulders. Your palms should be facing **away** from you.
- Pull your body up high enough so that your chin is slightly above the bar.
- Lower yourself slowly back to the starting position.
- Complete 3 to 5 sets of 8 to 12 repetitions.

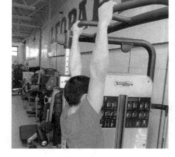
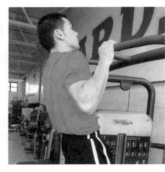

CHIN-UPS

muscle focus: latissimi dorsi and biceps

- Find a bar that is secure enough to hold your body weight.
- Hold onto the bar with your hands shoulder-width apart. Your palms should be facing toward you.
- Pull your body up high enough so that your chin is slightly above the bar.
- Lower yourself slowly back to the starting position.
- Complete 3 to 5 sets of 8 to 12 repetitions.

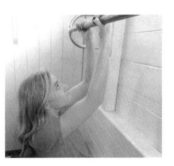
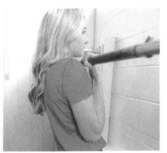

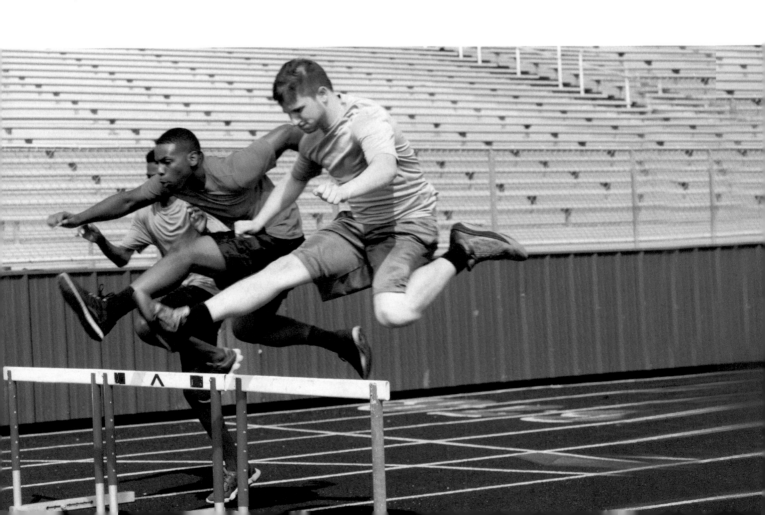

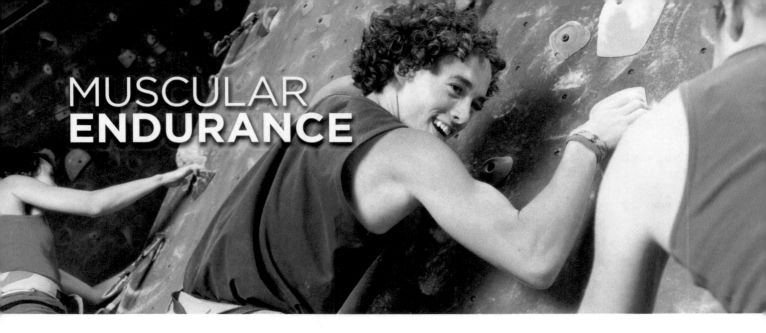

MUSCULAR ENDURANCE

MUSCULAR ENDURANCE

Muscular endurance is the ability of your muscles to exert force for an extended period of time, such as by sustaining repeated movements against resistance. As a main component of fitness, muscular endurance is important for everyone, not just people who play sports.

Some examples of muscular endurance include lifting weight for more repetitions or running for an extended period of time. Muscular endurance helps you do everyday activities such as carrying a small child through a store or walking up several flights of stairs.

Muscular strength and muscular endurance go hand in hand in that your strength can affect the measure of your endurance. It is vital to maintain good muscular endurance to be able to perform activities of daily living and more.

Muscular Endurance Tips
- Muscular endurance relies on muscular strength.
- Muscular endurance exercises are characterized by lower resistance with more repetitions or sets.
- Generally, to improve muscular endurance, complete 4 to 6 sets of 10 to 20 repetitions.
- Change up your resistance; it is okay to lift a little heavier on some days and lighter on others.
- Keep yourself hydrated.
- Warm up before beginning an endurance workout and cool down after.

PUSH-UPS

muscle focus: pectoralis majors, pectoralis minors, deltoids, triceps, biceps, and abdominal muscles

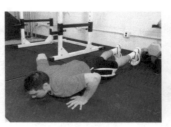
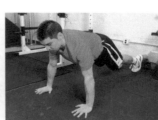

- Lie face down on a mat or the floor.
- Bending your elbows, place your hands next to your shoulders.
- Push with your hands to lift your body up off the mat or floor. Straighten your elbows when you come up.
- Keep your feet on the floor.
- Lower yourself slowly back to the floor, keeping your elbows close to your body.
- Complete 4 to 6 sets of 10 to 20 repetitions.

INCLINE PUSH-UPS

muscle focus: lower pectoralis muscles, deltoids, triceps, biceps, and abdominal muscles

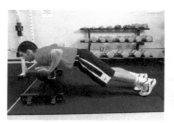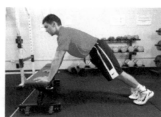

- Face a weight bench with your hands on the bench and your feet on the floor.
- Your hands should be just outside your shoulders and your elbows should be bent.
- Push with your hands so that your elbows are straight but not locked.
- Lower yourself slowly back to the starting position.
- Complete 4 to 6 sets of 10 to 20 repetitions.

DECLINE PUSH-UPS

muscle focus: pectoralis majors, deltoids, triceps, biceps, and abdominal muscles

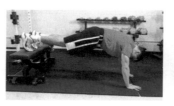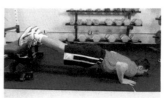

- Place your feet on a weight bench and your hands on the ground.
- Place your hands just outside of your shoulders.
- Push with your hands so that your elbows are straight but not locked.
- Lower yourself back to the starting position.
- Complete 4 to 6 sets of 10 to 20 repetitions.

TRICEP DIPS

muscle focus: triceps

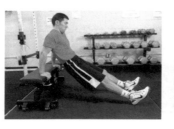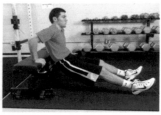

- Place your hands behind you on a weight bench or other safe elevated surface with your fingers pointing forward.
- Place your feet out in front of you so that you are in an inclined position.
- Bending your elbows, lower yourself slowly to the ground.
- Straightening your elbows, lift yourself slowly back up to the starting position.
- Complete 4 to 6 sets of 10 to 20 repetitions.

CRUNCHES

muscle focus: abdominal muscles

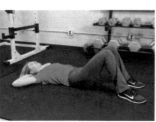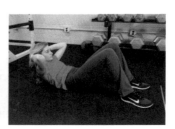

- Lie flat on your back either on a yoga mat or the floor with your knees bent.
- Place your hands behind your head.
- Lift your torso straight up until your shoulder blades are off the mat or floor. Tighten your abdominal muscles.
- Lower your torso back onto the mat or floor.
- Complete 4 to 6 sets of 10 to 20 repetitions.

SIDE CRUNCHES

muscle focus: abdominal muscles and oblique muscles

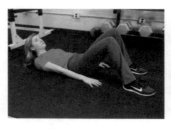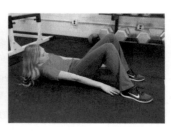

- Lie flat on your back either on a yoga mat or the floor with your knees bent.

- Place your arms and hands at your sides.

- Lift your shoulders slightly off the mat or floor.

- Bend to the right side so that your fingertips touch the heel of your right foot.

- Keep your lower back on the mat or floor.

- Complete 4 to 6 sets of 10 to 20 repetitions.

- Repeat this on the left side.

PLANKS

muscle focus: abdominal muscles

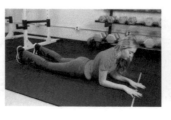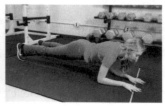

- Lie face down on either a mat or the floor.

- Bend your elbows and place them just under your shoulders. Your back should be in an extension position.

- Place your feet straight out behind you hip-width apart.

- Lift your body so that all of your weight is in your elbows, forearms, and feet.

- Keep your back flat and your abdomen tight.

- Hold this for 30 seconds.

- Lower yourself slowly back to the ground.

- Once 30 seconds starts to get easy, increase your time gradually.

BACK EXTENSIONS (MACHINE OR FITNESS BALL)

muscle focus: erector spinae

Machine

- Using a back-extension machine if you are at a gym, sit so that the padded bar is just below your shoulder blades.

- Adjust the weight rack to a weight that you can handle. Do not attempt a weight that is too heavy for you.

- Place your arms at your sides or on your thighs. Push the padded bar with your back so that your back is extended.

- Bring yourself slowly back to the starting position.

- Complete 4 to 6 sets of 10 to 20 repetitions.

Fitness Ball

- If you are at home and do not have a back-extension machine, you can use a fitness ball. Lie flat with your abdomen on the ball. Place your hands behind your head. Lift your upper body off the ball so that only your lower abdomen is on the ball.

- Complete 4 to 6 sets of 10 to 20 repetitions.

LUNGES

muscle focus: glutei maximi, hamstrings, and quadriceps

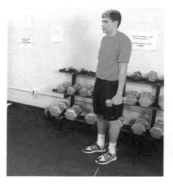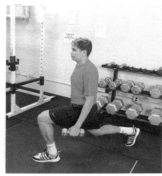

- Hold a dumbbell in each hand.

- Stand with your feet hip-width apart.

- Step forward with a foot and bend your knee at a 90-degree angle. Make sure that your knee does not go over your toes. Your back leg should almost be straight behind you.

- Bend your back knee to lower yourself to almost touching the ground.

- Come back up slowly, bringing your front leg back to the starting position.

- Switch legs.

- Complete 4 to 6 sets of 10 to 20 repetitions.

SQUATS

muscle focus: glutei maximi, hamstrings, and erector spinae

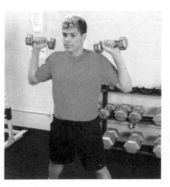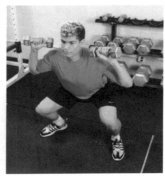

- Stand with your feet shoulder-width apart.

- Hold a dumbbell up near your shoulders with each hand.

- Bending your knees, lower your buttocks toward the ground. Keep your back straight.

- Do not let your knees go past your toes. If they do, you are going down too low or your legs are too close together.

- Straightening your knees, bring yourself back to the starting position.

- Complete 4 to 6 sets of 10 to 20 repetitions.

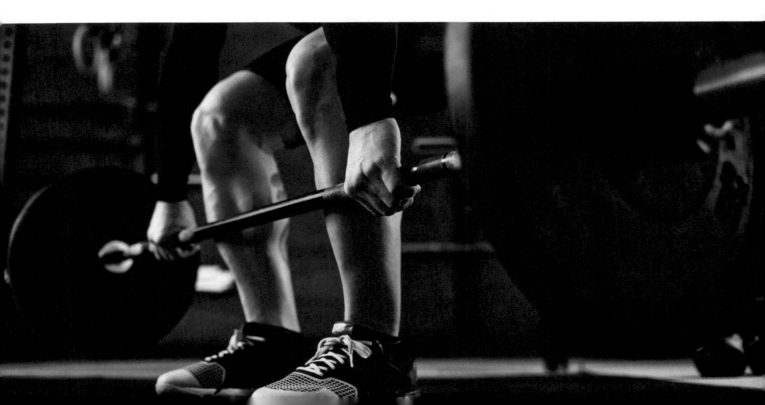

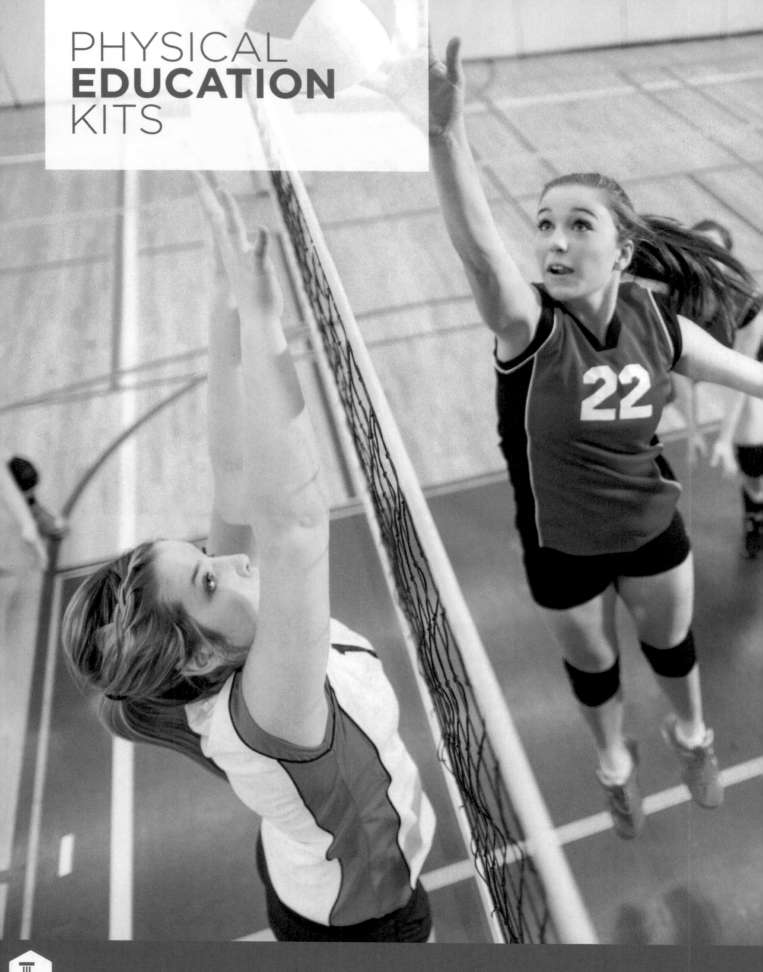

PHYSICAL
EDUCATION
KITS

PHYSICAL EDUCATION KITS

Physical Education is critical to developing the whole child. The National Association of Sport and Physical Education (NASPE) recommends that children have 60 minutes per day of physical activity. The Physical Education Kit has been designed to help create activities for each age. The kit includes various equipment that is designed to enhance your physical skills and fitness based on your age group. Equipment instructions are provided in the PE manual, online course and USB.

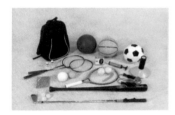

GRADE 7 EQUIPMENT KIT

- Backpack
- Badminton Set
- Playground Ball
- Basketball
- Disc Cones
- Golf Iron/ Golf Balls
- 9' Jump Rope
- Movement Band
- Pump
- 22" Tennis Racket
- 3 Foam Tennis Balls
- Soccer Ball
- 2 Stretch Bands
- Wiffle Ball Bat/Balls

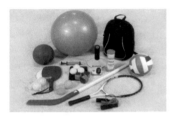

GRADE 8 EQUIPMENT KIT

- Backpack
- 30" Fitness Ball
- Playground Ball
- Disc Cones
- Juggle Pack
- 9' Jump Rope
- Movement Band
- Pickleball Paddles/ Balls
- Pump
- Tennis Racket
- 3 Tennis Balls
- Volleyball
- Hockey Stick/Puck/ Ball

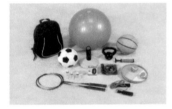

GRADE 9 EQUIPMENT KIT

- Backpack
- 30" Fitness Ball
- Badminton Set
- Basketball
- Disc Cones
- 9' Jump Rope
- Kettlebell
- Movement Band
- Pump
- Resistance Band/ Handles
- Soccer Ball
- Velcro Catch Set

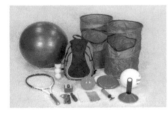

GRADE 10 EQUIPMENT KIT

- Backpack
- 30" Fitness Ball
- Weighted Ball
- Can Jam Set
- Disc Cones
- 9' Jump Rope
- Movement Band
- Pump
- 2 Stretch Bands
- Tennis Racket
- 3 Tennis Balls
- Volleyball

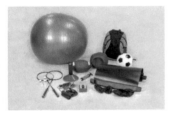

GRADE 11 EQUIPMENT KIT

- Backpack
- 35" Fitness Ball
- Badminton
- Disc Cones
- Double Grip Medicine Ball
- Football
- 9' Jump Rope
- Movement Band
- Pump
- Resistance Band/ Handles
- 8' Slider/Boots
- Soccer Ball

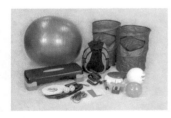

GRADE 12 EQUIPMENT KIT

- Backpack
- 35" Fitness Ball
- Weighted Ball
- Can Jam Set
- 9' Jump Rope
- Movement Band
- Pickleball Paddles/ Balls
- Pump
- Push-up Handles
- 2 Resistance Bands
- Stepper
- Volleyball

ELECTRONIC MOVEMENT BAND

Welcome! However you may choose to move, you will have fun watching your moves add up as your electronic movement band records all of your physical activity—not just steps. The electronic movement band keeps you aware of your daily physical activity so that you can make healthy decisions to keep moving. So, what are you waiting for? It is time to get started!

The instructions to set up your electronic movement band are included with the device.

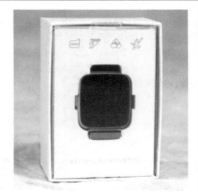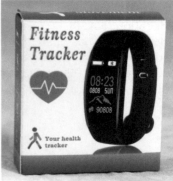

DID YOU KNOW?

Learning and using all this information is great; but, if you do not understand why it is important to take care of yourself both physically and mentally, the odds of you staying active as an adult will decrease. Lack of activity as an adult can result in many problems and illnesses. You might not think about it now, but the habits that you create as a child and young adult will affect you as an adult. Consider the information below.

- Lack of physical activity can lead to a greater risk of developing high blood pressure, cardiovascular disease, and other conditions.

- As you transition into adulthood and start a career, activity can help you manage stress and anxiety and can limit work burnouts.

  - Depending on your career choice, your opportunity to be active during the day can be significantly limited by your schedule, so finding exercise or activity that you thoroughly enjoy is imperative to your health and wellness.

  - On the other hand, if you have a career that is physically demanding, you want to make sure that you can perform at that job to the best of your ability.

- On a less obvious but more important scale, maintaining your physical and mental health is vital to being able to complete activities of daily living. Such activities include getting in and out of bed, getting yourself dressed and ready, climbing stairs, stepping onto a ladder or stepstool, walking through an amusement park, and so on.

  - These activities may seem minor and you might take for granted that you can do these things with ease now; but, if you are in poor health, these activities can be very difficult, if not impossible.

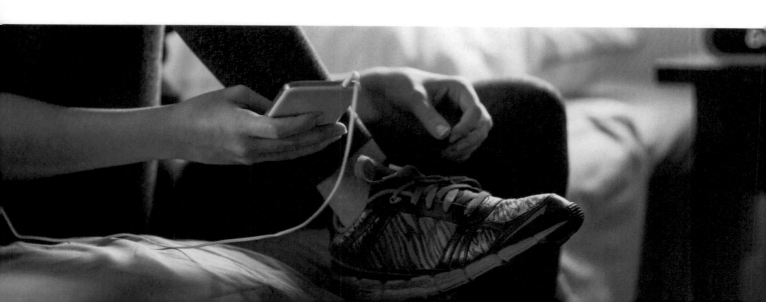

GRADE 7
PE EQUIPMENT KIT

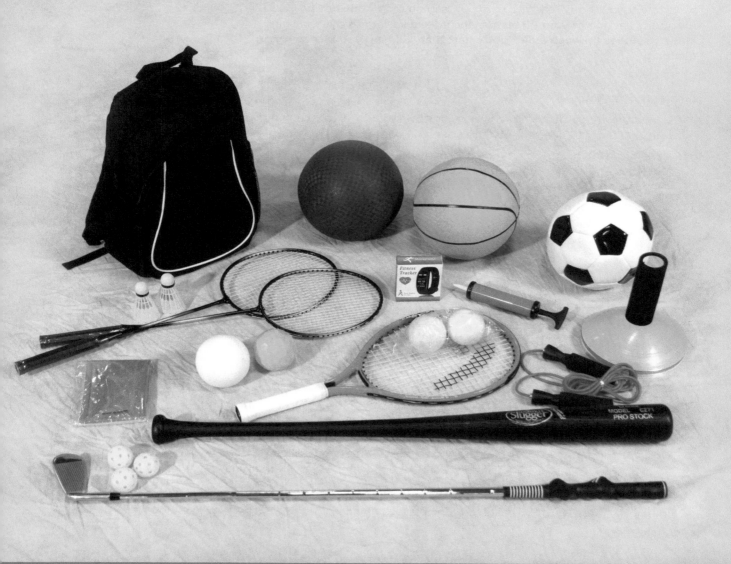

WARM-UP AND COOL-DOWN

⚠ **CAUTION:** Stretching should not be painful; ease up if stretching hurts. See the Flexibility section of your PE Manual for more information.

WARM-UP

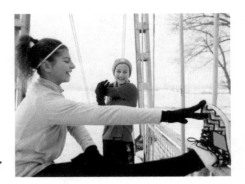

The purpose of a warm-up is to gradually increase heart rate, breathing rate, body temperature, and muscle temperature. Warming up prior to exercising increases circulation and blood flow to your muscles. When your muscles are warmed up, their performance—such as in the areas of strength and speed—is enhanced and risk of injury is decreased.

Before you begin any workout, you should always warm up. Getting your heart and muscles prepared for exercise is important. There are numerous ways to get your body ready to participate in physical activity. **The Flexibility section of your PE Manual includes a variety of dynamic and static stretches for each major body part that will help you increase your flexibility.**

Elements of a Warm-Up

1. **Low-intensity cardio**: Walk, slow jog, or slow swim for 5 to 10 minutes to increase your heart rate, breathing rate, and body temperature before your workout.

2. **Dynamic stretch**: Perform a repeated motion—such as kicks, high knees, lunges, or arm circles—that will loosen up your joints and prepare your muscles for the exercise that you are about to do. Perform each dynamic stretch for at least 30 seconds.

3. **Static stretch**: Stretch your muscles slowly and hold each stretch for 20 to 30 seconds without bouncing in order to lengthen your muscles and increase your flexibility. Some important areas to stretch as a part of your warm-up are your neck, sides, shoulders, triceps, back, hamstrings, quadriceps, and groin.

Example 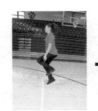 **+** 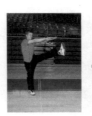 **+** 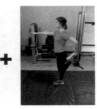 **= EFFECTIVE WARM-UP**

PERSONAL WARM-UP ACTIVITY

1. Select an exercise activity to participate in.

2. Design your personal warm-up plan for the activity that you selected. Any dynamic and static stretches that you choose to complete should be specific to the exercise activity that you chose.

3. Have a trusted adult or friend assess your stretches to make sure that you are using proper form.

4. Explain how the warm-up will decrease your risk of injury for this activity. _____

Procedure	Enter your personal warm-up regimen below.
1. **Low-intensity cardiovascular exercise:** Exercise for 5 to 10 minutes.	
2. **Dynamic stretches:** Perform dynamic stretches specifically for the selected activity.	
3. **Static stretches:** Perform static stretches specifically for the selected activity.	

COOL-DOWN

After you have finished your workout, exercise, or activity, it is imperative that your body returns to its normal state. You want to avoid stopping immediately and sitting down **unless you are in pain, dizzy, or injured**. Be sure to slow your heart rate and breathing rate back to or slightly above their resting rates. There are several ways to do this. You can simply walk or slow down your exercise for a few minutes, or you can find your own way to slow your body back down. You also may want to incorporate static stretches to increase flexibility and to avoid your muscles tightening. **The Flexibility section of your PE Manual includes a variety of static stretches for each major body part.** Always keep hydrated by drinking water before, during, and after exercise.

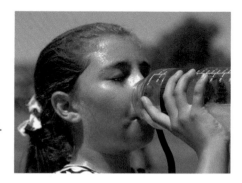

Elements of a Cool-Down

1. **Slow down**: Walk or gradually slow down your exercise—such as returning to a slow swim if you are swimming—until your heart rate, breathing rate, and body temperature are back to normal.

2. **Static stretch**: Stretch your muscles slowly and hold each stretch for 20 to 30 seconds without bouncing in order to lengthen your muscles and increase flexibility. Some important areas to stretch as part of your cool-down are your neck, sides, shoulders, triceps, back, hamstrings, quadriceps, and groin.

WALK + STATIC STRETCHES = EFFECTIVE COOL-DOWN

Design your personal cool-down plan. You can perform the same cool-down each time you finish a physical activity or you can change each time in order to reflect the exercise activity, such as by slowing your pedaling if you are biking.

Procedure	Enter your personal cool-down regimen below.
1. **Slow down:** Perform this slowed activity for 5 to 10 minutes.	
2. **Static stretches:** Perform several lower-body and upper-body stretches.	

AEROBIC EXERCISE

Aerobic exercise—also referred to as cardio or cardiovascular exercise—is any exercise that is done in your target heart rate zone and is performed for an extended period. Aerobic exercise is important for strengthening your heart muscle. The stronger your heart muscle, the longer you can perform physical activity before getting tired. Being able to perform physical activity without tiring is often referred to as being in shape.

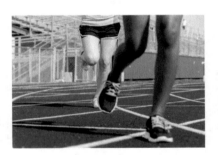

The purpose of this lesson is to encourage you to do an aerobic workout for at least 30 minutes 3 to 5 days per week in order to experience health benefits.

 CAUTION: Wear proper equipment and follow activity-specific safety rules.

AEROBIC EXERCISE

BENEFITS OF AEROBIC EXERCISE

- strengthens your heart and lung functions
- lowers blood pressure
- controls sugar in your blood
- burns calories and fat

- increases your energy
- reduces stress
- decreases your risk of cardiovascular diseases
- increases mental ability

After reviewing the benefits of aerobic exercise, discuss them with a trusted adult. Ask for help setting up an aerobic exercise program that works for you.

There are a variety of exercises to choose from. Choose aerobic exercises that will fit into your lifestyle and that you enjoy. Limit excuses and make a commitment to exercise!

Write down an excuse that you have used to avoid aerobic exercise and how you overcame or will overcome that obstacle.

My Excuse for Not Exercising	What I Did to Overcome That Excuse

TYPES OF AEROBIC EXERCISE

Sports: Examples include soccer, basketball, volleyball, swimming, hockey, lacrosse, tennis, badminton, pickleball, handball, gymnastics, dance, martial arts, wrestling, track and field, and so on.

Outdoor pursuits: Examples include walking, jogging, biking, canoeing, kayaking, golfing, fly fishing, hiking, rock climbing, horseback riding, skiing, and so on.

Fitness gyms: Find a gym that is convenient for you to attend where you can complete circuit exercises, use aerobic machines, take classes, and more.

Stationary exercise equipment: Examples include using a jump rope, treadmill, elliptical trainer, bike, mini trampoline, and so on.

Exercise apps or videos: Use a workout tutorial on an app, website, video, or other digital source.

Your own sequence workouts: You can also design your own workout sequences by following the steps below.

- Create your personal aerobic workout routines by blending activities that involve basic locomotor skills such as jogging in place, jumping jacks, high knees, and so on.
- Design the intensity and duration of the exercise according to your level of fitness.
- Perform your personal routine for some or all your aerobic workouts.

SAMPLE WORKOUT

The following is a sample workout that you can complete on your own and that does not require equipment. When you are beginning any exercise program, begin with workouts that match your fitness level and then build accordingly. You want to feel refreshed after each exercise session, not exhausted. Use your pulse rate to monitor aerobic workouts.

Each exercise is performed for 30 seconds: 10 seconds using a light force and slow pace, 10 seconds using a moderate force and moderate pace, and 10 seconds using a strong force and fast pace.

Practice each of the following exercises, concentrating on proper form, prior to engaging in a workout.

JUMPING JACKS:

Jump out so that your feet are apart and your arms are in a V above your head; then, jump in so that your feet are together and your arms are down by your sides. Continue this movement pattern.

MARCH:

Walk, lifting your knees to waist height and swinging your arms.

HIGH KNEES:

Alternate lifting your knees to waist height.

VERTICAL JUMPS:

Bend your knees and jump up. Swing your arms behind you at the start of the jump. Swing your arms forward and up while you are jumping.

BURPEES:

Stand with your feet shoulder-width apart. Bend your knees and place your hands on the floor. Extend your legs back so that you are in a push-up position. Return to the bent-knee position. Return to standing. Repeat this movement pattern.

FLOOR RUNS:

From a push-up position, run your legs in toward your chest and then back out.

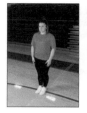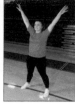

Jumping jacks

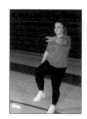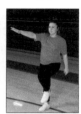

March

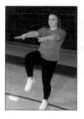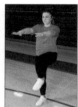

High knees

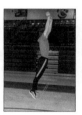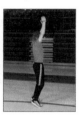

Vertical jumps

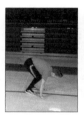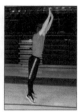

Burpees

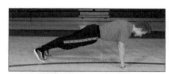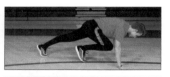
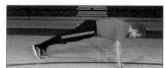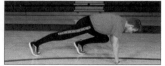

Floor runs

JOGGING IN PLACE:

Run slowly in place.

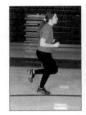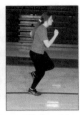

Jogging in place

SIDE SLIDES:

Step to the side with your right foot. Bring your left foot to your right foot in a step-together motion. Repeat this to the left.

REAR KICKS:

Alternate lifting the heels of your feet toward your upper thighs. Do not let your feet make contact with your body.

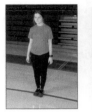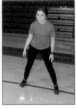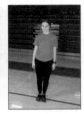

Side slides

KNEE TUCKS:

While standing, jump up and tuck your knees. Try to touch your knees with your extended hands. Gently land with your knees slightly bent.

¼-SQUAT JUMPS:

With your legs apart, lower your body by bending your knees and hips until your hips are even with your knees. Jump to the right, making a quarter turn and landing gently in a squat position. Continue until you are back to the starting position. Repeat the exercise to the left. For a challenge, try half turns and full turns.

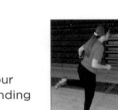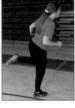

Rear kicks

CARIOCAS (GRAPEVINE):

Step to the side with your right foot and then cross your left foot in front of your right foot. Uncross your right foot and step to the right and then cross your left foot behind your right foot. Repeat this step-cross-step-cross movement.

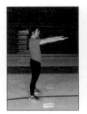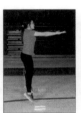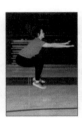

Knee tucks

Rest by walking slowly for 30 seconds. Hydrate as necessary.

Repeat all of the exercises 3 more times for a 24-minute aerobic workout.

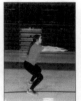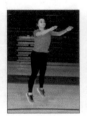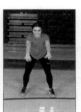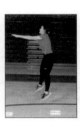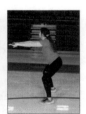

¼-squat jumps

EXTENSION: Use the above information to create a workout that you would enjoy.

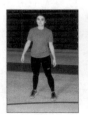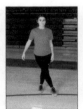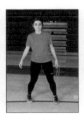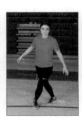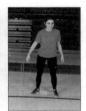

Cariocas (grapevine)

Record at least 3 aerobic exercise sessions that you participated in outside of PE class for 1 week. Record the time of each session.

An exercise can be any of the following.

1. a sport-related game

2. an outdoor pursuit

3. a self-created workout routine set to music

	Monday	Tuesday	Wednesday	Thursday	Friday	Saturday	Sunday
Exercise							
Time							
Exercise Heartrate							

List at least 1 response to each the following questions about aerobic exercise.

Question	Response
What positive emotional response did you experience by participating in aerobic exercise?	
What aerobic exercise activity did you enjoy the most?	
Why would the enjoyment of your favorite aerobic exercise activity lead to a lifetime of fitness for you?	

RESEARCH INTEGRATION

Research Newton's laws of motion and their connection to movement. How does the sample workout apply Newton's second law of motion?

HEALTH INTEGRATION

Use available technology to monitor your pulse rate and workout intensity. Apply the results to your overall fitness plan.

DANCE

Dancing is an exercise option for aerobic workout, for competition, or just for fun. You can dance on your own or with others. Dancing is expressing yourself through repeated patterns of movement which are usually set to music. Some forms of dance include creative, tap, ballet, hip-hop, modern, folk, square, jazz, line, Latin, ballroom, and social.

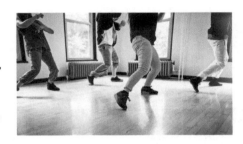

The purpose of this lesson is for you to perform basic locomotor movements using common dance concepts in rhythmic patterns to create your own dance for aerobic exercise.

PERSONAL DANCE ROUTINE

COMMON CONCEPTS OF DANCE TO USE FOR YOUR PERSONAL DANCE

- The concept of space includes the following.
  - ○ high, medium, or low **levels**
  - ○ forward, backward, right, or left **directions**
  - ○ curved, zigzag, straight, circle, or square **pathways**
- The concept of time includes the following.
  - ○ slow, medium, or fast **speeds**
  - ○ a pattern for **rhythm**
- The concept of force includes the following.
  - ○ applying light, moderate, or strong **weights**

CREATE A DANCE

Start with the 3 dance steps below. Then, complete the routine by adding your own dance steps. Set your dance to music.

1. Learn a sidestep.
   - Step to the right with your right foot.
   - Bring your left foot in to meet your right foot.
   - Touch your left toes to the floor with a light force, but do not put weight on them.
   - Repeat this to the left.

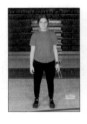
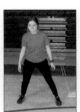
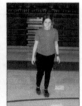

Sidestep

2. Learn a step-hop.
   - Step out to the right side with your right foot.
   - Bring your left foot in and simultaneously jump with a medium force.
   - Land with both feet together.
   - As you land, clap your hands.
   - Repeat this to the left.

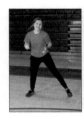
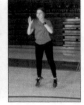

Step-hop

3. Combine the sidestep and step-hop for a double step (step together, step-hop, clap).
   - Step to the right with your right foot.
   - Bring your left foot in to meet your right foot.
   - Step out to the right side with your right foot.
   - Bring your left foot in and simultaneously jump, land, and clap.
   - Repeat this to the left.

4. Perform the double step 4 times.

5. Next, add your dance steps to complete the dance.

   - Choose locomotor skills to blend (slides, cariocas, turns, and so on).
   - Use your arms to accompany the footwork, for example: step, cross, step, clap.
   - Perform the skills at different levels.
   - Move in different directions.
   - Move in different pathways.
   - Move at slow, medium, and fast speeds.
   - Use light, moderate, and strong force to move your body.
   - Create a pattern.
   - Use an 8 count for each move.

Option: Dance with a partner or small group for a social experience.

RATE YOUR ENJOYMENT OF DANCE

On a scale from 1 to 4, where 1 is not enjoyable and 4 is very enjoyable, rate this activity.

1	It was not enjoyable, and I will not participate again.
2	It was not enjoyable, but I will participate again for exercise.
3	It was enjoyable, and I will dance again.
4	It was very enjoyable, and I will create more dances.

RESEARCH INTEGRATION

1. Research creative dance.
2. Join a dance class or dance to a dance video.
3. Join a dance from the USB if provided in your PE program.

HEALTH INTEGRATION

Count your pulse to determine if you are exercising in your personal target heart rate zone. Apply the results to your overall fitness plan. Many people choose to complete aerobic workouts through dance.

JUMP ROPE

Jumping rope is an exercise that meets components of both skill-related fitness and health-related fitness. It helps you develop coordination, balance, rhythm, agility, and timing. Jumping rope is an efficient way to perform aerobic exercise and build muscular strength and endurance in your legs. It can be done daily and in a small space almost anywhere there is a safe, stable surface.

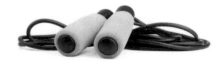

The purpose of this lesson is to provide you with the skills that you need to establish and implement your goal: to improve sport-related skills, to improve cardiovascular endurance, or both.

JUMP ROPE BASICS

FITTING THE JUMP ROPE TO YOUR HEIGHT

- Place a jump rope handle in each hand.
- Stand on the middle of the rope with 1 foot.
- Move the handles straight up, making sure that the rope is straight and pulled tight.
- The tops of the handles should reach close to your shoulders.

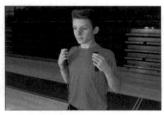

Fitting The Jump Rope To Your Height

ELEMENTS OF JUMP ROPE

- Keep your eyes forward.
- When you are turning the rope, keep your elbows near your sides, maintaining a 45-degree angle and making 2-inch circles with your wrists.
- Leave just enough space for the rope to pass under your feet when you jump.
- Stay on the balls of your feet.
- Land softly, keeping your knees slightly bent.

BASIC SKILLS

Practice each of the following exercises, concentrating on proper form, prior to engaging in a workout.

BASIC JUMP

- Pick up the rope. Holding a handle in each hand, rest the rope behind your feet. Stand on the balls of your feet. This is the ready position.
- Your hands should be just above the height of your waist.
- Swing the rope up and over your head.
- Jump over the rope when it approaches your toes.
- Continue as long as you can without stopping.

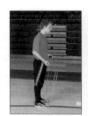 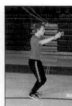 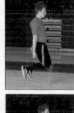
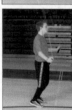 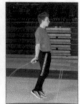

Basic jump

BACKWARD JUMP

- Begin with the rope in front of your feet.
- Swing the rope up and over your head.
- Jump over the rope when it approaches your feet.

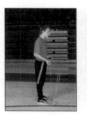 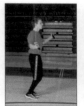 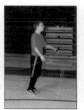 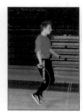 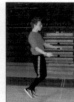

Backward jump

SAMPLE OF A CARDIOVASCULAR CONDITIONING WORKOUT	SAMPLE OF A WORKOUT TO IMPROVE FOOTWORK SPEED
• basic jump 2 minutes • march or jog in place 30 seconds • basic jump 2 minutes • march or jog in place 30 seconds • backward jump 2 minutes • march or jog in place 30 seconds • backward jump 2 minutes • march or jog in place 30 seconds • repeat for a 20-minute workout	• basic jump 1 minute at a medium pace • basic jump 30 seconds at a fast pace • rest 30 seconds • back jump 1 minute at a medium pace • back jump 30 seconds at a fast pace • rest 30 seconds • basic jump 30 seconds at a medium pace • basic jump 1 minute at a fast pace • rest 30 seconds • back jump 30 seconds at a medium pace • back jump 1 minute at a fast pace • rest 30 seconds • repeat as needed
DESIGN YOUR PERSONAL CARDIOVASCULAR JUMP ROPE ROUTINE	DESIGN YOUR PERSONAL FOOTWORK SPEED ROUTINE

CHALLENGE SKILLS

The following challenges are for students who have mastered the basic jump rope skills. The challenge level is recommended for you if you want to improve agility and further explore jump rope activities.

JUMP ROPE CHALLENGE SKILLS

Practice each of the following exercises, concentrating on proper form, prior to engaging in a workout.

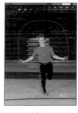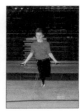

Hop on 1 foot (switch)

HOP ON 1 FOOT (SWITCH)

- Perform the basic jump on 1 foot instead of 2 feet.

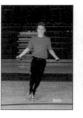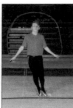

Skier

SKIER

- With both feet together, hop from side to side while turning the rope.

CROSSOVERS

- After the rope moves over your head, cross the rope in front of you, jump, and uncross the rope.

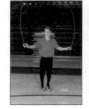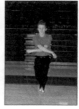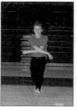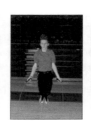

Crossovers

FRONT KICKS

- Kick 1 foot forward as the rope passes under your feet with a skip-step between.
- Alternate kicks.

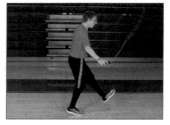

Front kicks

Design your personal jump rope routine by blending the basic skills and the challenge skills.

BLENDING: Perform a jump rope skill and transition smoothly to another jump rope skill without stopping between moves.

Check off the blended challenge skills that you have successfully completed at least 3 consecutive times.

_____ Blend forward consecutive jumps, crossovers, and skiers.

_____ Blend backward consecutive jumps, right-foot hops, and left-foot hops, all while backward turning.

_____ Blend forward consecutive jumps, front kicks, and skiers.

_____ Create your personal blend.

PARTNER SKILLS

Jump rope can have a social component. Individual jumping with a friend may motivate you and may make your workout more fun. Partner or long jump rope requires 2 or more participants.

PARTNER JUMP ROPE SKILLS

Practice each of the following exercises, concentrating on proper form, prior to engaging in a workout.

PARTNER CHAIN JUMP

- Make sure that each person has their own rope.
- Standing side by side, face forward in the ready position.
- Exchange inside handles with your partner; hold your handle with your outside hand and your partner's handle with your inside hand.
- Turn the rope over your head and jump together.
- Establish a rhythm with your partner. Jump rope together to that rhythm.

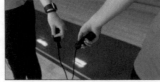
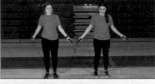
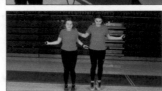
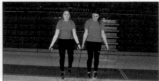

Partner chain jump

FACING YOUR PARTNER JUMP

- You will need 1 rope.
- Stand face-to-face with your partner.
- Have 1 person hold the rope.
- If you are holding the rope, stand facing your partner and turn the rope.
- If you are not holding the rope, stand facing your partner and jump rope with your partner as they turn the rope.
- No matter who is holding and turning the rope, establish a rhythm with your partner and jump rope together.

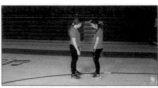
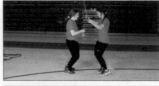
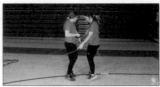
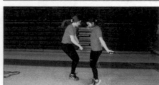

Facing your partner jump

SIDE BY SIDE JUMP

- You will need 1 rope.
- Stand beside your partner.
- Hold a handle of the rope with your outside hand. Your partner should hold the other handle in their outside hand.
- Jump rope together as you work together to turn the rope.

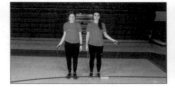
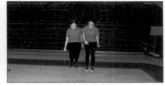

Side by side jump

List at least 1 response to each of the following questions about jumping rope.

Question	Response
What jump rope activity do you enjoy the most?	
Why did you enjoy the above-mentioned activity the most?	

 RESEARCH INTEGRATION

Research competitive jump rope.

HEALTH INTEGRATION

Count your pulse to determine if you are exercising in your personal target heart rate zone.

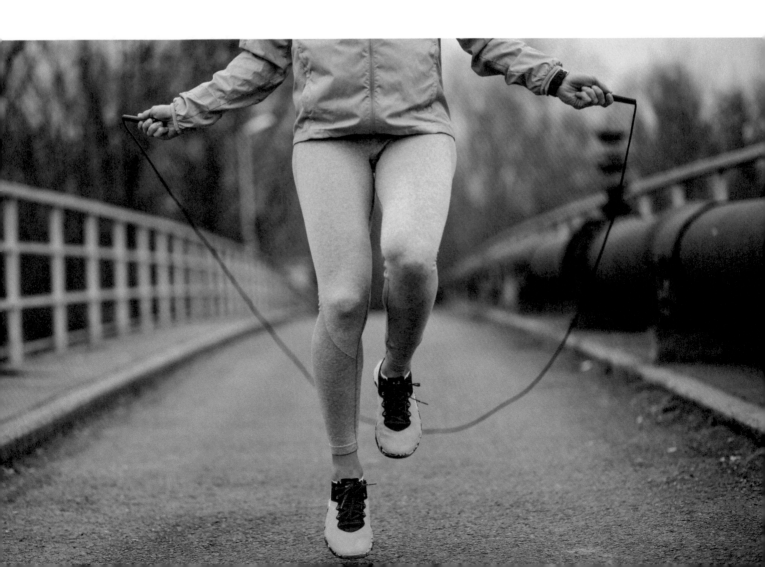

STRENGTH BUILDING

Skeletal muscles are soft tissues that are attached to bones and are responsible for moving the body. Your body is made up of over 600 muscles. Muscles work in pairs to pull on bones to create movement. Opposing muscles, or antagonistic muscles, should be equally trained because they work together. For example, when you bend your elbow, your triceps relaxes while your biceps contracts.

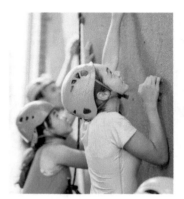

Muscles that are not used and not exercised become weak. Strength training, or resistance training, builds muscular strength and endurance.

The purpose of this lesson is to encourage you to perform strength-training exercises 2 or more days per week in order to experience health benefits. A certified trainer should help you set up a balanced, effective strength program.

⚠ **CAUTION: Have a certified trainer plan for you and supervise you when you are working with weights.**

STRENGTH TRAINING

BENEFITS OF STRENGTH TRAINING

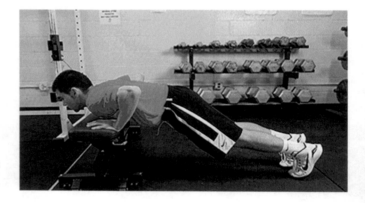

- strengthens your skeletal muscles
- strengthens your heart muscle
- strengthens your bones
- improves your posture
- lowers your risk of exercise-related injury
- burns calories and fat
- reduces stress

After reviewing the benefits of strength training, discuss them with a trusted adult. Ask for help setting up a program that works for you and for help staying committed to that program.

There are a variety of exercises from which to choose. Do strength exercises for the muscles of your upper body, lower body, and core. Choose the intensity of each exercise to fit your fitness level. For example, if you are struggling to do a right-angle push-up, switch to a knee push-up. Limit excuses and make a commitment to exercise!

STRENGTH-TRAINING EXERCISE IDEAS

Weightlifting machines: You can use large stationary machines like those typically found in gyms.

Free weights: You can use free-weight equipment such as dumbbells, barbells, medicine balls, kettlebells, resistance bands, and weighted ropes to perform strength-training exercises.

Pilates or yoga: Pilates and yoga sessions are excellent workouts for muscle lengthening and muscle strengthening.

Personal workouts: You can use your own body weight as a source of resistance and create your own strength-training workouts. Create a personal workout by blending basic strength-building exercises such as sit-ups, push-ups, pull-ups, planks, and so on, and design the intensity and duration of each exercise according to your level of fitness. Include upper-body, lower-body, and core exercises in your workout. Perform your personal routine for some or all your strength-training workouts.

The following is a sample personal strength-training workout that uses personal body weight as resistance. Practice each of the following exercises, concentrating on proper form, prior to engaging in a workout.

IN-OUT ABS

muscle focus: abdominal muscles

Intensity Level 1

Sit on a cushioned surface with your elbows flat on the ground slightly behind your hips. Keeping your knees bent, lift both legs until they are parallel to the ground. Extend your legs straight out in front of you and then return to the bent-knee position.

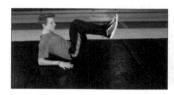

In-out abs: Intensity Level 1

Intensity Level 2

Sit on a cushioned surface with your hands flat on the ground slightly behind your hips. Keeping your knees bent, lift both legs until they are parallel to the ground. Extend your legs straight out in front of you and then return to the bent-knee position.

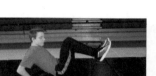
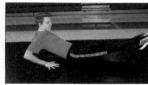

In-out abs: Intensity Level 2

Intensity Level 3

Sit on a cushioned surface with your arms held straight above your head. Keeping your knees bent, lift both legs until they are parallel to the ground. Extend your legs straight out in front of you and then return to the bent-knee position.

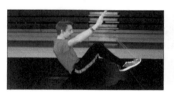
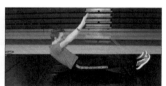

In-out abs: Intensity Level 3

FORWARD LUNGES

muscle focus: glutei maximi, hamstrings, and quadriceps

Intensity Level 1

Perform alternate forward lunges. Start with your feet together. Step 1 foot forward and bend your knee as low as you comfortably can. Do not exceed a 90-degree angle. Return to the starting position and then repeat the exercise with your other leg.

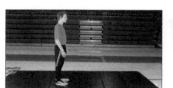
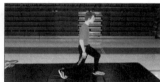

Forward lunges: Intensity Level 1

Intensity Level 2

Perform alternate forward lunges. Start with your feet together. Step 1 foot forward and bend your knee to a 90-degree angle. Return to the starting position and repeat the exercise with your other leg.

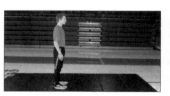
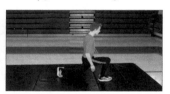

Forward lunges: Intensity Level 2

Intensity Level 3

Start with your feet together. Step your right foot forward and bend your knee to a 90-degree angle. Go back to the starting position. Continue lunging with your right foot until you have completed the repetitions. Next, lunge by stepping forward with your left foot until you complete the repetitions.

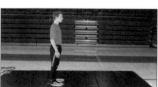
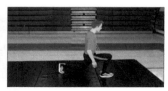

Forward lunges: Intensity Level 3

RIGHT-ANGLE PUSH-UPS

muscle focus: pectoralis majors, deltoids, triceps, biceps, and abdominal muscles

Intensity Level 1

Perform knee push-ups. Kneel on a cushioned surface with your back straight and your hands on the ground under your shoulders. Bend your elbows 90 degrees and then return to the straight-arm position, or plank position.

Intensity Level 2

Lie on your stomach. Place your hands under your shoulders. Straighten your arms to lift up your body. Make sure that your back and legs are straight from head to toe. Lower your body by bending your elbows as far as you can without exceeding 90. Straighten your arms to lift your body back up to the plank position, keeping your back and legs straight.

Intensity Level 3

Lie on your stomach. Place your hands under your shoulders. Straighten your arms to lift up your body. Make sure that your back and legs are straight from head to toe. Lower your body by bending your elbows 90 degrees. Straighten your arms to lift your body back up to the plank position, keeping your back and legs straight.

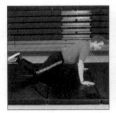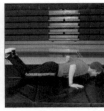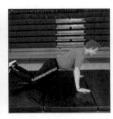

Right-Angle Push-ups: Intensity Level 1

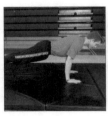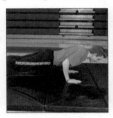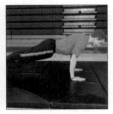

Right-Angle Push-ups: Intensity Level 2

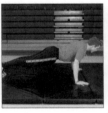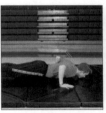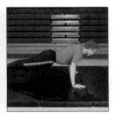

Right-Angle Push-ups: Intensity Level 3

ALTERNATE 6 INCHES

muscle focus: abdominal muscles

Intensity Level 1

Lie on your back on a cushioned surface. Pull 1 knee toward your chest. Extend your other leg straight out in front of you and parallel to the floor. Hold your extended leg 6 to 10 inches above the ground for 3 seconds. Switch legs.

Intensity Level 2

Lie on your back on a cushioned surface. Extend 1 leg up toward the ceiling with your knee bent. Extend your other leg straight out in front of you and parallel to the floor. Hold your extended leg 6 to 10 inches above the ground for 6 seconds. Switch legs.

Intensity Level 3

Lie on your back on a cushioned surface. Extend 1 leg straight up toward the ceiling. Extend your other leg straight out in front of you and parallel to the floor. Hold your extended leg 6 inches above the ground for 6 seconds. Switch legs.

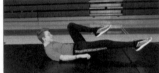

Alternate 6 inches: Intensity Level 1

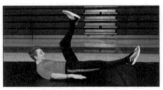

Alternate 6 inches: Intensity Level 2

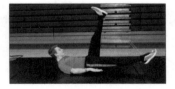

Alternate 6 inches: Intensity Level 3

SQUATS

muscle focus: glutei maximi, hamstrings, and quadriceps

Intensity Level 1

Stand with your legs shoulder-width apart and your hands on your hips. Lower your body by bending your knees and hips as low as you comfortably can. Do not lower your hips below knee level.

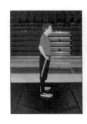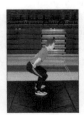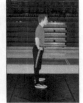

Squats: Intensity Level 1

Intensity Level 2

Stand with your legs shoulder-width apart and your arms extended out in front of you at shoulder height. With your legs apart, lower your body by bending your knees and hips until your hips are even with your knees.

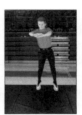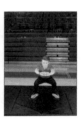

Intensity Level 3

Perform ¼-squat jumps. Standing with your legs shoulder-width apart, lower your body by bending your knees and hips until your hips are even with your knees. Jump to the right, making a quarter turn and landing gently in a squat position. Continue until you are back to the starting position. Repeat the exercise to the left.

Squats: Intensity Level 2

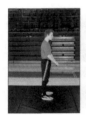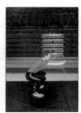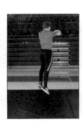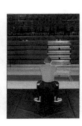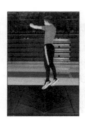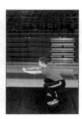

Squats: Intensity Level 3

TRICEPS PUSH-UPS (NARROW PUSH-UPS)

muscle focus: pectoralis majors, pectoralis minors, deltoids, triceps, biceps, and abdominal muscles

Intensity Level 1

Perform knee push-ups. Kneel on a cushioned surface with your back straight and your hands on the ground inside your shoulders. Bend your elbows 90 degrees and return to straight arms.

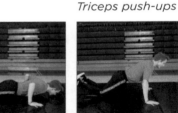

Triceps push-ups

Intensity Level 2

Lie on your stomach. Place your hands on the floor close to your body at chest level. Lift your body up with your triceps until you return to the straight-arm position. Make sure that your back and legs are straight from head to toe. Lower your body by bending your elbows as far as you can without exceeding 90 degrees. Return to the straight-arm position.

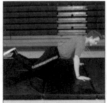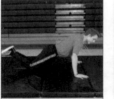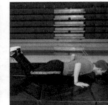

Triceps push-ups: Intensity Level 1

Intensity Level 3

Lie on your stomach. Place your hands on the floor close to your body at chest level. Lift your body up with your triceps until you return to the straight-arm position. Make sure that your back and legs are straight from head to toe. Lower your body by bending your elbows 90 degrees. Return to the straight-arm position.

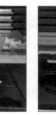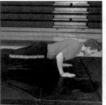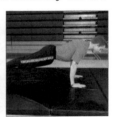

Right-Angle Push-ups: Intensity Level 2

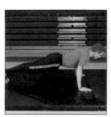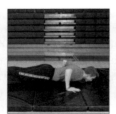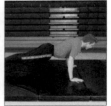

Right-Angle Push-ups: Intensity Level 3

SIT-UPS

muscle focus: abdominal muscles

Intensity Level 1

Perform fitness curl-ups. Lie on a cushioned surface with your knees flexed and your feet about 12 inches from your buttocks. With your arms at your sides, slide your fingertips 3 to 4 inches forward along the ground, simultaneously lifting your head and shoulders off the ground. Slowly lower your head and shoulders back to the ground.

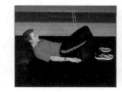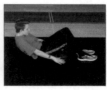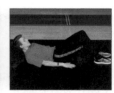

Sit-ups: Intensity Level 1

Intensity Level 2

Perform sit-ups. Lie on a cushioned surface with your knees flexed and your feet about 12 inches from your buttocks. A partner may hold your feet. Cross your arms, placing your hands on opposite shoulders and holding your elbows close to your chest. Raise your body until your elbows touch your thighs; then, lower your body until your shoulder blades touch the ground.

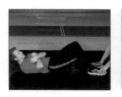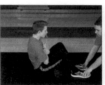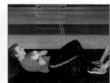

Sit-ups: Intensity Level 2

Intensity Level 3

Perform sit-ups. Lie on a cushioned surface with your knees flexed and your feet about 12 inches from your buttocks. Cross your arms, placing your hands on opposite shoulders and holding your elbows close to your chest. Raise your body until your elbows touch your thighs; then, lower your body until your shoulder blades touch the ground.

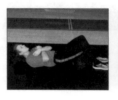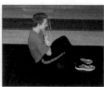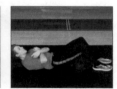

Sit-ups: Intensity Level 3

STEP-BACK LUNGES

muscle focus: glutei maximi, hamstrings, and quadriceps

Intensity Level 1

Perform alternate step-back lunges. Start by standing with your feet together and your hands on your hips. Step back with 1 foot and lower your knee as low as you comfortably can. Go back to the starting position and repeat this with your other leg.

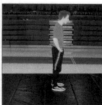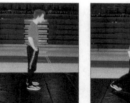

Step-back lunges: Intensity Level 1

Intensity Level 2

Perform alternate step-back lunges with high arms. Start by standing with your feet together and your arms extended straight above your head. Step back with 1 foot and lower your knee as far as you comfortably can. Return to the starting position and repeat this with your other leg.

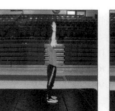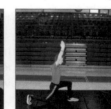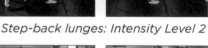

Step-back lunges: Intensity Level 2

Intensity Level 3

Start by standing with your feet together. Step back with your right foot and lower your knee as far as you comfortably can. Return to the starting position and continue lunging back with your right foot until you have completed the repetitions. Next, step back with your left foot until you complete the repetitions. Your hands may remain on your hips or remain extended.

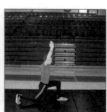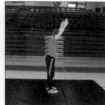

Step-back lunges: Intensity Level 3

WIDE PUSH-UPS

muscle focus: pectoralis majors, deltoids, triceps, biceps, and abdominal muscles

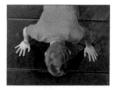

Wide push-ups

Intensity Level 1

Kneel on a cushioned surface with your back straight and your hands on the ground outside your shoulders. Bend your elbows 90 degrees. Return to the straight-arm position.

Intensity Level 2

Lie on your stomach. Place your hands outside your shoulders. Lift your body up to a straight-arm position. Make sure that your back and legs are straight from head to toe. Lower your body by bending your elbows as far as you can without exceeding 90 degrees. Return to the straight-arm position.

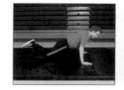 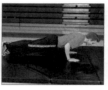 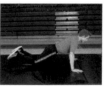

Wide push-ups: Intensity Level 1

Intensity Level 3

Lie on your stomach. Place your hands outside your shoulders. Lift your body up to a straight-arm position. Make sure that your back and legs are straight from head to toe. Lower your body by bending your elbows 90 degrees. Return to the straight-arm position.

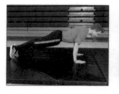 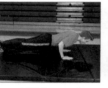 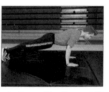

Wide push-ups: Intensity Level 2

HOW TO USE YOUR BODY WEIGHT IN A STRENGTH-TRAINING WORKOUT

- Warm up before your workout. Cool down after your workout.

- Choose the appropriate level of intensity for you.

- Perform each exercise 2 to 3 days per week.

- Begin with 1 set of 10 repetitions of each exercise. Increase sets and repetitions when the exercise becomes easy for you.

- Your goal should be to reach 3 sets of 15 repetitions of each exercise.

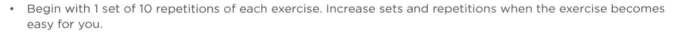

Wide push-ups: Intensity Level 3

List at least 1 response to each of the following questions about strength training.

Question	Response
What positive emotional response did you experience by participating in strength training?	
Why would the enjoyment of strength training lead you to a lifetime of fitness?	

💻 RESEARCH INTEGRATION

Research and compare skeletal muscles with muscles that work your heart, digestion, and eye focus.

RESISTANCE BANDS

Resistance bands are elastic bands that are used to improve flexibility, muscular strength, muscular endurance, and body composition. When you first use resistance bands, start with the lightest resistance and then gradually increase to a higher resistance as you get stronger.

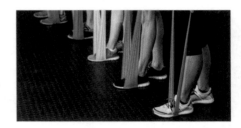

The purpose of this lesson is to encourage you to use resistance bands for strength training.

FITNESS TIP: Secure the resistance band in a way that the length is appropriate to give resistance for the entire exercise. Wrap the band around your hands if you need to increase your resistance level.

CAUTION: Check the resistance band for damage or wear before exercising. When you are exercising, secure the band before adding any resistance.

BENEFITS OF STRENGTH TRAINING WITH RESISTANCE BANDS

- is an effective overall strength workout that does not require weights
- offers a variety of resistance adjustments for beginner through advanced levels
- requires inexpensive pieces of equipment
- requires equipment that is easy to carry with you when you are traveling

Practice each of the following exercises, concentrating on proper form, prior to engaging in a workout.

SQUATS

muscle focus: quadriceps, hamstrings, and glutei maximi

- Stand on the middle of the band with your feet shoulder-width apart.
- Hold an end of the band in each hand. Bend your elbows and place your hands by your ears.
- Bend your legs as if you were sitting in a chair. Bend until your legs are at 90-degree angles. Do not let your knees go past your toes.
- Stand back up to the starting position. Do not lock your knees.

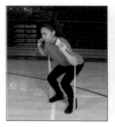
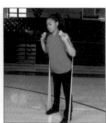

Squats

LEG EXTENSIONS

muscle focus: quadriceps, hamstrings, and glutei maximi

- Lay with your back flat on the ground and with your right knee bent to your chest.
- Wrap your band around the bottom of your right foot, holding an end in each hand.
- Keep your left leg flat on the ground.
- Hold the band firmly in your hands and push your right leg straight out without fully straightening your knee.
- Bring your leg slowly back to the starting position.
- After completing the set, switch to your left leg.

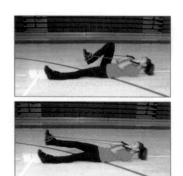

Leg extensions

OVERHEAD PRESSES

muscle focus: pectoralis majors, anterior deltoids, and triceps

- Sit in a chair on the middle of the resistance band so that you have an even amount of space on either side.
- Sit up straight and place an end of the band in each hand.
- Bend your elbows, bringing your hands up to your ears. The band should run parallel to your triceps.
- Extend both hands straight up and above your head.
- Bend your elbows, lowering your hands slowly back to the starting position.

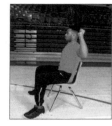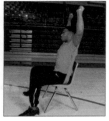

Overhead presses

LATERAL RAISES

muscle focus: pectoralis majors, pectoralis minors, biceps, triceps, and front fibers of deltoids

- Place an end of the band under your right foot and the other end in your right hand.
- Keeping your right arm straight at your side, make sure that the tension of the band is at a good level. If the resistance is not enough, wrap the band around your hand until it feels comfortable.
- Keeping your right arm straight, raise it out to your side so that it is parallel to the ground.
- Bring your right arm slowly back to your side. Keep your arm straight during the entire exercise.
- After completing the repetitions, repeat the exercise with your left arm.

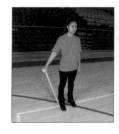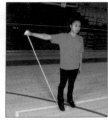

Lateral raises

TRICEPS EXTENSIONS

muscle focus: biceps and triceps

- Stand with your feet shoulder-width apart.
- Hold the band with an end in each hand.
- Bring the band behind your back so that your left hand is resting on your lower back and your right hand is just above your head with your elbow bent. The band should be parallel to your spine.
- Holding your left arm in place, extend your right arm straight above your right shoulder.
- Bend your right arm back to the starting position.
- After completing the repetitions, repeat the exercise with your left arm.
- If you need more resistance, wrap the band around your hands until it feels comfortable.

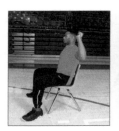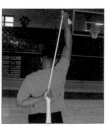

Tricep extensions

BICEPS HAMMER CURLS

muscle focus: biceps and triceps

- Stand on the middle of the exercise band with your feet shoulder-width apart.
- Hold both ends of the exercise band with your palms facing in toward your body.
- Bend at your elbows and slowly bring both hands toward the respective shoulder while keeping your elbows by your sides and your palms turned in toward your body.
- Return your arms slowly back to the starting position without fully straightening your elbows.

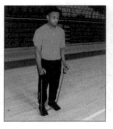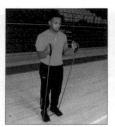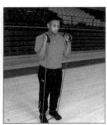

Biceps hammer curls

Have a trusted adult or friend evaluate you for correct form for the previous exercises. Did you respond positively to the feedback?

Reciprocate and evaluate your friend. Were you able to provide feedback in a positive manner?

How to Use Resistance Bands in a Strength-Training Workout

- Warm up before your workout. Cool down after your workout.
- Perform each resistance band exercise 2 to 3 days per week. Do not exercise the same muscle group on consecutive days.
- Begin with 1 set of 10 repetitions for each exercise. Increase sets and repetitions when the exercise becomes easy for you.
- Your goal should be to reach 3 sets of 10 to 15 repetitions.
- Wrap the band to increase resistance as necessary.

💻 RESEARCH INTEGRATION

Research and discuss with a trusted adult the role of exercise and nutrition in weight management.

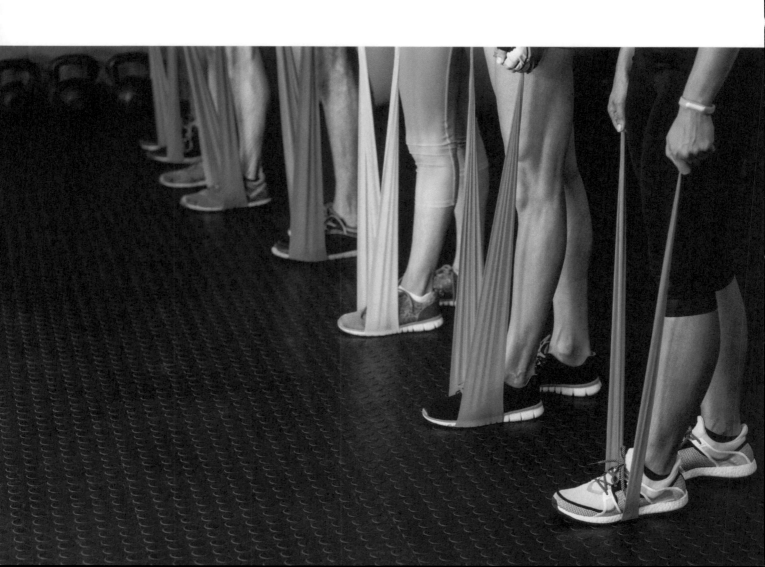

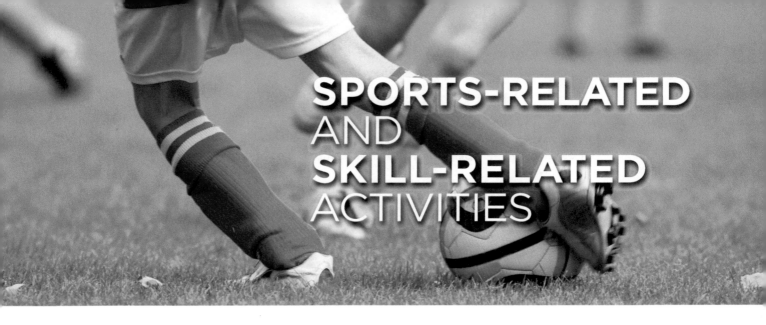

SPORTS-RELATED AND SKILL-RELATED ACTIVITIES

FITNESS TIP: Prior to beginning your physical education activities, read the following safety information that applies to every lesson, review the timeline, and review the assessment rubric.

SAFETY ALERT: Before you exercise, make sure that you are properly warmed up and have enough room to perform each activity. Wear proper equipment and follow activity-specific safety rules. Stay hydrated and take breaks as needed. Exercise only if you are healthy, and always exercise at your own pace. If an exercise starts to hurt, if you feel dizzy, or if you feel light-headed, stop the exercise completely and get help. Upon completion of any workout, cool down and stretch.

TIMELINE

Review all of the activity information before beginning. Use the scoring rubrics as assessment tools. You may ask a trusted adult or friend to observe your performance and provide feedback. Progress according to your skill level. The time that it takes you to complete a module will depend on your personal progress.

Practice and assess the first skill until competent.

Continue to progress until you have practiced and assessed each skill until competent.

Apply skills in a game situation.

ASSESSMENT RUBRIC

You will find a rubric assessment tool following some of the basic skills. Use this tool to evaluate and score your progress in learning the elements of a new skill.

SKILL	PROGRESSING	COMPETENT	PROFICIENT
skill 1	1 or 2 of the elements	3 or 4 out of 5 elements	all elements met

BADMINTON

Badminton is a sport that is played by striking a shuttlecock, or birdie, with a racket over a net. This striking activity helps you develop concentration, hand-eye coordination, and footwork. You may play badminton as a competitive sport or as an opportunity for social play.

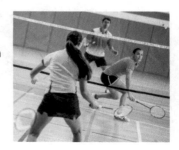

The purpose of this lesson is for you to practice badminton skills, participate in a badminton game, follow game rules, and communicate with others in a positive and effective manner.

⚠ **CAUTION: Make sure that nobody is close to you before you swing your racket. Do not walk into the path of another person who is swinging a racket.**

BADMINTON STROKES

READY POSITION

- Bending your knees, stand with your feet shoulder-width apart.
- Keep your head up and your weight on the balls of your feet.
- Hold the racket in your dominant hand.
- React quickly.
- Anticipate direction.

SKILL	PROGRESSING	COMPETENT	PROFICIENT
ready position	1 or 2 of the elements	3 or 4 out of 5 elements	all elements met

HANDSHAKE GRIP (V GRIP)

- Hold the handle of the racket in your dominant hand in a handshake grip.
- Form a V with your thumb and forefinger.
- Point the racket away from your body at waist height.
- Placing the head of the racket vertical to the ground, point the handle toward your belly button.
- Support the throat of racket lightly with your non-dominant hand.

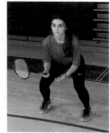

SKILL	PROGRESSING	COMPETENT	PROFICIENT
handshake grip	1 or 2 of the elements	3 or 4 out of 5 elements	all elements met

UNDERHAND STROKE

- Hold the racket so that the head is facing the ground and is under the birdie.
- Step forward with your non-dominant foot.
- Flick your wrist to hit the birdie with the center of the racket.
- Rotate your forearm so that it faces upward on contact.
- Follow through to your target.

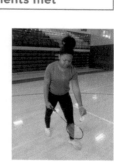

SKILL	PROGRESSING	COMPETENT	PROFICIENT
underhand stroke	1 or 2 of the elements	3 or 4 out of 5 elements	all elements met

OVERHAND STROKE

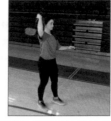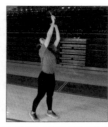

- Bend your elbow so that your racket is in a back-scratching position.
- Reach up and position the racket under the birdie.
- Flick your wrist to hit the birdie with the center of the racket. Extend your arm when you make contact.
- Follow through to your target.

SKILL	PROGRESSING	COMPETENT	PROFICIENT
overhand stroke	1 or 2 of the elements	3 out of 4 elements	all elements met

FOREHAND STROKE

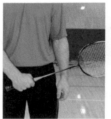

- The racket should be on the same side of your body as your dominant hand.
- Face the palm of your hand forward.
- Rotate your hips in the direction that you are hitting.
- Extend your arm and flick your wrist to hit the birdie.
- Point the face of the racket up to get the birdie over the net.
- Follow through to your target.

SKILL	PROGRESSING	COMPETENT	PROFICIENT
forehand stroke	1, 2, or 3 of the elements	4 or 5 out of 6 elements	all elements met

BACKHAND STROKE

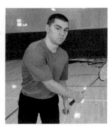

- Rotate the racket and extend it across your body.
- Rotate your feet, hips, and shoulders in the same direction as the racket.
- Face the back of your hand forward.
- Flick your wrist when you are hitting the birdie with the center of the racket.
- Follow through to your target.

SKILL	PROGRESSING	COMPETENT	PROFICIENT
backhand stroke	1 or 2 of the elements	3 or 4 out of 5 elements	all elements met

UNDERHAND SERVE

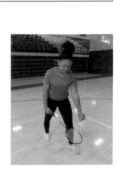

- Hold the racket in your dominant hand with the head of the racket pointed down toward the ground.
- Hold the birdie by the feathers in your non-dominant hand.
- Step forward with your non-dominant foot.
- Drop the birdie slightly below your waist.
- Hit the birdie with the center of the racket. Flick your wrist when you make contact.
- Follow through to your target.

SKILL	PROGRESSING	COMPETENT	PROFICIENT
underhand serve	1, 2, or 3 of the elements	4 or 5 out of 6 elements	all elements met

PRACTICE THE STROKES

Practice independently by holding the birdie by the feathers in your non-dominant hand. Hold the racket appropriately for the stroke. Drop the birdie and make contact with the racket.

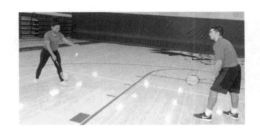

- First, practice each stroke without using the birdie.

- Then, practice each stroke using the birdie.

- Practice the underhand stroke by holding the head of the racket down toward the floor. Drop the birdie and make contact with the racket slightly below your waist. Flick your wrist and make contact with the birdie. How many times you can hit the birdie in a row?

- Strike the birdie toward a target using the various strokes.

- Strike the birdie toward a target using different levels of force.

- Aim and strike the birdie to the left of a target.

- Aim and strike the birdie to the right of a target.

- Practice with a partner. Hit the birdie back and forth with a partner. How many times can you hit it back and forth?

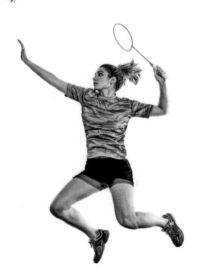

BADMINTON SHOTS

CLEAR SHOT	DROP SHOT	SMASH SHOT

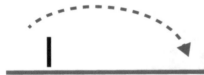 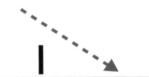

The overhead and underhand defensive clear shots arc or lob the birdie high and push your opponent to the rear of the court. This slows down the game to give you a chance to get ready for your opponent's shot.

The overhand drop shot keeps the pace of the game the same. It is sent at a steep angle, forcing your opponent to rush forward.

The overhand smash shot is a powerful hit at a severe angle. You need to contact the birdie high, which may even require you to jump to hit the birdie. This shot is often used to end a game.

PRACTICE THE SHOTS

Practice the shots independently by tossing the birdie at the appropriate height for each shot. Practice with a set-up net.

- Practice the clear shot with both the underhand and overhand strokes.

- Practice the drop shot.

- Practice the smash shot.

- Practice with a partner. Have a partner toss the birdie for you. Practice each shot and then switch roles. Be supportive and encouraging to your partner.

BADMINTON GAME

- Badminton is usually a singles game with 2 players or a doubles game with 4 players.

- Start with an underhand serve from the right side of the court. Serve from behind the end line to your opponent on the left.

- If you hit the birdie onto your opponent's side and your opponent cannot return it, you win the rally—which is the series of consecutive strokes back and forth until a point is earned—and get a point.

- Now, serve from the left side of the court.

- When your score is an even number, serve behind the right end line. When your score is an odd number, serve behind the left end line.

- In a doubles game, the same player on a team serves throughout a rally, alternating serving sides until losing the rally. The opponent then serves until the rally is lost. Partners alternate turns serving.

- You may only hit the birdie 1 time on each side.

- You lose a rally if you or your racket touch the net.

- You lose a rally if you hit the birdie into the net, hit it out of bounds, or miss it when you swing.

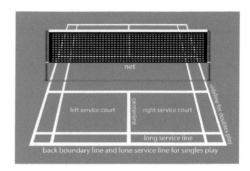

DEMONSTRATE POSITIVE GAME BEHAVIOR

- Follow rules.

- Call for the shot, when appropriate, to identify that you are going to hit the shot. This is for safety and game efficiency.

- Be supportive and encouraging to your teammate.

- Treat your opponents with respect.

SKILL	PROGRESSING	COMPETENT	PROFICIENT
game behavior	1 or 2 of the elements	3 or 4 out of 5 elements	all elements met

HOW TO SCORE

- You score a point when you hit the birdie over the net and onto your opponent's side before your opponent can return it. You also score a point when your opponent hits the birdie either into the net or out of bounds.

- A match consists of 3 games of 21 points.

- If you win a rally, you score 1 point.

- If the score is tied at 20 points, the first team to score 2 points wins the game.

- If the score is tied at 29 points, the first team to score its 30th point wins the game.

- The winning team serves first in the next game.

RATE YOUR ENJOYMENT OF BADMINTON

On a scale from 1 to 4, where 1 is not enjoyable and 4 is very enjoyable, rate this activity.

1	It was not enjoyable, and I will not participate again.
2	It was not enjoyable, but I will participate again for exercise.
3	It was enjoyable, and I will play again.
4	It was very enjoyable, and I will initiate future games.

💻 RESEARCH INTEGRATION

Research badminton's country of origin, who invented the game, where badminton is played throughout the world, and the official rules of the game.

♥ HEALTH INTEGRATION

Count your pulse during and after playing badminton to determine if you are exercising in your personal target heart rate zone. Apply the results to your overall fitness plan. Keep in mind that many people choose to complete aerobic workouts by playing in casual games with friends.

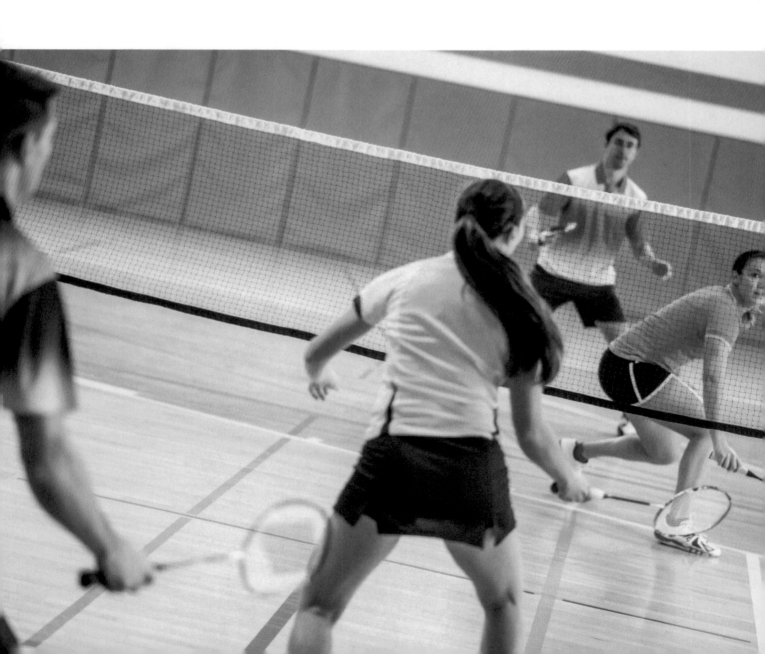

BASKETBALL

Learning and practicing basketball helps you develop the skills necessary for playing games outside of PE class. Basketball enhances health-related and skill-related components of fitness. Learning basketball skills will not only help improve your basketball game but may also enhance your skills in other sports and activities. Playing basketball is a great aerobic workout.

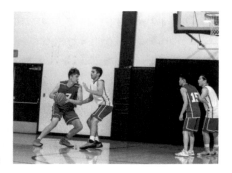

The official game of basketball is played by 2 opposing teams that are each made up of 5 players. The players play on a basketball court. Points are scored when the ball goes through a basketball hoop. There are also other basketball games and activities that you can enjoy, such as independent shooting and dribbling challenges, shooting games, and half-court games of 1-on-1, 2-on-2, and 3-on-3 versions of the official game.

The purpose of this lesson is for you to participate in aerobic exercise and in skill-building activities. Game participation will depend upon the availability of a facility and players. Any time you play a game of basketball, be sure to follow game rules, communicate with teammates in a positive and effective manner, and exhibit appropriate behavior with your team and the opposing team.

 CAUTION: Do not overinflate the basketball.

DRIBBLING SKILLS

Learning to dribble efficiently with both your right hand and left hand is necessary for playing basketball.

BASIC STATIONARY DRIBBLING

- Using your dominant hand, spread your fingers and push the ball down gently toward the ground with your finger pads. Do not slap the ball.
- Let the ball bounce on the ground and come back to your hand. Do not let the ball bounce higher than your waist.
- Flex your wrist and push the ball back to the ground with your finger pads. This is a continuous movement; do not catch the ball after every bounce.
- Dribble with your head up.
- Keep your eyes looking forward, not watching the ball.
- Repeat dribbling the ball with your non-dominant hand.

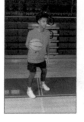 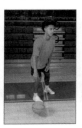 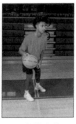

Basic stationary dribbling

SKILL	PROGRESSING	COMPETENT	PROFICIENT
right-handed dribble	1 or 2 of the elements	3 or 4 out of 5 elements	all elements met
left-handed dribble	1 or 2 of the elements	3 or 4 out of 5 elements	all elements met

STATIONARY DRIBBLING

- See how many times you can dribble the ball with your dominant hand without losing control of the ball.
- Push the ball down with different amounts of force to make it bounce at different levels.
- Try pushing the ball with a soft force so that it bounces at a low level.
- Try pushing the ball with a hard force so that it bounces at a high level.
- Dribble with your dominant hand.
- Dribble with your non-dominant hand.
- Dribble the ball from 1 hand to the other.

DRIBBLING WHILE MOVING

- Dribble from 1 hand to the other while moving.
- Dribble while moving, increasing and decreasing speed.
- Dribble while moving and change directions.

CROSSOVER DRIBBLING

- Set up disc cones about 2 feet apart in a zigzag pattern.
- Start at the first cone and dribble the basketball to the next cone using the hand with which you are most comfortable.
- Reach the second cone and do a crossover (switch hands) in order to move on to the next cone.
- Complete a crossover at each cone until you have reached the last cone.
- Turn around and do the same thing back to the first cone.
- Continue this until you feel comfortable with dribbling and crossing over.

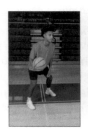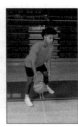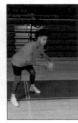

Crossover dribbling

CHALLENGE SKILLS

The following challenge skills are for those who are proficient in basic stationary dribbling. The challenge drills reinforce dribbling effectively with both the right hand and left hand. Practice as appropriate to your needs.

FIGURE-8 DRIBBLE

- Stand with your legs wide and your knees bent.
- Dribble the ball through your legs and around your ankles in a figure-8 pattern.
- Alternate hands while dribbling.
- Reverse directions for an advanced challenge.

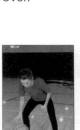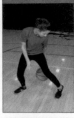
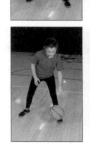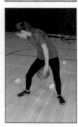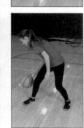

Figure-8 dribble

FRONT 2, BACK 2 DRIBBLE

- Stand with your legs shoulder-width apart and your knees bent.
- Dribble twice in front of your body. Alternate hands while dribbling, but do not put both hands on the ball at the same time.
- Switch hands behind you, and dribble twice behind your body. This is a 1, 2, 3, 4 count.
- Move while making quarter turns for an advanced challenge.

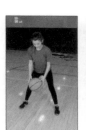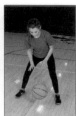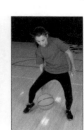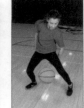

Front, back 2 dribble

2-BALL DRIBBLE

- Dribble 2 balls at the same time.
- Keep the balls at the same height.

2-ball dribble

2-BALL HIGH-LOW DRIBBLE

- Dribble a ball with each hand.
- Dribble the ball on the right high while simultaneously dribbling the ball on the left low.
- Dribble the ball on the right low while simultaneously dribbling the ball on the left high.

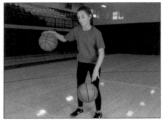

2-ball high-low dribble

2-BALL FIGURE-8 DRIBBLE

- Dribble 1 ball between your legs while circling the other ball around 1 of your legs.
- When the ball that is circling your leg reaches the middle point between your legs, switch it with the ball between your legs.

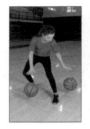 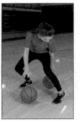 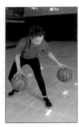

2-ball figure-8 dribble

Check off the challenge skills that you have mastered.

_____**FIGURE-8 DRIBBLE**

_____**FRONT 2, BACK 2 DRIBBLE**

_____**2-BALL DRIBBLE**

_____**2-BALL HIGH-LOW DRIBBLE**

_____**2-BALL FIGURE-8 DRIBBLE**

PASSING SKILLS

There are 2 common passes that are used in the game of basketball. The bounce pass and chest pass are used to move the ball to your teammates. You can practice these passes with a partner or against a wall.

BOUNCE PASS AND CATCH

BOUNCE PASS

- Stand facing the target.
- Hold the ball with both hands at chest level and your elbows out.
- Step toward the target.
- Extend both arms toward the target. The ball should bounce on the floor between you and the target before it reaches the target.

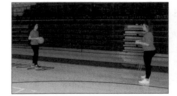 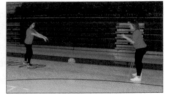

2-ball dribble

CATCH

- When you are catching, watch the ball all the way until it reaches your hands.
- Move your hands toward the ball.
- Give with the ball (pull the ball slightly toward you) as it hits your hands to make a soft catch.

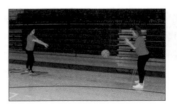 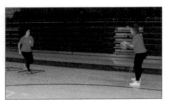

Catch

SKILL	PROGRESSING	COMPETENT	PROFICIENT
bounce pass	1 or 2 of the elements	3 out of 4 elements	all elements met
bounce-pass catch	1 of the elements	2 out of 3 elements	all elements met

CHEST PASS AND CATCH

CHEST PASS

- Stand facing the target.
- Hold the ball with both hands at chest level and your elbows out.
- Step toward the target.
- Extend both arms toward the target. The ball should not bounce on the floor.

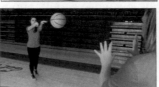
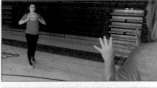
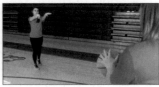

Chest pass

CATCH

- When you are catching, watch the ball all the way until it reaches your hands.
- Move your hands toward the ball.
- Give with the ball (pull the ball slightly toward you) as it hits your hands to make a soft catch.

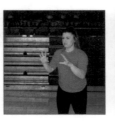
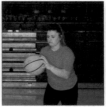
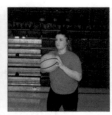

Catch

SKILL	PROGRESSING	COMPETENT	PROFICIENT
chest pass	1 or 2 of the elements	3 out of 4 elements	all elements met
chest-pass catch	1 of the elements	2 out of 3 elements	all elements met

PRACTICE PASSING WITH A PARTNER

- How many bounce passes can you and your partner do in a row?
- How many chest passes can you and your partner do in a row?
- Bounce pass to your partner. Your partner will send a chest pass back. Switch roles.
- Bounce pass as you and your partner move down the court.
- Chest pass as you and your partner move down the court.

BASIC SHOOTING SKILLS

BASIC SHOOTING

- Stand facing the hoop with your feet shoulder-width apart and your knees slightly bent.
- Place your dominant hand on the back of the basketball and bend your wrist. Place your non-dominant hand on the side of the ball.
- Place the ball on the finger pads of your dominant hand.
- Use your non-dominant hand as your guide.
- Position your elbow so that it is behind the ball, not out to the side.
- Look at the target—the front of the rim.
- Push your dominant hand toward the target while straightening your legs to give you more power to shoot.
- Shoot the ball toward the target and follow through with your arm and wrist. Snap your wrist as the ball leaves your hand.

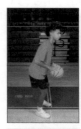
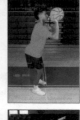
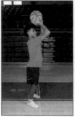
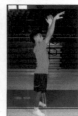

Basic shooting skills

- Remember BEEF.
  - **Balance** the ball in your dominant hand.
  - Place your **elbow** behind the ball, not out to the side.
  - Keep your **eyes** on the target.
  - **Follow** through with a snap of your wrist.

SKILL	PROGRESSING	COMPETENT	PROFICIENT
BEEF elements	1 or 2 of the elements	3 out of 4 elements	all elements

SHOOTING DRILLS

PRACTICE SHOOTING

- Practice some shooting drills after you become comfortable shooting the basketball.
- Pick different spots on the court, both closer and farther away from the hoop.
- Map out a pattern in your mind as to what spots you will go to first, second, third, and so on.
- Practice shooting from each spot.
- Start on 1 side of the hoop and move around to the other side.
- Work back around to the starting position.

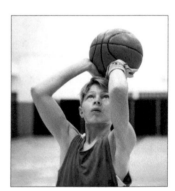

FOUL LINE SPELLING GAME

- You will need 2 or more players.
- Line up behind the foul line.
- The goal of the game is to be the first player to spell A-E-R-O-B-I-C.
- The first person takes a shot from behind the foul line.
- If the player makes the basket, the player gets a letter and goes to the back of the line to wait for their next turn.
- If the player misses, the player does not get a letter and goes to the back of the line.
- The next player in line repeats the above procedure.
- Continue to play until a player spells A-E-R-O-B-I-C.

OFFENSIVE AND DEFENSIVE SKILLS

Agile footwork is an essential component of basketball. Practice footwork skills to improve your offensive and defensive play.

OFFENSIVE SKILLS

Practice each of the following skills, concentrating on proper form, prior to using them in a game or other competition.

OFFENSIVE READY POSITION

The ready position allows a player to move quickly in any direction. It is used for both offense and defense.

- With your elbows out, hold the ball with both hands to the dominant side of your chest.
- Bend your knees to keep your body low.
- Stand with your feet shoulder-width apart.
- Keep your head up and your weight on the balls of your feet.

SKILL	PROGRESSING	COMPETENT	PROFICIENT
offensive ready position	1 or 2 of the elements	3 out of 4 elements	all elements met

PIVOT

The purpose of the pivot in a basketball game is for you to look around and decide to dribble, pass, or shoot.

- Plant 1 foot, which will be your pivot foot, in place on the ground.
- Place your weight on the balls of your feet.
- Slide your non-pivot foot and rotate your body 180 degrees.
- Repeat this exercise with your other foot.

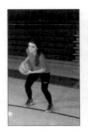 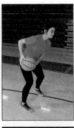 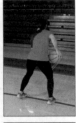
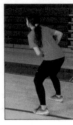 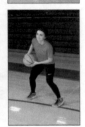

SKILL	PROGRESSING	COMPETENT	PROFICIENT
pivot	1 of the elements	2 out of 3 elements	all elements

FAKE

- Look in 1 direction, and then pass or move in another direction.
- Stay on the balls of your feet.
- Move quickly.

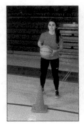 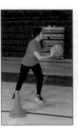 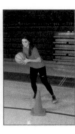 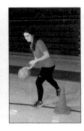

SKILL	PROGRESSING	COMPETENT	PROFICIENT
fake	1 of the elements	2 out of 3 elements	all elements

GIVE AND GO

The purpose of the give and go in a basketball game is to for you to pass the ball to a teammate and to quickly relocate so that you can receive a pass.

- Pass the ball to a teammate.
- Move quickly to relocate and support your offense.
- Indicate (call out) that you are ready and open to receive the ball.
- Catch the ball.

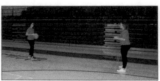 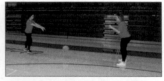
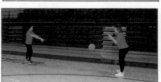 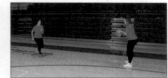
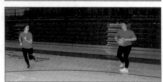

SKILL	PROGRESSING	COMPETENT	PROFICIENT
give and go	1 or 2 of the elements	3 out of 4 elements	all elements

DEFENSIVE SKILLS

Practice each of the following skills, concentrating on proper form, prior to using them in a game or other competition.

DEFENSIVE SLIDES

The purpose of defensive slides in basketball is to keep up with your opponent and to legally take the ball or legally disrupt the opponent's pass or shot.

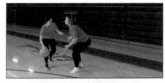

- Place your weight on the balls of your feet.

- Slide to the side with quick steps.

- Do not cross your feet.

- Keep your knees bent.

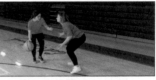

- Face your hips toward your opponent.

- Hold your hands up at chest level.

- Keep your eyes on your opponent's waistline.

- Stay with your opponent.

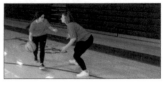

- Anticipate and react quickly to your opponent's movements.

SKILL	PROGRESSING	COMPETENT	PROFICIENT
defensive slides	1, 2, 3, 4, or 5 of the elements	6, 7, or 8 out of 9 elements	all elements met

PRACTICE OFFENSIVE AND DEFENSIVE SKILLS

- Practice the **pivot** by planting your right foot and rotating your left foot until you feel comfortable with the movement.

- Practice the **pivot** by planting your left foot and rotating your right foot until you feel comfortable with the movement.

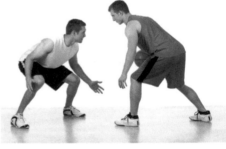

- Practice the **give and go** with a partner and a defender. Pass the ball, quickly relocate, and then receive the pass, avoiding the defender.

- Practice the **fake** independently. Set up a cone as a decoy. Fake the pass toward the cone and then pass to your partner until you feel comfortable with the movement.

- Practice the **fake** with a partner defending you. Dribble, fake, and move in another direction to get around the defensive player. Do this until you feel comfortable with the fake.

- Practice the **defensive slide** with a partner. As your partner dribbles, defensive slide to try to prevent them from making a successful pass or shot. Do this until you feel comfortable with the defensive slide.

BASKETBALL GAME

- The game is played by 2 opposing teams of 5 players each. Each team has a point guard, a shooting guard, a small forward, a power forward, and a center.

- The game is played on a basketball court 92 feet long and 50 feet wide.

- A 10-foot-high basketball hoop with a net is at each end of the court.

- The object of the game is to move the ball down the court by passing or dribbling and to score by shooting the ball through the opposing team's hoop.

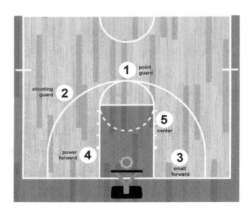

- A high school game is divided into 8-minute quarters of play time with a rest period after 2 quarters of play.
- The team with the most points is the winning team.
- The game begins with a jump ball at mid-court. A referee tosses the ball between 2 opposing players.
- The team that possesses the ball is on offense, and the other team is on defense.
- The player with the ball must dribble, pass, or shoot.
- When they are moving with the ball, the player must dribble. When the player stops dribbling, they cannot take any more steps.
- If a player walks without dribbling, the ball is turned over to the opposing team.
- The players on defense try to intercept, or take away, the ball.

DEMONSTRATE POSITIVE GAME BEHAVIOR

- Follow the rules of the game.
- Do not commit a foul or make illegal physical contact against an opposing player.
  - A foul against a non-shooting player results in a turnover, which is a change in possession of the ball between teams.
  - A foul against a shooting player results in the team getting free shots—2 shots for a foul on a player shooting a 2-point shot and 3 shots for a player shooting a 3-point shot.
  - A player who commits 5 fouls is removed from the game.
- Be supportive and encouraging to your teammates.
- Treat your opponents with respect.

SKILL	PROGRESSING	COMPETENT	PROFICIENT
game behavior	1 or 2 of the elements	3 out of 4 elements	all elements met

HOW TO SCORE

- An arc line, referred to as a 3-point line, is marked on the basketball court.
  - A player who makes a basket from behind the 3-point line is awarded 3 points.
  - A player who makes a basket from inside the 3-point line is awarded 2 points.
- Foul shots are worth 1 point each.

OPTIONAL 1-ON-1 GAME

Playing 1-on-1 allows you to play basketball and complete an aerobic workout when you only have 2 players. This is an example of how to break down the barrier of not having enough players for an official game and create a solution.

- You can play a 1-on-1 half-court game with 2 players.
- Determine the boundaries.
- Determine who starts with the ball.
- Begin behind the half-court line of your established boundary.
- After a score, the opposing player takes the ball out to the half-court line and tries to score.
- Scoring is the same as in the official rules.
- You will have to call your own fouls or have another person referee.
- Treat your opponent with respect.
- If there are more players, you can play 2-on-2 or 3-on-3 games.

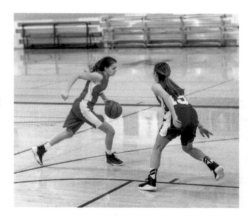

Prior to playing 1-on-1, establish and review the game rules so that you and your opponent understand them. If problems arise, work to solve them in a positive and effective manner. Appreciate different players' abilities. An example of a rule that you may want to decide upon is the boundaries.

Below are our game rules for safety and fairness.
1.
2.
3.
4.
5.

RATE YOUR ENJOYMENT OF THE BASKETBALL ACTIVITY THAT YOU ENJOYED MOST

On a scale from 1 to 4, where 1 is not enjoyable and 4 is very enjoyable, rate this activity.

1	It was not enjoyable, and I will not participate again.
2	It was not enjoyable, but I will participate again for exercise.
3	It was enjoyable, and I will play again.
4	It was very enjoyable, and I will initiate future games.

RESEARCH INTEGRATION

1. Research the official rules and regulations of high school basketball for additional official basketball information.
2. Attend a basketball game or watch a basketball game on television. It can be men's, women's, or co-ed basketball at any level—youth, high school, college, or professional. Identify the basketball skills you have learned that are used by the players throughout the game.

HEALTH INTEGRATION

Count your pulse during and after playing basketball to determine if you are exercising in your personal target heart rate zone. Apply the results to your overall fitness plan. Many people choose to complete aerobic workouts by playing in fast-paced games like basketball.

GOLF

The game of golf can be played as a competitive sport or as a casual game. Golf is played around the world by people of all ages for exercise and for the enjoyment of the social and competitive aspects of the game. The object of the game is to use clubs to hit a ball into each hole in a course. The player who hits their ball the fewest times is the winner of the game.

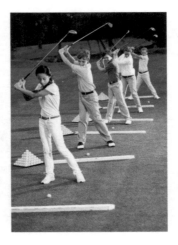
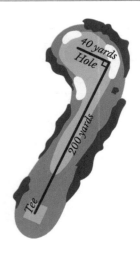

Golf is played on an open outdoor course. A typical course has 18 holes. A hole consists of a starting tee, a putting green of short and smooth grass where the hole is located, and a long area of grass between the tee and putting green called a fairway. A variety of up to 14 long-handled clubs are used to hit a small, hard ball into the holes. Common types of clubs include drivers, woods, irons, hybrids, and putters. Part of the game is knowing which club to use for each hit.

The mechanics of a golf swing are similar for most clubs, with adjustments for distance and direction. The clubs are used to launch the ball into the air toward the hole. The putter is a club that is used differently than the other clubs. It is used to hit the ball when it is on a green into the hole with a stroke called a putt, which is a small, close, controlled strike that causes the ball to roll on the ground.

The purpose of this lesson is for you to learn the mechanics of the full golf swing and to encourage you to participate in the game of golf.

⚠ **CAUTION: Make sure that nobody is close to you before you swing a golf club. Do not walk into the path of another person who is swinging a golf club.**

GOLF SKILLS

GRIP AND STANCE

OVERLAPPING GRIP: RIGHT-HANDED

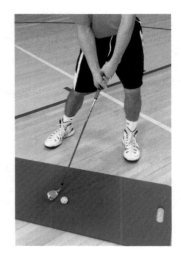

- Hold the golf club with the head of the club on the ground.
- Grasp the grip of the golf club with your left hand as if you were shaking hands with the club, laying your left thumb flat on the front of the grip and pointing it toward the head of the golf club. If you were looking at direction like the face of a clock, your thumb would be pointing at 1:00.
- Place your right hand over your left hand, covering your left thumb with your right middle fingers.
- Overlap your right pinky so that it is behind your left hand and between the pointer finger and middle finger of your left hand.
- When you are gripping the golf club, the back of your left hand and the palm of your right hand should be facing the target.

OVERLAPPING GRIP: LEFT-HANDED

- Hold the golf club with the head of the club on the ground.
- Grasp the grip of the golf club with your right hand as if you were shaking hands with the club, laying your right thumb flat on the front of the grip and pointing it toward the head of the golf club. If you were looking at direction like the face of a clock, your thumb would be pointing at 11:00.
- Place your left hand over your right hand, covering your right thumb with your left middle finger.
- Overlap your left pinky so that it is behind your right hand and between the pointer finger and middle finger of your right hand.

- When you are gripping the golf club, the back of your right hand and the palm of your left hand should be facing the target.

SKILL	PROGRESSING	COMPETENT	PROFICIENT
grip	1, 2, or 3 of the elements	4 out of 5 elements	all elements met

STANCE

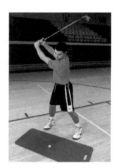

- Stand with your feet shoulder-width apart with your knees slightly bent. Bend at your waist, but keep your back straight.
- Your head should be angled down slightly to see the ball.
- Maintain balance, keeping your center of gravity over your feet.

SKILL	PROGRESSING	COMPETENT	PROFICIENT
stance	1 of the elements	2 out of 3 elements	all elements met

GOLF SWING

THE FULL GOLF SWING IN 3 PARTS

Practice each step of the full swing without golf balls repeatedly before using golf balls.

1. BACKSWING

- Position the clubhead so that it is on the ground and slightly behind the ball.
- In the backswing, the clubhead, your hands, and your shoulders must start in a single motion.
- Bring your head back slowly to make sure that your left shoulder is slightly higher than your right shoulder. During the backswing, rotate at your hips, keeping your arms straight and your upper body and shoulders in line.
- The weight of your feet in the stance shifts laterally from your front foot to your back foot. This helps with hip rotation.
- As your weight is shifted to your back foot, lateral rotation at your left hip turns your pelvis away from the ball.
- Keep your head forward and your eyes on the ball.

These steps are for a right-handed golfer. Switch directions in each step for a left-handed golfer.

SKILL	PROGRESSING	COMPETENT	PROFICIENT
backswing	1, 2, or 3 of the elements	4 or 5 out of 6 elements	all elements met

2. DOWNSWING

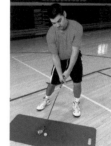

- Swing the club forward by first twisting your hips toward the target and then following through with your arms.
- As your body shifts to uncoil, make sure that your weight starts to shift from your right foot to your left foot.
- Your arms should return to their original position at the point of contact with the ball.
- Your wrists should stay strong but should rotate in the direction of your swing when the club contacts the ball; so, you should finish your swing with the back of your wrist slightly more toward your target than the front of your wrist.

These steps are for a right-handed golfer. Switch directions in each step for a left-handed golfer.

SKILL	PROGRESSING	COMPETENT	PROFICIENT
downswing	1 or 2 of the elements	3 out of 4 elements	all elements met

3. FOLLOW-THROUGH

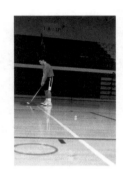

- The follow-through is what your body and club do after making contact with the ball.
- Bring your club all the way through the swing, with the club finishing over your front shoulder.
- Twist your upper body so that it ends up being squared with your target. Keep your front leg in the starting position. The knee of your back leg should be bent, and your toes should be on the ground.
- Turn your hips enough to allow your belly button to face your target.
- The club itself should wrap behind your shoulders while you maintain a straight back.
- Freeze your body in a finishing position for a few seconds while watching the flight of the ball.

SKILL	PROGRESSING	COMPETENT	PROFICIENT
follow-through	1, 2, or 3 of the elements	4 or 5 out of 6 elements	all elements met

TARGET PRACTICE

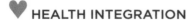

- For this activity, make sure that you are in a large, open space.
- Set up discs so that they are spread out at a variety of distances, like shown in the picture.
- Stand about 10 feet from the closest disc. From that spot, practice chipping the ball as close to the different discs as you can.
- As you get better, increase your distance from the discs.
- Make a game by assigning a point value to each of the different discs. The closer discs can be worth 1 or 2 points each, and the further discs can be worth 3 to 5 points each.

RATE YOUR ENJOYMENT OF GOLF

On a scale from 1 to 4, where 1 is not enjoyable and 4 is very enjoyable, rate this activity.

1	It was not enjoyable, and I will not participate again.
2	It was not enjoyable, but I will participate again for exercise.
3	It was enjoyable, and I will play again.
4	It was very enjoyable, and I will initiate future games.

🖥 RESEARCH INTEGRATION

1. Research the 3 common golf grips: the overlapping (Vardon) grip, the interlocking grip, and the baseball grip. Try each grip to determine the grip that you prefer.
2. Play a round of golf with a seasoned golfer or watch golf on television.

♥ HEALTH INTEGRATION

Discuss with a trusted adult or friend how someone could reduce their stress levels by playing golf through concentrating on the task, socializing, exercising, and so on.

PLAYGROUND BALL GAMES

You can use a playground ball to play many fun games and activities that can help you develop your skills and participate in cardiovascular conditioning.

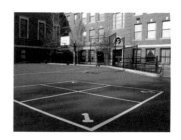

A popular playground game is 4 square. This game is played on a square court that is divided into 4 quadrants and with a playground ball.

Playing the game utilizes and improves the skill-related components of agility, balance, coordination, speed, and reaction. Playing 4 square with moderate intensity also serves as an aerobic workout. Finally, the game provides the opportunity to interact with others in a competitive and social manner.

The purpose of this lesson is to encourage you to participate in a game of 4 square with other players, follow game rules, and exhibit appropriate behavior.

 CAUTION: Do not overinflate the ball.

4 SQUARE GAME

Using chalk or ropes, divide a 10-foot by 10-foot space into 4 even squares. You will need 4 players for this game. Number the squares 1, 2, 3, and 4. The goal of the game is to reach square 4 and be the server. Players move in numerical order to get to square 4.

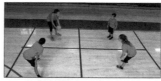
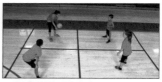
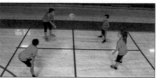
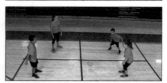
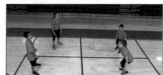

RULES

- Each player stands in a square. Extra players stand in the waiting line near square 1.

- The player in square 4 is the server.

- If you are the server, serve underhand to the square of your choice. You must bounce the ball before you strike it to serve.

- Serve again if the ball lands on a line.

- A miss results in the player who missed moving to the end of the waiting line or to square 1 if there are only 4 players total.

- Misses include double bounces, out of bounds bounces, and catches.

Prior to playing the game, establish and review the game rules so that all participants understand them. If problems arise, work as a group to solve them in a positive and effective manner. Appreciate different players' abilities. An example of a rule that you that may want to decide upon is whether or not overhand strikes are allowed in your game.

Below are our game rules for safety and fairness.
1.
2.
3.
4.
5.

RATE YOUR ENJOYMENT OF 4 SQUARE

On a scale from 1 to 4, where 1 is not enjoyable and 4 is very enjoyable, rate this activity.

1	It was not enjoyable, and I will not participate again.
2	It was not enjoyable, but I will participate again for exercise.
3	It was enjoyable, and I will play again.
4	It was very enjoyable, and I will initiate future games.

RESEARCH INTEGRATION

Research 4 square's country of origin, who invented the game, where it is played throughout the world, and the official rules of the game.

HEALTH INTEGRATION

Count your pulse during and after playing 4 square to determine if you are exercising in your personal target heart rate zone. Many people choose to complete aerobic workouts by playing in casual games with friends.

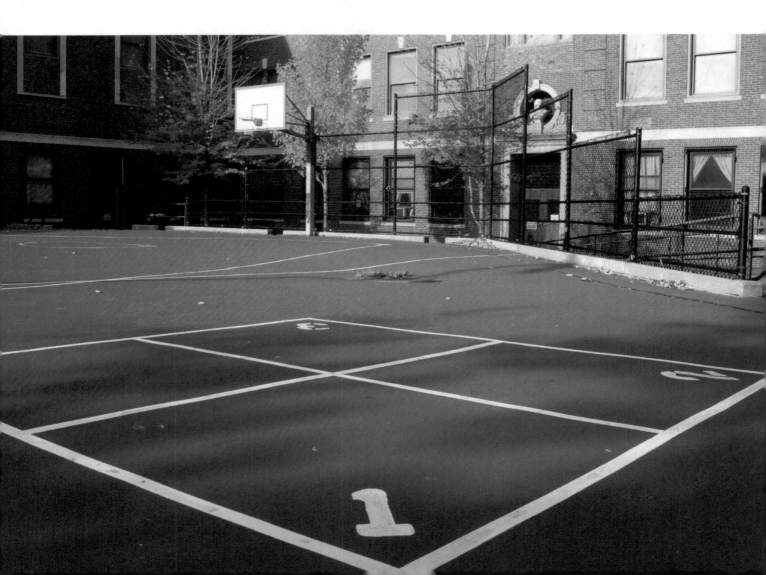

TEAM HANDBALL: A PASSING GAME

Team handball is a game that is played by 2 teams of 7 players on a rectangular court with a lightweight ball. The object of the game is to pass the ball into the goal to score more points than your opponent in 2 periods of 30 minutes. It is an Olympic sport and is gaining popularity worldwide.

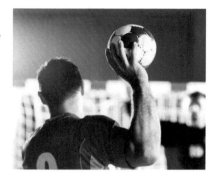

Playing the game requires you to utilize and helps you to make improvements in the skill-related components of agility, balance, coordination, speed, power, and reaction. Playing team handball at a moderate intensity level is an aerobic workout. The game also provides the opportunity to work as a team to develop offensive and defensive strategies and the ability to transition quickly from each. It is a game that improves mental focus.

The purpose of this lesson is for you to participate in aerobic exercise and in skill-building activities. Game participation will depend upon the availability of a facility and players. Any time you play team handball, be sure to follow game rules, communicate with teammates in a positive and effective manner, and exhibit appropriate behavior with your team and the opposing team.

OFFICIAL TEAM HANDBALL COURT

Court dimensions: 20m by 40m (22 yd. by 44 yd.)

Goal line: 6m (6.2 yd.)

Goal net: 3m by 2m (3.2 yd. by 2.2 yd.)

Penalty line: 9m (9.3 yd.)

 CAUTION: Do not overinflate the ball.

TEAM HANDBALL SKILLS

The following skills are used to play team handball. Practice each skill prior to playing a game. Practicing the skills will lead to better performance and more confidence when you are playing the game.

OVERHEAD PASS

- Grip the ball with your hands.
- Step toward your target and transfer your weight to your front foot.
- Move your arms forward in the direction of your target.
- Snap your wrists.

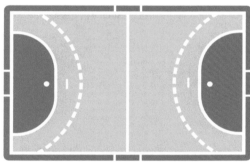
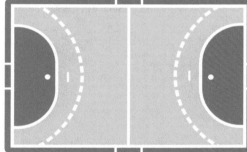

- Aim and pass to your target by releasing the ball, using the appropriate force to reach your target.

SKILL	PROGRESSING	COMPETENT	PROFICIENT
overhead pass	1 or 2 of the elements	3 or 4 out of 5 elements	all elements met

RECEIVING

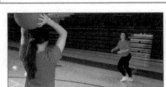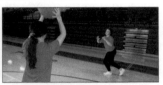

- Spread your fingers to catch the ball.
- Catch the ball firmly using only your hands.
- Gain control of the ball.
- Maintain your balance throughout the catch.
- Make the necessary pass or run with the ball after the catch.

SKILL	PROGRESSING	COMPETENT	PROFICIENT
receiving	1 or 2 of the elements	3 or 4 out of 5 elements	all elements met

RECEIVING WHILE RUNNING

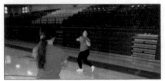

- Keep your eyes on the ball.
- Anticipate the throw. Change your speed and direction to accommodate the throw.
- Use speed and direction to create an opening.
- Catch the majority of throws.

SKILL	PROGRESSING	COMPETENT	PROFICIENT
receiving while running	1 or 2 of the elements	3 out of 4 elements	all elements met

PIVOT

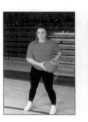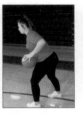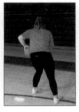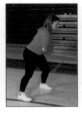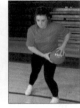

The purpose of the pivot in a handball game is for you to look around and decide to pass or to attempt to score.

- Plant 1 foot, which will be your pivot foot, in place on the ground.
- Place your weight on the balls of your feet.
- Slide your non-pivot foot and rotate your body 180 degrees.

Repeat this exercise with your other foot.

SKILL	PROGRESSING	COMPETENT	PROFICIENT
pivot	1 of the elements	2 out of 3 elements	all elements

DEFENSIVE SLIDES

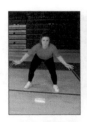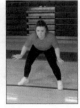
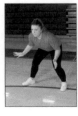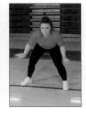

The purpose of performing defensive slides is to keep up with your opponent and to legally disrupt your opponent's pass or shot on goal.

- Place your weight on the balls of your feet.
- Slide to the side with quick steps.
- Do not cross your feet.
- Keep your knees bent.
- Square your hips so that they are facing your opponent.
- Hold your hands at chest level.
- Keep your eyes on your opponent's waistline.

- Stay with your opponent.
- Anticipate and react quickly to your opponent's movements.

SKILL	PROGRESSING	COMPETENT	PROFICIENT
defensive slides	1, 2, 3, 4, or 5 of the elements	6, 7, or 8 out of 9 elements	all elements met

TEAM HANDBALL PICK-UP GAME

OBJECT OF THE GAME

A pick-up game is like an official game except that it has adjustments to accommodate your environment. Team handball is a passing game that is played by 2 teams. Players can take up to 3 steps while in possession of the ball and can hold onto the ball for 3 seconds before passing to a teammate or shooting. Players continue passing to each other until a goal is scored, the ball is turned over to the other team, or a penalty occurs.

HANDBALL SETUP

- It is recommended that you have a trusted adult supervise the game.
- Use a playground ball to play the game.
- There are 7 players on each team including 1 goalie. Player numbers can be adjusted for pick-up games according to how many players are available.
- A rectangular handball court is comparable to a basketball court; however, you have the option of playing indoors on a court or outdoors on a field. No matter where you play, establish the size and boundaries for a safe play area.
- Set up 2 goals, each with a marked semicircle boundary from the goal line that only the goalie can be in. A net or cones can be used to mark off each goal. Also mark a penalty area beyond each semicircle.
- The above lines aren't bulleting for whatever reason, but they should be bulleted just as the points in the other sections are.

RULES OF THE GAME

- Establish the time of your game or the total points of your game.
- Establish who will be the goalie on your team.
- The other 6 players on your team should be arranged in 2 lines of 3 on your side of the court—a front line and a back line. Establish who will play on the right and left sides and who will cover the middle of the court.

	X back	X wing
X goalie	X center back	X center line
	X back	X wing

- Begin the game at midcourt with a jump ball. A neutral person should toss the ball between 2 designated opposing players.
  - o In the event that there is not a neutral person available to toss the ball, use a coin toss to decide who has first possession of the ball.
- The goalies are the only players who are allowed to touch the ball with their feet.
- A goalie can come out of their goal area only without possession of the ball.
- The goalie throws the ball back into play immediately after a score.

- A player can only hold onto the ball for 3 seconds before moving or passing.
- A player can only take 3 steps while in possession of the ball.
- A turnover, which is a change in possession of the ball between teams, occurs whenever an incomplete pass or an interception is made.
- Players are not allowed to make physical contact.
- Physical contact that is made by the team on defense is a penalty that results in a throw-in by the player on offense.
- Physical contact that is made by the team on offense is a penalty that results in a turnover.

Prior to playing the game, establish and review the game rules so that all participants understand them. If problems arise, work as a group to solve them in a positive and effective manner. Appreciate different players' abilities. An example of a rule that you may want to decide upon is when to switch out the player in the goalie position so that everyone has equal play time.

Below are our game rules for safety and fairness.
1.
2.
3.
4.
5.

RATE YOUR ENJOYMENT OF HANDBALL

On a scale from 1 to 4, where 1 is not enjoyable and 4 is very enjoyable, rate this activity.

1	It was not enjoyable, and I will not participate again.
2	It was not enjoyable, but I will participate again for exercise.
3	It was enjoyable, and I will play again.
4	It was very enjoyable, and I will initiate future games.

RESEARCH INTEGRATION

Research the official rules and regulations of handball and compare them to the pick-up game rules that are given in this lesson.

HEALTH INTEGRATION

Count your pulse during and after playing handball to determine if you are exercising in your personal target heart rate zone. Predict and then compare the difference between your heart rate after playing in the goalie position and your heart rate after playing in a running position. Apply your results to your overall fitness plan. Many people choose to complete aerobic workouts by playing in fun pick-up games of sports like handball.

SOCCER

Soccer is a sport that is popular around the globe. The object of the game is to use your feet to dribble, pass, and kick a ball in order to score goals by getting the ball into your opponent's net.

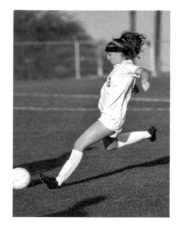

People of all skill levels enjoy playing casual or competitive games of soccer. In most communities, there are soccer leagues for everyone from preschoolers to adults. Playing soccer is a great way to improve footwork, interact with others, have fun, and complete an aerobic workout.

The purpose of this lesson is for you to participate in soccer activities. Students who practice soccer skills are more likely to join a game and exercise outside of PE class. You will practice skills, learn game rules, be encouraged to communicate with teammates in a positive and effective manner, and be reminded to exhibit appropriate behavior with your team and the opposing team.

 CAUTION: Wear appropriate safety equipment. Do not overinflate the ball.

SOCCER SKILLS

DRIBBLING

Use your peripheral vision, or your side vision, to watch the ball as you dribble it. Dribbling is a series of small, controlled touches that you complete in order to move with the ball in your possession. Dribble the ball with the insides and outsides of your feet as well as with the tops of your feet, where your shoelaces lay. Do not dribble the ball with your toes, otherwise, you risk losing control of the ball.

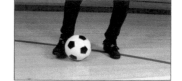

- Start with the ball positioned in front of you on the ground.
- Dribble forward, keeping the ball close—no more than 3 to 5 feet in front of you.
- Move the ball with the insides, outsides, and/or tops of both of your feet.
- Keep your head up.
- Match your speed to your skill.
- Change directions.

SKILL	PROGRESSING	COMPETENT	PROFICIENT
dribbling	1, 2, or 3 of the elements	4 or 5 out of 6 elements	all elements

PASSING

Passing the ball is an important part of soccer. Players pass the ball to each other in order to keep the other team from gaining control of the ball and to progress the ball up the field toward the other team's goal.

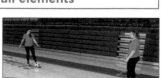
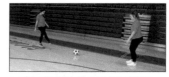
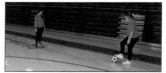

- Start with the soccer ball on the ground, next to the inside of your dominant foot.
- Position the inside of your kicking foot behind the middle of the soccer ball.
- Establish your non-kicking foot slightly behind you.
- Swing your kicking leg back, keeping it straight throughout your entire kick.
- Contact the middle of the ball with the inside of your foot. Follow through your kick with your foot and leg.
- Use appropriate force and direction to keep your pass on target.

SKILL	PROGRESSING	COMPETENT	PROFICIENT
passing	1, 2, or 3 of the elements	4 or 5 out of 6 elements	all elements

TRAPPING: OPTION 1

Trapping is a way of stopping the ball, receiving a pass, or gaining control of the ball.

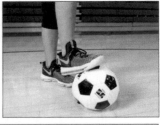

- Start with the ball positioned in front of you on the ground.
- Place your dominant foot on top of the ball. To do this, lift your foot slightly off the ground, keeping your ankle locked and your toes up.
- Repeat this with your non-dominant foot.

SKILL	PROGRESSING	COMPETENT	PROFICIENT
trapping: option 1	1 of the elements	2 out of 3 elements	all elements

TRAPPING: OPTION 2

Trapping is also a way to stop the ball in order to quickly gain control and transition to your next move.

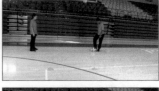

- When the soccer ball comes toward you, turn the ankle of whichever foot you are trapping with so that your instep, or the inside of your foot, is facing forward.
- Cushion the ball with your foot as you stop it lightly, as if you were catching an egg.
- Repeat this with your other foot.

SKILL	PROGRESSING	COMPETENT	PROFICIENT
trapping: option 2	1 of the elements	2 out of 3 elements	all elements

SHOOTING

The purpose of shooting is to get the soccer ball into your opponent's goal by striking it with your foot.

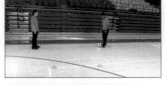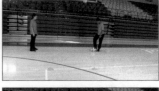
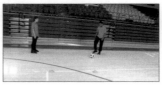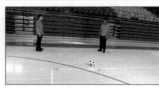

- Place 2 discs about 4 feet apart and 5 feet in front of you. Place the soccer ball on the ground in front of you.
- Stand so that your dominant leg, or kicking leg, is pulled back behind you.
- Place your non-kicking foot alongside the soccer ball, with your toes pointing at the goal that you made.
- Bend the knee of your kicking leg by pulling your foot back. Then, in a single motion, swing your leg forward, straightening your leg and pointing your toes to kick the soccer ball with the top of your foot. Kick the center of the soccer ball with the laces of your shoe, pointing your toes down. You do not want to kick the soccer ball with your toes.
- Follow through your kick, making sure that you finish with your toes pointing toward the goal.

SKILL	PROGRESSING	COMPETENT	PROFICIENT
shooting	1 or 2 of the elements	3 or 4 out of 5 elements	all elements

PRACTICE THE SKILLS

After mastering the basic soccer skills, put them all together in practice activities.

DRIBBLE

- Practice dribbling by placing discs in various locations around your practice area. As you are dribbling, weave in and out of the discs.

TRAP

- Place 2 discs about 4 feet apart to create a goal. Make your goal 10 to 20 feet away from you.
- Toss the ball up in the air, trapping it with your foot and guiding it to the ground just in front of you.
  - After mastering trapping the soccer ball with your feet, try trapping it using your thigh. Throw the soccer ball up in the air and bend your knee so that your thigh is just under the soccer ball. As the soccer ball comes back down, cushion it with your thigh. Allow the ball to hit your thigh and then guide it with your thigh as it falls to the ground.
- Dribble the soccer ball toward the goal.
- When you get about 5 feet away from the goal, shoot the ball through the discs.

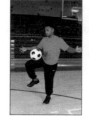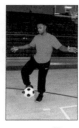

Trap

PASS

- Set up 2 discs about 3 feet apart. Aim to kick the soccer ball between the discs.
- If you kick the soccer ball in the middle, the soccer ball will go straight.
- Move to the left of the discs. Try passing the soccer ball between the discs from the left. Kick the right side of the ball with the instep of your right foot to make the soccer ball go to the left.
- Move to the right of the discs. Try passing the soccer ball between the discs from the right. Kick the left side of the ball with the instep of your left foot to make the ball go to the left.

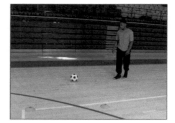

Pass

SHOOT ON GOAL

- Place 2 discs about 4 feet apart to use as your goal.
- Shoot the soccer ball between the discs that you set up as a goal.
- Dribble the soccer ball toward the goal and shoot. You can add extra discs between you and the goal to act as pathways that you can dribble through or points where you can change directions before shooting on goal.

STRATEGIES TO REMEMBER

- When you are dribbling the soccer ball, keep it close to you.
- When you are passing the ball, kick with the instep of your foot.
- When you are trapping the ball, cushion it as if you were catching an egg.
- When you are shooting the soccer ball, point your toes down and kick the middle of the ball with the top of your foot. Your non-kicking foot should be next to the ball, pointing toward the target. When you follow through, make sure that your kicking toes end up pointing toward the target as well.

CHALLENGE SKILLS

The following advanced skills are for those who have mastered the basic skills. The challenge skills are recommended for those who want to improve their footwork.

TOE TAPS

With the ball stationary on the ground, hop onto your right foot and tap the top of the ball with the toes of your left foot. Then, hop onto your left foot and tap the top of the ball with the toes of your right foot. Continue this pattern. How fast can you go?

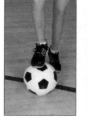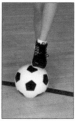

Toe taps

SIDE TO SIDE

With the ball between your feet, move the ball from side to side with the insteps of your feet while taking small hops.

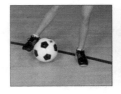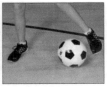

Side to side

PULL BACK/REVERSE DIRECTION

Place your foot on top of the ball. Pull your foot back so that the ball rolls along the bottom of your foot from back to front. This will pull the ball back so that you can make a quick turn to dribble or pass in the opposite direction.

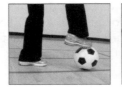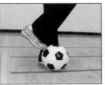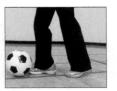

Pull back/Reverse direction

BACKSPIN/CATCH

Position your toes on the top of the ball to start. In a single motion, roll your toes backward and down along the ball to roll the ball back onto your toes.

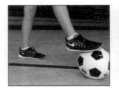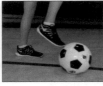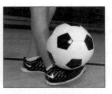

Backspin/Catch

SCISSORS

Swing 1 foot around the ball. Then, swing your other foot around the ball in the opposite direction. Try again, switching the directions that you swing your feet.

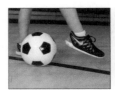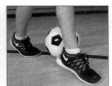

Scissors

KNEE JUGGLE

Drop the ball onto your knee, softly bouncing it back up. Use the same knee or your other knee to bounce the ball. See how many times you can bounce the ball on your knees to keep it from hitting the ground.

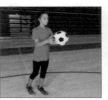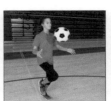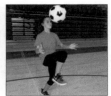

Knee juggle

INSIDE FOOT JUGGLE

Hold up 1 of your feet, bending at the knee to angle the instep of your foot up. Drop the ball and bounce it back up with the instep of your foot. Use the same foot or the instep of your other foot to bounce the ball back up again before it hits the ground. How many times can you juggle the ball with the insides of your feet before it touches the ground?

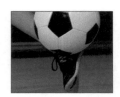

Inside food juggle

OUTSIDE FOOT JUGGLE

Drop the ball softly. Use the outside of 1 of your feet, angling your ankle down, to kick the ball back up. Repeat this with 1 or both of your feet. How long can you juggle the ball without it hitting the ground?

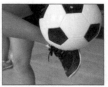

Outside food juggle

TOE JUGGLE

Drop the ball slightly in front of you. Gently kick the ball back up with the top part of your foot. Continue this with 1 or both of your feet to juggle the ball without letting it hit the ground for as long as you can.

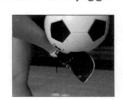

Toe juggle

COMBINATION JUGGLE

Use a combination of your knees and the insides, outsides, and tops of your feet to keep the ball up for as long as you can.

OFFENSIVE AND DEFENSIVE SKILLS

Quick, fast, agile footwork is an essential component of a soccer game. Practice footwork skills to improve offensive and defensive play.

OFFENSIVE SKILLS

FAKE

- Look 1 direction, but pass or move the ball in another direction.
- Stay on the balls of your feet.
- Move quickly.

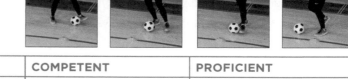

SKILL	PROGRESSING	COMPETENT	PROFICIENT
fake	1 of the elements	2 out of 3 elements	all elements

GIVE AND GO

The purpose of the give and go in a soccer game is for you to pass the ball to a teammate and quickly relocate so that you can receive a pass.

- Pass the ball to a teammate.
- Move quickly to relocate and support your offense.
- Indicate (call out) that you are ready and open to receive the ball.
- Receive the ball.

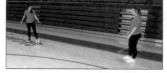
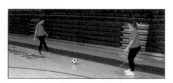
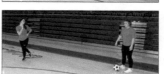
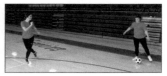

SKILL	PROGRESSING	COMPETENT	PROFICIENT
give and go	1 or 2 of the elements	3 out of 4 elements	all elements

THROW-IN

The only time that a player other than a goalie can use their hands to touch the ball in a game is to perform a throw-in. A throw-in occurs when the ball goes out of bounds on either of the long sides of the field. The team that sends the ball out of bounds loses possession of the ball. The other team gains control of the ball and throws it in from the point where it went out of bounds.

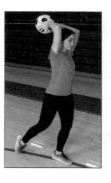
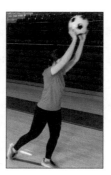
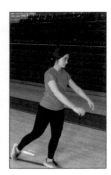

- Hold the ball in front of your body with both hands.
- Lift the ball over and behind your head.
- Step forward and throw the ball to a teammate. You cannot be the first person to touch the ball after you throw it in; or, you cannot throw-in to yourself.
- Follow through toward your target.
- Both of your feet must remain on the ground when you complete a throw-in. You can drag your back foot, but you cannot hop.

SKILL	PROGRESSING	COMPETENT	PROFICIENT
throw-in	1 or 2 of the elements	3 or 4 out of 5 elements	all elements

DEFENSIVE SKILLS

DEFENSIVE READY POSITION

The ready position allows a player to move quickly in any direction. It is used for both offense and defense.

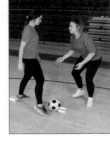

- Bend your knees to keep your body low.
- Stand with your feet shoulder-width apart.
- Keep your head up and your weight on the balls of your feet.
- Hold your arms extended out above waist height.
- Be ready to move and react quickly.
- Anticipate direction.

SKILL	PROGRESSING	COMPETENT	PROFICIENT
defensive ready position	1, 2, or 3 of the elements	4 or 5 out of 6 elements	all elements met

DEFENSIVE SLIDES

The purpose of the defensive slides in soccer is to keep up with your opponent and to legally take the ball or legally disrupt the opponent's pass or shot.

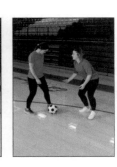

- Place your weight on the balls of your feet.
- Slide to the side with quick steps.
- Do not cross your feet.
- Keep your knees bent.
- Square your hips so that they face your opponent.
- Hold your hands up at chest level.
- Keep your eyes on your opponent's waistline.
- Stay with your opponent.
- Anticipate and react quickly to your opponent's movements.

SKILL	PROGRESSING	COMPETENT	PROFICIENT
defensive slides	1, 2, 3, 4, or 5 of the elements	6, 7, or 8 out of 9 elements	all elements met

PRACTICING OFFENSIVE AND DEFENSIVE SKILLS

- Practice the **give and go** with a partner and a defender. Pass the ball, quickly relocate, and then receive the pass, avoiding the defender.
- Practice the **fake** independently. Set up a cone as a decoy. Fake the pass toward the cone, and then pass to your partner. Practice until you feel comfortable with the movement.
- Practice the **fake** with a partner defending you. Dribble, fake, and then move in another direction to get around the defensive player. Practice until you feel comfortable with the fake.
- Practice the **defensive slides** with a partner. As your partner dribbles, defensive slide to try to prevent the player from making a successful pass or shot. Practice until you feel comfortable with the defensive slide.

SOCCER GAMES

KEEP AWAY

Keep away is an activity that lets you practice your soccer skills, even if you do not have enough players to play a full game of soccer.

- You need at least 5 players to play this game.
- Make a circle with all but 1 of the players. The remaining 1 person goes in the middle of the circle.
- The players on the outside, or making up the circle, can touch the ball twice to keep it away from the person in the middle.
- If the person in the middle touches the ball, they switch with the person the ball was stolen from.
- If the players on the outside touch the ball 21 times before the person in the middle touches it, the outside players win and the person in the middle stays in the middle for another round.

ABOUT THE GAME

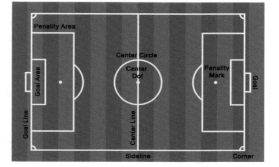

- To begin, 2 opposing teams of 11 players each including a goalie are established.
- All players must wear shin guards, socks that cover their shin guards, and appropriate cleats.
- The game is played on a rectangular grass or turf field.
- A goal is located at each end of the field.
- The object of the game is to move the ball down the field by passing or dribbling with your feet and to score by getting the ball into your opponent's goal.
- A game is divided into 45-minute halves.
- A goal is worth 1 point.
- The team with the most points at the end of the second half wins.

PLAYING THE GAME

- The game begins with a coin toss made by a referee at midfield.
- The team that possesses the ball is on offense and the other team is on defense.
- The first player to touch the ball at kickoff can only touch the ball once. They must kick the ball or pass it to another player who can dribble, pass, or kick the ball.
- No players except for the goalies or a player who is performing a throw-in can touch the ball with their hands. The entire arm counts as a hand in soccer, which means that a player cannot touch the ball anywhere from their fingertips to their upper arm.
- It is legal to use any body part other than a hand to contact the ball.
- If a player illegally uses their hands, which is referred to as a handball, the ball is turned over to the opposing team.
- The players on defense try to intercept, or take away, the ball from the offensive team to gain possession of the ball.

DEMONSTRATE POSITIVE GAME BEHAVIOR

- Follow all game rules.
- Do not conduct any fouls against another player (do not make illegal physical contact) and do not exhibit any unsportsmanlike behavior.
    - Fouls and unsportsmanlike behavior can result in a free kick, a yellow card warning, or a red card ejection from the game for the offending player.
- Be supportive and encouraging to your teammates.
- Treat your opponents with respect.

SKILL	PROGRESSING	COMPETENT	PROFICIENT
game behavior	1 or 2 of the elements	3 out of 4 elements	all elements met

MODIFIED 5-ON-5 GAME

Play a casual game of soccer according to the number of available players. Play a game of 3-on-3, 4-on-4, 5-on-5, or whatever you are able with your available players. The following information is for a 5-on-5 game.

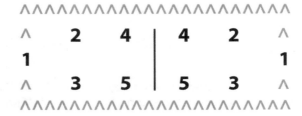

- Establish 2 teams, each consisting of 1 goalie, 2 defensive players, and 2 offensive players.
- Establish boundaries and set up a goal for each team.
- Establish the perimeters that the 5 players on each team adhere to. Establishing perimeters encourages teamwork and passing. The following are suggestions.
    - The goalie remains in the goalie area.
    - The defenders are allowed up to midfield.
    - The offensive players are allowed from ¾ of the way back on their side to the opposing goal.
- Establish rules for your game. The following are suggestions.
    - For out-of-bounds balls, a player from the opposing team throws the ball back into play.
    - Goalies throw the ball in after a score.
    - Goalie and players may use their hands to throw the ball in.

RATE YOUR ENJOYMENT OF THE SOCCER ACTIVITY THAT YOU ENJOYED MOST

On a scale from 1 to 4, where 1 is not enjoyable and 4 is very enjoyable, rate this activity.

1	It was not enjoyable, and I will not participate again.
2	It was not enjoyable, but I will participate again for exercise.
3	It was enjoyable, and I will play again.
4	It was very enjoyable, and I will initiate future games.

💻 RESEARCH INTEGRATION

1. Research soccer's country of origin, who invented soccer, where soccer is played throughout the world, alternate names for soccer, and the official rules and regulations of soccer.

2. Attend a soccer game or watch a soccer game on television. It can be men's, women's, or co-ed soccer at any level—youth, high school, college, or professional. Identify the soccer skills you have learned that are used by the players throughout the game.

❤️ HEALTH INTEGRATION

1. Count your pulse after practicing skills and after playing in a game to determine if you are exercising in your personal target heart rate zone. Predict and then compare the difference between your heart rate after playing in the goalie position and your heart rate after playing in a running, or field, position. Apply the results to your overall fitness plan. Many people choose to complete aerobic workouts by playing in fast-paced games like soccer.

2. Have a discussion about the protective gear that is worn by a soccer player and why they wear this gear.

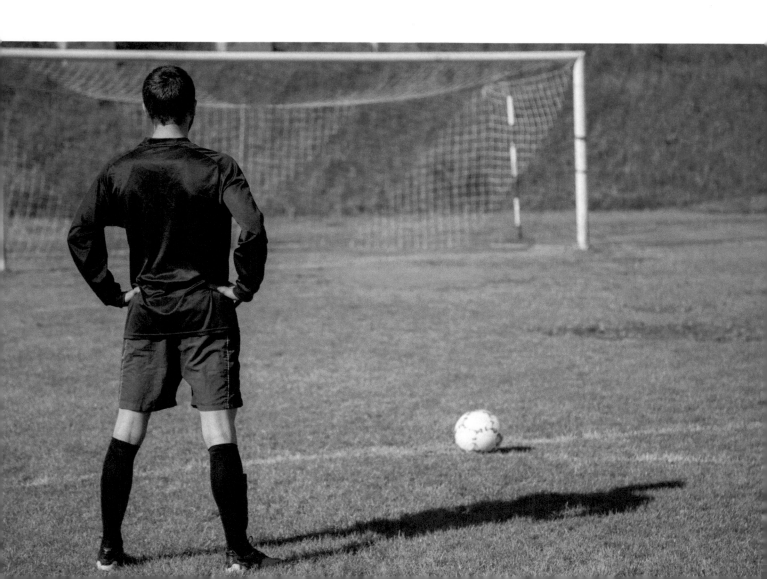

SHORT-HANDLED RACKET TENNIS

Tennis is a sport that is played by striking a ball with a racket over a net. It is played by 2 opposing players or by 2 teams of 2 as a doubles game. The required striking activity helps you develop concentration, hand-eye coordination, and footwork. You can play tennis as a competitive sport or as an opportunity for social play.

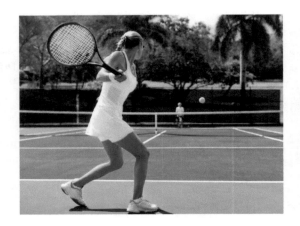

The purpose of this lesson is for you to learn to use a short-handled tennis racket by learning the mechanics of the tennis strokes, to participate in tennis games, and to get an aerobic workout.

⚠ **CAUTION: Make sure that nobody is close to you before you swing the racket. Do not walk into the path of another person who is swinging a racket.**

RACKET SKILLS

READY POSITION

The ready position allows a player to move quickly in any direction.

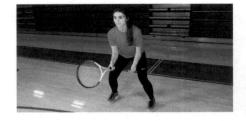

- Bending your knees, stand with your feet shoulder-width apart.
- Keep your head up.
- Keep your weight on the balls of your feet.
- Hold the racket in your dominant hand.

SKILL	PROGRESSING	COMPETENT	PROFICIENT
ready position	1 or 2 of the elements	3 out of 4 elements	all elements met

HANDSHAKE GRIP

- Hold the racket in your dominant hand as if you were about to shake someone's hand.
- Place your 4 fingers around the racket; then, wrap your thumb around the racket in the opposite direction.
- Hold the racket so that the head is vertical to the ground. Make sure that the strings on the racket head are facing front and back.
- Point the handle toward your belly button.

SKILL	PROGRESSING	COMPETENT	PROFICIENT
handshake grip	1 or 2 of the elements	3 out of 4 elements	all elements met

FOREHAND STROKE

- Begin in the ready position.
- Pivot to bring the racket back on the same side of your body as your dominant hand.
- Face the palm of your hand forward.
- While swinging the racket with your dominant hand, shift your weight from your back foot to your front foot as you step forward.
- Extend your arm and flick your wrist to hit the ball, pointing the face of the racket up to get the ball over the net.
- Follow through to your target.

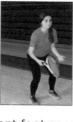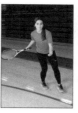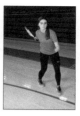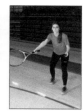

SKILL	PROGRESSING	COMPETENT	PROFICIENT
forehand stroke	1, 2, or 3 of the elements	4 or 5 out of 6 elements	all elements met

BACKHAND STROKE

- Begin in the ready position.
- Rotate the racket and extend it across your body.
- Rotate your feet and shoulders in the same direction as the racket.
- Face the back of your hand (the side that your knuckles are on) forward.
- As you swing the racket, step forward with your non-dominant foot.
- Flick your wrist as you are hitting the ball with the center of the racket.
- Follow through to your target.

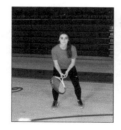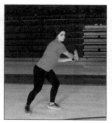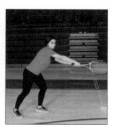

SKILL	PROGRESSING	COMPETENT	PROFICIENT
backhand stroke	1, 2, or 3 of the elements	4, 5, or 6 out of 7 elements	all elements met

2-HANDED BACKHAND STROKE

- Place your non-dominant hand below your dominant hand on the racket handle.
- Rotate the racket and extend it across your body.
- Rotate your feet and shoulders in the same direction as the racket.
- Flick your wrists when you are hitting the ball with the center of the racket.
- Follow through to your target.

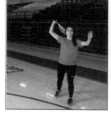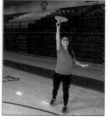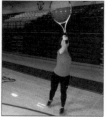

OVERHAND STROKE

- Bend your elbow slightly and position the racket under the ball.
- Flick your wrist to hit the ball with the center of the racket.
- Extend your arm as you are making contact.
- Follow through to your target.

SKILL	PROGRESSING	COMPETENT	PROFICIENT
overhand stroke	1 or 2 of the elements	3 out of 4 elements	all elements met

SERVES

Every game starts with a serve.

PUNCH SERVE

Stand behind the service line at a 45-degree angle to the net. A punch serve is an excellent stroke to use as a beginner.

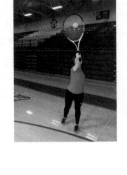

- If you are right-handed, place your left foot forward; if you are left-handed, place your right foot forward. Put your weight on your back foot.

- Hold the racket with a forehand grip in your dominant hand. Raise the racket over your head and slightly back.

- Hold the ball with your fingertips in your non-dominant hand.

- Toss the ball slightly in front of you and high above the racket. Look up at the ball.

- As the ball comes back down, hit it up and forward with the racket. Extend your arm and the racket while you are hitting the ball.

- Follow through to your target. Swing out, across, and down.

SKILL	PROGRESSING	COMPETENT	PROFICIENT
punch serve	1, 2, or 3 of the elements	4 or 5 out of 6 elements	all elements met

OVERHAND SERVE

- Hold the racket with your dominant hand.

- Place your non-dominant foot so that it is pointing toward the opposite post of the net and your dominant foot so that it is parallel to the court.

- Toss the ball into the air just above your head.

- Bring your dominant arm back with the head of the racket pointing toward the sky.

- Watch for the ball to begin to fall.

- Extend your arm up over your head and contact the ball with the head of the racket.

SKILL	PROGRESSING	COMPETENT	PROFICIENT
overhand serve	1, 2, or 3 of the elements	4 or 5 out of 6 elements	all elements met

SKILL PRACTICE

AGAINST A WALL

- Practice the various strokes and serves by hitting the ball against a wall with the racket. Catch the ball each time and repeat.

- Allow the ball to bounce before hitting it against the wall.

- Volley against the wall, aiming and hitting different spots on the wall.

WITH A PARTNER

You can use a jump rope to separate each side if a net is unavailable.

- Have a partner stand on 1 side of the net and toss the ball toward your forehand. Return with a proper forehand stroke.

- Have a partner stand on 1 side of the net and toss the ball toward your backhand. Return with a proper backhand stroke.

- Have a partner stand on 1 side of the net and toss the ball, mixing up forehand and backhand shots. Return with proper forehand strokes or backhand strokes.
- Use the various strokes to hit the ball back and forth with a partner. Stand 15 feet away from your partner when you are volleying back and forth.

GAMES

INDEPENDENT RACKET DRIBBLE CHALLENGE

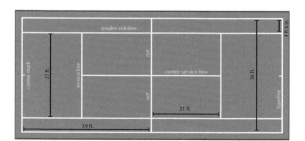

- Place the palm of your dominant hand on top of the racket and turn the face of the racket toward the ground.
- Hold the ball in your non-dominant hand.
- Bump the ball with the racket.
- Let the ball bounce back up to the racket.
- Continue dribbling the ball. How many consecutive dribbles can you do in a row?
- To increase difficulty, stand near a line and try to make the ball hit the line each time you dribble it. How many consecutive line dribbles can you do in a row?
- Practice air dribbling. Hit the ball consecutively up in the air with the racket. Do not let the ball touch the ground between hits. How many hits can you do in a row?

COOPERATIVE SCORING GAME

- Begin with 1 person standing on either side of the net. If a net is unavailable, separate the sides with a jump rope.
- Conduct a coin toss to determine who will serve first.
- Rally the ball back and forth following the serve.
- Count each time a player strikes the ball and keeps it in play, not counting the serve.
- The ball can only be hit once per side. So, each player can only use 1 hit on their own side of the court to return the ball to the other side of the court.
- The ball can be returned after 1 bounce or on a fly, which means that the player can strike the ball before it hits the ground.
- Continue until the ball is not in play.
- Indicate the score.
- Switch servers.
- Play again and try to beat your previous score.

OFFICIAL SINGLES GAME

You will need traditional tennis balls for this game.

- Start with an overhand serve from the right side of the court. Serve from behind the baseline to your opponent on the left.
- You must get the ball into your opponent's service box. You have 2 tries to get the ball into the service box.
- If you hit the ball into your opponent's service box and your opponent cannot return it, you win that volley and get a point.
- Now, serve from the left side of the court.

- When your score is an even number, serve from the right side of the court. When your score is an odd number, serve from the left side of the court.
- Continue serving the ball until the game is over. The receiver becomes the server during the next game.
- You may only hit the ball 1 time on each side.
- You score if your opponent does not have a successful serve, fails to return a serve, or hits the ball out of bounds.
- You lose a volley if you or the racket touch the net.

SCORING

- The server's score is always announced first.
- The point system is given below.
    - 0 points (love) = 0 points
    - 1 point = 15 points
    - 2 points = 30 points
    - 3 points = 40 points
    - 4 points = win
- To win a game, you must lead by at least 2 points.
- If the score is tied at 40 points (a deuce), you must earn 2 consecutive points (an advantage point) to win the game.
- You must win at least 6 games in a set. You must lead by 2 sets to win a match.

RATE YOUR ENJOYMENT OF THE TENNIS ACTIVITY THAT YOU ENJOYED MOST

On a scale from 1 to 4, where 1 is not enjoyable and 4 is very enjoyable, rate this activity.

1	It was not enjoyable, and I will not participate again.
2	It was not enjoyable, but I will participate again for exercise.
3	It was enjoyable, and I will play again.
4	It was very enjoyable, and I will initiate future games.

RESEARCH INTEGRATION

1. Research tennis's country of origin, who invented tennis, and the official rules and regulations of tennis.
2. Attend a tennis game or watch a tennis game on television.

HEALTH INTEGRATION

Count your pulse to determine if you are exercising in your personal target heart rate zone. Count your pulse after practicing skills and after playing a game. Apply the results to your overall fitness plan. Many people choose to complete aerobic workouts by playing in social, competitive games with friends.

WIFFLE® BALL

Wiffle® ball is a game played by 2 teams of 1 to 10 players each on a small version of a baseball field with a plastic bat and ball. The object of the game is to scores more runs than the opposing team. People of all ages play Wiffle® ball to get exercise and to enjoy the social aspect of the game.

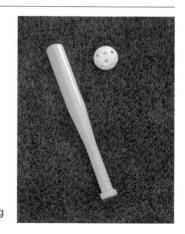

Playing the game allows you to utilize and improve the skill-related components of agility, balance, coordination, speed, power, and reaction. Wiffle® ball also provides the opportunity to work as a team to develop offensive and defensive strategies as well as the ability to transition quickly between them.

The purpose of this lesson is to practice the skills necessary for you to participate in a team game, follow game rules, communicate with teammates in a positive and effective manner, and exhibit appropriate behavior with your team and the opposing team.

⚠ CAUTION: Make sure that nobody is close to you before you swing the bat. Do not walk into the path of another person who is swinging a bat. Do not throw the bat.

WIFFLE® BALL SKILLS

STRIKING AND BASE-RUNNING SKILLS

GRIP AND STANCE

GRIP

- If you are right-handed, wrap your left hand below your right hand at the bottom of the bat. If you are left-handed, wrap your right hand below your left hand at the bottom of the bat.
  - o Smaller batters may benefit from choking up on the bat, or holding the bat a little higher up from the base of the handle.
- Your hands should be touching each other.

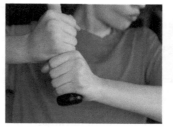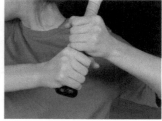

STANCE

- Position your body perpendicular to the plate.
- Bending your knees slightly, place your feet so that they are shoulder-width apart. Your hips, knees, and shoulders should be squared. This stance should be comfortable.
- Once your feet are inside the batter's box, face your shoulder toward the pitcher and point the tip of the bat up toward the sky. If you are right-handed, face your left shoulder toward the pitcher. If you are left-handed, face your right shoulder toward the pitcher.

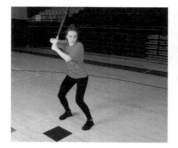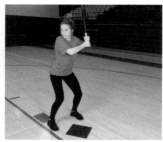

SKILL	PROGRESSING	COMPETENT	PROFICIENT
grip and stance	1 or 2 of the elements	3 or 4 out of 5 elements	all elements met

STRIKING A BALL FROM A PITCH

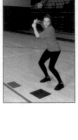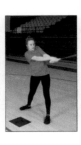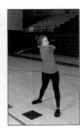

- Check your position to see if your swing will cross over the plate. Stand in the batter's box and touch the opposite side of the plate with the bat. Adjust your stance if necessary.
- While in the correct position, practice swinging all the way through, keeping the bat level with the ground and twisting your body as you hit the ball.
- The whole swing should be in your hips. Try to get in the habit of twisting your whole body rather than just swinging your arms.
- Take a small step toward the pitcher as they throw the ball. Rotate your hips toward the pitcher, moving your hands through the strike zone and over the plate. Watch the ball as it comes toward you and over the plate before you hit it into the outfield.
- After swinging the bat, face your hips toward the pitcher. Pivot your back foot, but do not let it come off the ground.
- During a game, after you hit the ball, drop the bat to the ground and run to first base.

SKILL	PROGRESSING	COMPETENT	PROFICIENT
striking	1 or 2 of the elements	3 or 4 out of 5 elements	all elements met

BASE RUNNING

- Drop the bat to the ground after you hit the ball.
- Immediately sprint as fast as you can to first base.
- Run on and through the base.

SKILL	PROGRESSING	COMPETENT	PROFICIENT
base running	1 of the elements	2 out of 3 elements	all elements met

THROWING, CATCHING, AND FIELDING SKILLS

OVERHAND THROW

An overhand throw can be used by the field players and the pitcher.

- Take a first step, such as a hop or shuffle step, toward your target.
- Bring your throwing arm back, up, and around.
- Step with your opposite foot.
- Rotate your hips as you twist with your throw.
- Release the ball high in your throw, when your throwing arm is in an L shape near your ear.
- Follow through your throw to make it accurate.

SKILL	PROGRESSING	COMPETENT	PROFICIENT
overhand throw	1, 2, or 3 of the elements	4 or 5 out of 6 elements	all elements met

CATCHING

- Track the ball with your eyes.
- Step toward your target.
- Extend your hands to the level of the ball.
- Give with the ball (pull it slightly toward you) as it hits your hands for a soft catch.

SKILL	PROGRESSING	COMPETENT	PROFICIENT
catching	1 or 2 of the elements	3 out of 4 elements	all elements met

FIELDING GROUND BALLS

- Keep your body low and ready.
- Scoop up the ball as it rolls.
- Look to your target.
- Throw accurately to your target.

SKILL	PROGRESSING	COMPETENT	PROFICIENT
fielding	1 or 2 of the elements	3 out of 4 elements	all elements met

SKILL PRACTICE

THROW AND CATCH

- Throw and catch a ball against a wall.
- Throw and catch a ball with a partner.
- Throw and catch a ball with a partner while moving.

BATTING FOR DISTANCE

- As a batter, hit a pitch that is thrown to you by a partner.
- The pitcher will place a disc cone where the ball landed, marking the distance it traveled.
- Hit another pitch, trying to increase the distance you hit the ball from your last hit.
- Take turns batting and pitching with your partner.

BATTING FOR DIRECTION

- Place disc cones in the right, left, and center field.
- Before you bat, call out the direction in which your hit will go: right field, left field, or center field.
- Hit a pitch from your partner in the determined direction.
- Take turns batting and pitching with your partner.

BATTING FOR FORCE

- Before you bat, call out what the force of your hit will be—soft, medium, or hard.
- Hit a pitch from your partner with the force that you called out.
- Take turns batting and pitching with your partner.

3 PLAYERS PRACTICE GAME: STRIKING, FIELDING, AND BASE RUNNING

- Set up a playing field with first base, second base, third base, home base, and a pitching mound.
- Choose 1 player to be the pitcher, 1 player to be the batter, and the remaining players to be outfielders.
- If you are the pitcher, pitch the ball to the batter until the batter gets a hit. Retrieve the ball and run to home base before the batter gets there.
- If you are the batter, run the bases after you hit the ball. If the pitcher gets to home base before you, you are out.
- If you are an outfielder, retrieve the ball and give it back to the pitcher before the batter gets to home base.
- Take turns in the different positions.

WIFFLE® BALL GAME

- Wiffle® ball teams can range from being made up of 1 to 10 players.
- The pitcher throws 3 balls to each batter, and the batter must attempt to hit them.
- If you fail to hit the ball within 3 pitches, you strike out.
- Do not run to the next base until the batter hits the ball.
- If you hit the ball into the single zone, you advance 1 base. If you hit the ball into the double zone, you advance 2 bases. If you hit the ball past the triple zone, you get a home run.
- Every player who makes it around the bases scores a run for their team.
- You are out if the batted ball is caught in the air, a fielder tags you when you are running to a base, or the ball is fielded and thrown to a base before you get there.
- An inning is over when all the batters have had their turns or if 3 batters strike out.
- At the end of the game, the team with the most runs is the winner. Games may last a set time or last a set number of innings.

GAME NOTES

1. A **foul ball** is a ball that the batter hits outside of the baseline. The batter gets another pitch if this happens. There are unlimited foul balls unless a defensive player catches a fly ball.
2. The field is split up into different **zones**. The suggested sizes of these zones are given below, but the zones can be adjusted according to your play area.
    - The single zone is 24 feet from home base.
    - The double zone is 20 feet from the single zone.
    - The triple zone is 20 feet from the double zone.
    - The home run zone is 20 feet from the triple zone.

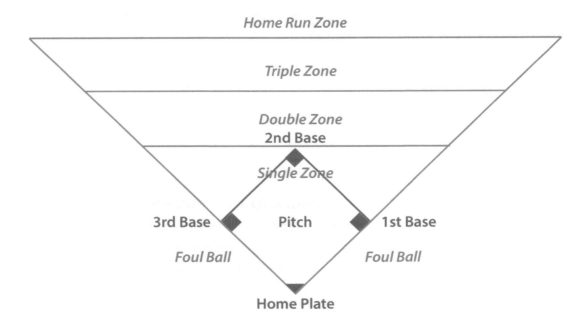

3. A **strike** occurs when the batter swings and misses the ball. The batter is out after 3 strikes.
4. A **fly ball** is a ball that is hit up in the air. Fly balls are often caught to strike a player out.
5. The **pitcher** is the defensive player who stands on the pitching mound and pitches (throws) the ball to the batter.

6. The **catcher** is the defensive player who plays behind home base. The catcher returns the ball to the pitcher and tags players out at home base.

7. An **outfielder** is a defensive player who plays behind the baseline to retrieve the ball when it is hit far.

8. A **baseman** is a defensive player who plays on first, second, or third base. The 3 basemen should stand near their bases. To prevent colliding with a runner, the basemen should not stand on their bases; however, the basemen can touch their bases to strike a runner out.

RATE YOUR ENJOYMENT OF WIFFLE® BALL

On a scale from 1 to 4, where 1 is not enjoyable and 4 is very enjoyable, rate this activity.

1	It was not enjoyable, and I will not participate again.
2	It was not enjoyable, but I will participate again for exercise.
3	It was enjoyable, and I will play again.
4	It was very enjoyable, and I will initiate future games.

RESEARCH INTEGRATION

1. Research who invented the game of Wiffle® ball and the rules and regulations of the game.

2. Attend a baseball game or watch a baseball game on television and compare the skills that you have practiced for the game of Wiffle® ball with the skills that the baseball players use.

HEALTH INTEGRATION

Count your pulse after practicing Wiffle® ball skills and after playing in a Wiffle® ball game to determine if you are exercising in your personal target heart rate zone. Apply the results to your overall fitness plan. Often, when you are playing in games that require you to take turns, you may find that your pulse rate is not in your aerobic target zone. If that is the case for you, remember that you still need to get your aerobic exercise in for the week. Enjoy the game and count it toward your 60 minutes per day of being active.

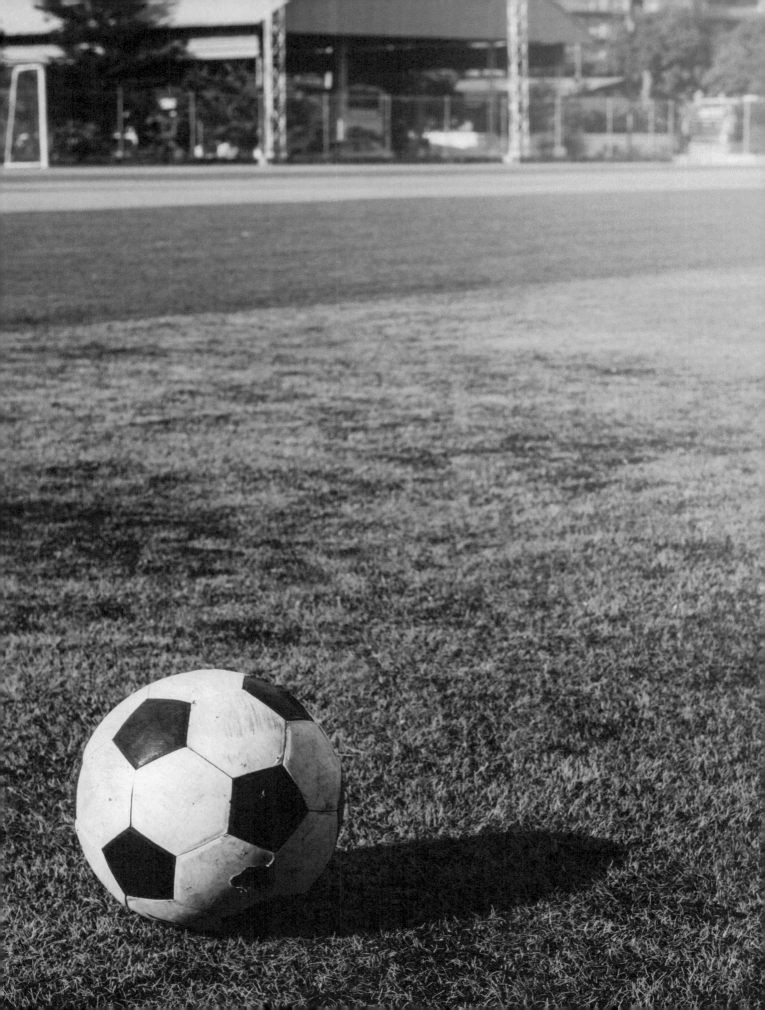

GRADE 8
PE EQUIPMENT KIT

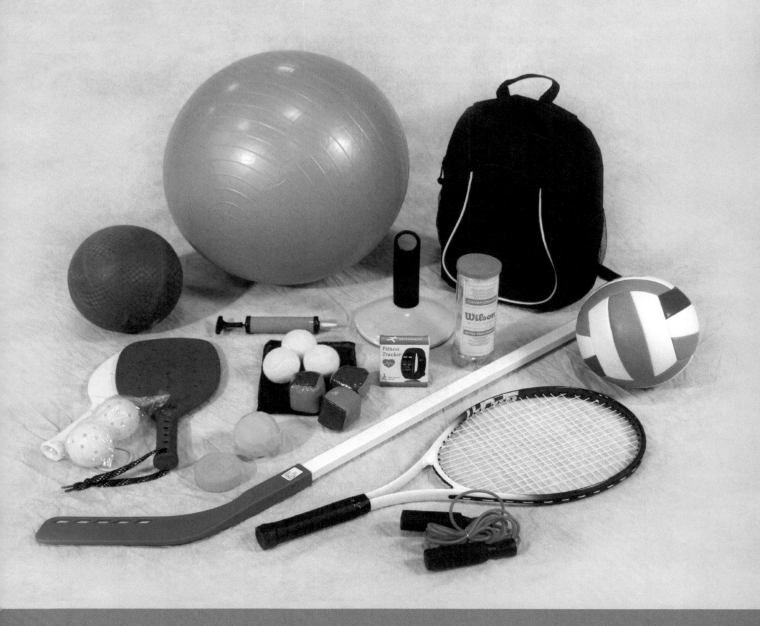

WARM-UP AND COOL-DOWN

⚠️ **CAUTION: Stretching should not be painful; ease up if stretching hurts. See the Flexibility section of your PE Manual for more information.**

WARM-UP

The purpose of a warm-up is to gradually increase heart rate, breathing rate, body temperature, and muscle temperature. Warming up prior to exercising increases circulation and blood flow to your muscles. When your muscles are warmed up, their performance—such as in the areas of strength and speed—is enhanced and risk of injury is decreased.

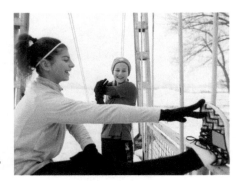

Before you begin any workout, you should always warm up. Getting your heart and muscles prepared for exercise is important. There are numerous ways to get your body ready to participate in physical activity. **The Flexibility section of your PE Manual includes a variety of dynamic and static stretches for each major body part that will help you increase your flexibility.**

Elements of a Warm-Up

1. **Low-intensity cardio**: Walk, slow jog, or slow swim for 5 to 10 minutes to increase your heart rate, breathing rate, and body temperature before your workout.

2. **Dynamic stretch**: Perform a repeated motion—such as kicks, high knees, lunges, or arm circles—that will loosen up your joints and prepare your muscles for the exercise that you are about to do. Perform each dynamic stretch for at least 30 seconds.

3. **Static stretch**: Stretch your muscles slowly and hold each stretch for 20 to 30 seconds without bouncing in order to lengthen your muscles and increase your flexibility. Some important areas to stretch as a part of your warm-up are your neck, sides, shoulders, triceps, back, hamstrings, quadriceps, and groin.

Example 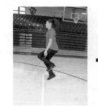 **+** 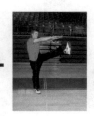 **+** 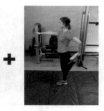 **= EFFECTIVE WARM-UP**

PERSONAL WARM-UP ACTIVITY

1. Select an exercise activity to participate in.

2. Design your personal warm-up plan for the activity that you selected. Any dynamic and static stretches that you choose to complete should be specific to the exercise activity that you chose.

3. Have a trusted adult or friend assess your stretches to make sure that you are using proper form.

4. Explain how the warm-up will decrease your risk of injury for this activity. _____

Procedure	Enter your personal warm-up regimen below.
1. **Low-intensity cardiovascular exercise:** Exercise for 5 to 10 minutes.	
2. **Dynamic stretches:** Perform dynamic stretches specifically for the selected activity.	
3. **Static stretches:** Perform static stretches specifically for the selected activity.	

COOL-DOWN

After you have finished your workout, exercise, or activity, it is imperative that your body returns to its normal state. You want to avoid stopping immediately and sitting down **unless you are in pain, dizzy, or injured**. Be sure to slow your heart rate and breathing rate back to or slightly above their resting rates. There are several ways to do this. You can simply walk or slow down your exercise for a few minutes, or you can find your own way to slow your body back down. You also may want to incorporate static stretches to increase flexibility and to avoid your muscles tightening. **The Flexibility section of your PE Manual includes a variety of static stretches for each major body part.** Always keep hydrated by drinking water before, during, and after exercise.

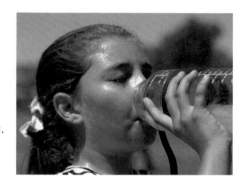

Elements of a Cool-Down

1. **Slow down**: Walk or gradually slow down your exercise—such as returning to a slow swim if you are swimming—until your heart rate, breathing rate, and body temperature are back to normal.

2. **Static stretch**: Stretch your muscles slowly and hold each stretch for 20 to 30 seconds without bouncing in order to lengthen your muscles and increase flexibility. Some important areas to stretch as part of your cool-down are your neck, sides, shoulders, triceps, back, hamstrings, quadriceps, and groin.

WALK + STATIC STRETCHES = EFFECTIVE COOL-DOWN

Design your personal cool-down plan. You can perform the same cool-down each time you finish a physical activity or you can change each time in order to reflect the exercise activity, such as by slowing your pedaling if you are biking.

Procedure	Enter your personal cool-down regimen below.
1. **Slow down:** Perform this slowed activity for 5 to 10 minutes.	
2. **Static stretches:** Perform several lower-body and upper-body stretches.	

AEROBIC EXERCISE

Aerobic exercise—also referred to as cardio or cardiovascular exercise—is any exercise that is done in your target heart rate zone and is performed for an extended period. Aerobic exercise is important for strengthening your heart muscle. Your heart pumps nutrient-rich, oxygenated blood to the cells of your body. Your skin, hair, bones, muscles, brain, and internal organs benefit from the increased nutrition and oxygen provided during regular aerobic workouts.

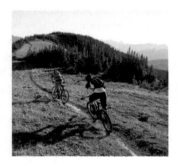

The purpose of this lesson is to encourage you to do an aerobic workout for at least 30 minutes 3 to 5 days per week in order to experience health benefits. An aerobic workout can be included as part of your recommended 60 minutes of daily physical activity. **The Cardiovascular Endurance section of your PE Manual includes the target heart rate zone formula and the Borg Rating of Perceived Exertion Scale to help you to determine if you are exercising for heart health.** You can also use available technology to monitor your pulse rate and workout intensity.

 CAUTION: Wear proper equipment and follow activity-specific safety rules.

AEROBIC EXERCISE

There are a variety of exercises to choose from. Choose aerobic exercises that will fit into your lifestyle and that you enjoy. Limit excuses and make a commitment to exercise!

TYPES OF AEROBIC EXERCISE

Sports: Playing a sport or sport-related game provides the opportunity to complete an aerobic workout and interact with others. Examples include soccer, basketball, volleyball, swimming, hockey, lacrosse, tennis, badminton, pickleball, handball, gymnastics, dance, martial arts, wrestling, track and field, and so on.

Outdoor pursuits: Examples include walking, jogging, biking, canoeing, kayaking, golfing, fly fishing, hiking, rock climbing, horseback riding, skiing, and so on.

Fitness gyms: Find a gym that is convenient for you to attend where you can complete circuit exercises, use aerobic machines, take classes, and more.

Stationary exercise equipment: Examples include using a jump rope, treadmill, elliptical trainer, bike, mini trampoline, and so on.

Exercise apps or videos: Use a workout tutorial on an app, website, video, or other digital source.

Your own sequence workouts: You can also design your own workout sequences by following the steps below.

- Create your personal aerobic workout routines by blending activities that involve basic locomotor skills such as jogging in place, jumping jacks, high knees, and so on.

- Design the intensity and duration of the exercise according to your level of fitness.

- Consider setting your routine to music.

- Perform your personal routine for some or all your aerobic workouts.

When you are beginning any exercise program, begin with workouts that match your fitness level and then build accordingly. You want to feel refreshed after each exercise session, not exhausted. Use your pulse rate to monitor aerobic workouts.

EXAMPLE OF HOW TO BUILD CARDIOVASCULAR ENDURANCE AT A STANDARD TRACK

Warm-up: Walk 1 lap and jog 1 lap. If your heart rate, breathing rate, and body temperature have not increased, repeat this.

Day of the Week	Monday/Wednesday/Friday		Tuesday/Thursday	
	Exercise	**Duration**	**Exercise**	**Duration**
	Walk the straight section of the track and sprint the curves.	4 laps	Walk or jog lightly.	3 laps
	Walk or jog lightly.	2 laps	Run or sprint.	1 lap
	Walk the straight section of the track and sprint the curves.	4 laps	Walk or jog lightly.	3 laps
	Walk or jog lightly.	2 laps	Run or sprint.	1 lap

Cool-down: Slowing your pace, continue to walk around the track until your heart rate, breathing rate, and body temperature have returned to baseline.

Record at least 3 aerobic exercise sessions that you participated in outside of PE class for 1 week. Record the time of each session.

An exercise can be any of the following.

1. a sport-related game
2. an outdoor pursuit
3. a self-created workout routine set to music

	Monday	**Tuesday**	**Wednesday**	**Thursday**	**Friday**	**Saturday**	**Sunday**
Exercise							
Time							
Exercise Heartrate							

List at least 1 response to each the following questions about aerobic exercise.

Question	**Response**
What positive emotional response did you experience by participating in aerobic exercise?	
What aerobic exercise activity did you enjoy the most?	
Why would the enjoyment of your favorite aerobic exercise activity lead to a lifetime of fitness for you?	

RESEARCH INTEGRATION

Review the 7th-grade Aerobic Exercise section in your PE Manual to practice the correct form for the basic locomotor skills before creating your movement sequence.

HEALTH INTEGRATION

Use available technology to monitor your pulse rate and workout intensity. Apply the results to your overall fitness plan.

HIP-HOP DANCE

Dancing is an exercise option for aerobic workout, for competition, or just for fun. You can dance on your own or with others. Dancing is expressing yourself through repeated patterns of movement which are usually set to music. Some forms of dance include creative, tap, ballet, hip-hop, modern, folk, square, jazz, line, Latin, ballroom, and social.

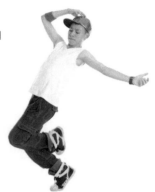

Hip-hop is an energetic dance type that originated when the hip-hop style of music surfaced. Hip-hop dancing was first performed within a subculture and is now also practiced in dance studios.

The purpose of this lesson is for you to perform basic hip-hop steps and locomotor movements using common dance concepts in rhythmic patterns to create your own dance for aerobic exercise.

HIP-HOP DANCE: CREATE YOUR PERSONAL DANCE ROUTINE

COMMON CONCEPTS OF DANCE TO USE FOR YOUR PERSONAL DANCE

- The concept of space includes the following.
  - high, medium, or low **levels**
  - forward, backward, right, or left **directions**
  - curved, zigzag, straight, circle, or square **pathways**
- The concept of time includes the following.
  - slow, medium, or fast **speeds**
  - a pattern for **rhythm**
- The concept of force includes the following
  - applying light, moderate, or strong **weights**

CREATE YOUR OWN DANCE

Start with the dance steps below. Then, complete the routine by adding your own dance steps. Set your dance to music.

1. Learn a scoop.
   - Face forward, with your feet a little more than shoulder-width apart.
   - Place your hands lightly on your thighs.
   - Simultaneously bend your knees and lean to the right.
   - Repeat this to the left.
   - Do these 4 times.

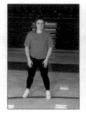 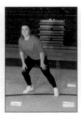 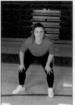 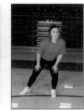

2. Learn a circle.
   - Face forward, with your feet a little more than shoulder-width apart.
   - Place your hands lightly on your thighs.
   - Simultaneously bend your knees, lean to the right, and do a complete circle to the right with your upper body.
   - Repeat this to the left.
   - Do these 4 times.

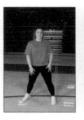 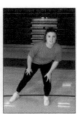 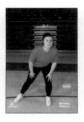 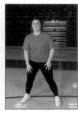

3. Learn a walk step with an arm pump.

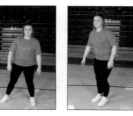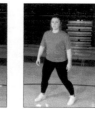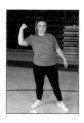

- Walk to the right with your right foot leading; step right, left, right, left.
- At the last left step, simultaneously pump your right arm; reach above your head and pull your hand down to shoulder level with your elbow bent.
- Repeat this to the left.
- Do these 4 times.

4. Combine the scoop, circle, and walk step, doing them 4 times each.

5. Next, choreograph your dance steps to complete the dance. Create the steps, write a description of each step, and practice the steps.

- Choose locomotor skills to blend (steps, jumps, slides, turns, and so on).
- Use your arms to accompany the footwork, for example: step, cross, step, clap.
- Perform each skill at different levels.
- Move in different directions.
- Move in different pathways.
- Move at slow, medium, and fast speeds.
- Use light, moderate, and strong force to move your body.
- Create a pattern.
- Use an 8 count for each move.

Option: Dance with a partner or small group for a social experience. You can also perform your dance for friends or family.

RATE YOUR ENJOYMENT OF HIP-HOP DANCE

On a scale from 1 to 4, where 1 is not enjoyable and 4 is very enjoyable, rate this activity.

1	It was not enjoyable, and I will not participate again.
2	It was not enjoyable, but I will participate again for exercise.
3	It was enjoyable, and I will dance again.
4	It was very enjoyable, and I will create more dances.

RESEARCH INTEGRATION

1. Research hip-hop dance and some hip-hop moves that you can safely use in your dance.
2. Join a dance class or dance with a dance video.
3. Join a dance from the USB if provided in your PE program.

HEALTH INTEGRATION

Count your pulse to determine if you are exercising in your personal target heart rate zone. Apply the results to your overall fitness plan. Many people choose to complete aerobic workouts through dance.

JUMP ROPE

Jumping rope is an exercise that meets components of both skill-related fitness and health-related fitness. It helps you develop coordination, balance, rhythm, agility, and timing. Jumping rope is an efficient way to perform aerobic exercise and build muscular strength and endurance in your legs. It can be done daily and in a small space almost anywhere there is a safe, stable surface.

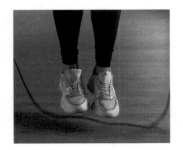

The purpose of this lesson is to provide you with the skills that you need to establish and implement your goal: to improve sport-related skills, to improve cardiovascular endurance, or both.

JUMP ROPE BASICS

FITTING THE JUMP ROPE TO YOUR HEIGHT

- Place a jump rope handle in each hand.
- Stand on the middle of the rope with 1 foot.
- Move the handles straight up, making sure that the rope is straight and pulled tight.
- The tops of the handles should reach close to your shoulders.

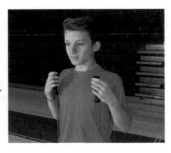

ELEMENTS OF JUMP ROPE

- Keep your eyes forward.
- When you are turning the rope, keep your elbows near your sides, maintaining a 45-degree angle and making 2-inch circles with your wrists.
- Leave just enough space for the rope to pass under your feet when you jump.
- Stay on the balls of your feet.
- Land softly, keeping your knees slightly bent.

BASIC SKILLS

BASIC JUMP

- Pick up the rope. Holding a handle in each hand, rest the rope behind your feet. Stand on the balls of your feet. This is the ready position.
- Your hands should be just above the height of your waist.
- Swing the rope up and over your head.
- Jump over the rope when it approaches your toes.
- Continue as long as you can without stopping.

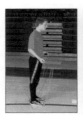 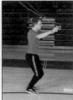 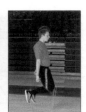
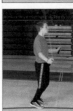 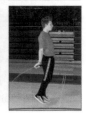

Basic jump

BACKWARD JUMP

- Begin with the rope in front of your feet.
- Swing the rope up and over your head.
- Jump over the rope when it approaches your feet.
- Continue as long as you can without stopping.

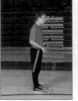 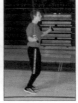 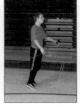 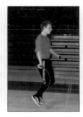 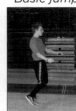

Backward jump

ALTERNATE-FOOT JUMP

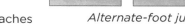

- Pick up the rope. Holding a handle in each hand, rest the rope behind your feet. Stand on the balls of your feet. This is the ready position. Note that 1 foot will be lifted off the ground during each turn of the rope before the other foot jumps.

- Turn the rope from behind you up over your head. When the rope reaches your toes, jump over it with your right foot.

- Turn the rope again from behind you up over your head. When the rope reaches your toes this time, jump over it with your left foot.

Alternate-foot jump

- Continue turning the rope and alternating feet as if you were running in place. Try it jumping backward.

SAMPLE OF A CARDIOVASCULAR CONDITIONING WORKOUT	SAMPLE OF A WORKOUT TO IMPROVE FOOTWORK SPEED
• basic jump 2 minutes • march or jog in place 30 seconds • backward jump 2 minutes • march or jog in place 30 seconds • alternate-foot jump 2 minutes • walk or jog in place 30 seconds • basic jump 2 minutes • march or jog in place 30 seconds • repeat for a 20-minute workout	• basic jump 1 minute at a medium pace • basic jump 30 seconds at a fast pace • rest 30 seconds • back jump 1 minute at a medium pace • back jump 30 seconds at a fast pace • rest 30 seconds • alternate-foot jump 1 minute at a medium pace • alternate-foot jump 30 seconds at a fast pace • rest 30 seconds • repeat as needed
DESIGN YOUR PERSONAL CARDIOVASCULAR JUMP ROPE ROUTINE AND SET IT TO MUSIC **(You can include basic, challenge, and partner skills after you have completed the module.)**	**DESIGN YOUR PERSONAL FOOTWORK SPEED ROUTINE**

CHALLENGE SKILLS

The following challenges are for students who have mastered the basic jump rope skills. The challenge level is recommended if you want to improve agility and further explore jump rope activities.

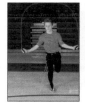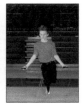

Hop on 1 foot (switch)

HOP ON 1 FOOT

Perform the basic jump on your right foot.

Perform the basic jump on your left foot.

SKIER

With both feet together, hop side to side while turning the rope.

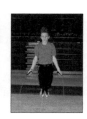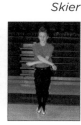

Skier

CROSSOVERS

- After the rope moves over your head, cross the rope in front of you, jump, and uncross the rope.

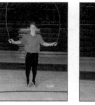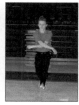

Crossovers

FRONT KICKS

- Kick 1 foot forward as the rope passes under your feet with a skip-step in between.
- Alternate kicks.

SIDE KICKS

- Kick 1 foot and then the other out to the side with a skip-step in between.

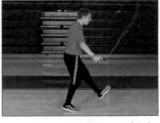

Front kicks

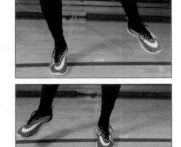

Side kicks

Practice the challenge jump rope skills until competent. Next, design your personal aerobic jump rope routine by blending the basic jump rope skills and the challenge skills. Set your routine to music. Monitor your pulse rate.

BLENDING: Perform 1 jump rope skill and transition smoothly to another jump rope skill without stopping between moves.

BLENDED 3 SKILLS CHECKLIST SAMPLE

Check off the blended challenge skills that you have successfully completed at least 3 consecutive times.

_____ Blend forward consecutive jumps, crossovers, and skiers.

_____ Blend backward consecutive jumps, right-foot hops, and left-foot hops, all while backward turning.

_____ Blend forward consecutive jumps, front kicks, and side kicks.

_____ Create your personal blend.

_____ Combine blends for an aerobic workout.

PARTNER SKILLS

Jump rope can have a social component. Individual jumping with a friend may motivate you and may make your workout more fun. Partner or long jump rope requires 2 or more participants.

PARTNER JUMP ROPE SKILLS

PARTNER CHAIN JUMP

- Make sure that each person has their own rope.
- Standing side by side, face forward in the ready position.
- Exchange inside handles with your partner; hold your handle with your outside hand and your partner's handle with your inside hand.
- Turn the rope over your head and jump together.
- Establish a rhythm with your partner. Jump rope together to that rhythm.

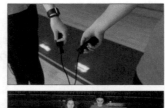
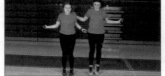
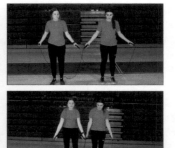

Partner chain jump

3-PERSON CHAIN JUMP

- This is like the partner chain jump except that 3 people participate.
- Try adding another person to the group of 3 to make it a 4-person chain jump.

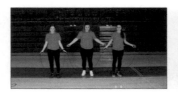
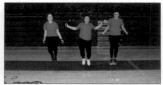

3-person chain jump

FACING YOUR PARTNER JUMP

- You will need 1 rope.
- Stand face-to-face with your partner.
- Have 1 person hold the rope.
- If you are holding the rope, stand facing your partner and turn the rope.
- If you are not holding the rope, stand facing your partner and jump rope with your partner as they turn the rope.
- No matter who is holding and turning the rope, establish a rhythm with your partner and jump rope together.

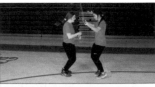
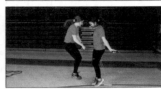

Facing your partner jump

FACE THE SAME WAY

- Either stand in front of your partner with your back turned to them or stand behind your partner and face their back. Both you and your partner should be facing the same way.
- If you are not holding the rope, stand in front of your partner and jump rope together.
- If you are holding the rope, stand behind your partner and turn the rope. Jump rope together.
- Establish a rhythm with your partner. Jump rope together to that rhythm.

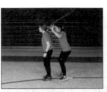

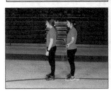
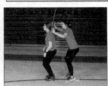
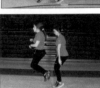
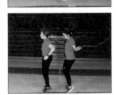

Facing the same way

SIDE BY SIDE JUMP

- You will need 1 rope.
- Stand beside your partner.
- Hold a handle of the rope with your outside hand. Your partner should hold the other handle in their outside hand.
- Jump rope together as you work together to turn the rope.

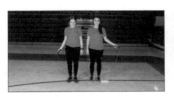
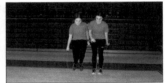

Side by side jump

List at least 1 response to each of the following questions about jumping rope.

Question	Response
What jump rope activity do you enjoy the most?	
Why did you enjoy the above-mentioned activity the most?	

 RESEARCH INTEGRATION

Research how jump rope is used in training for a sport.

 HEALTH INTEGRATION

Count your pulse to determine if you are exercising in your personal target heart rate zone. Apply the results to your overall fitness plan.

STRENGTH TRAINING

Your body is made up of over 600 muscles. Muscles work in pairs to pull on bones to create movement. Opposing muscles, or antagonistic muscles, should be equally trained because they work together. For example, the quadriceps and hamstring muscles work together, 1 contracting while the other relaxes to bend and straighten your knee.

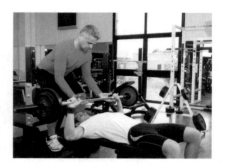

The saying "if you don't use it you will lose it" can be applied to your skeletal muscles. Muscles that are not used and not exercised become weak. Muscles are important for posture, movement, and maintaining body temperature. Strength training, also known as resistance training, builds muscular strength and endurance.

The purpose of this lesson is to encourage you to design your personal strength-training program and to perform exercises 2 to 3 days per week to experience health benefits.

 CAUTION: Have a certified trainer plan for you and supervise you when you are working with weights.

STRENGTH-TRAINING EXERCISES

There are a variety of exercises from which to choose. Do strength exercises for the muscles of your upper body, lower body, and core. Choose the intensity of each exercise to fit your fitness level. For example, if you are struggling to do a right-angle push-up, switch to a knee push-up. Limit excuses and make a commitment to exercise!

STRENGTH-TRAINING EXERCISE IDEAS

Weightlifting machines: You can use large stationary machines like those typically found in gyms.

Free weights: You can use free-weight equipment such as dumbbells, barbells, medicine balls, kettlebells, resistance bands, and weighted ropes to perform strength-training exercises.

Pilates or yoga: Pilates and yoga sessions are excellent workouts for muscle lengthening and muscle strengthening.

Personal workouts: You can use your own body weight as a source of resistance and create your own strength-training workouts. Create a personal workout by blending basic strength-building exercises such as sit-ups, push-ups, pull-ups, planks, and so on, and design the intensity and duration of each exercise according to your level of fitness. Include upper-body, lower-body, and core exercises in your workout. Perform your personal routine for some or all your strength-training workouts.

SAMPLE

The following is a sample personal strength-training workout that uses personal body weight as resistance.

Practice each of the following exercises, concentrating on proper form, prior to engaging in a workout.

IN-OUT ABS

muscle focus: abdominal muscles

Intensity Level 1

Sit on a cushioned surface with your elbows flat on the ground slightly behind your hips. Keeping your knees bent, lift both legs until they are parallel to the ground. Extend your legs straight out in front of you and then return to the bent-knee position.

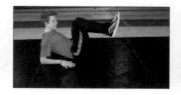 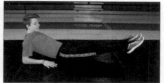

In-out abs: Intensity Level 1

Intensity Level 2

Sit on a cushioned surface with your hands flat on the ground slightly behind your hips. Keeping your knees bent, lift both legs until they are parallel to the ground. Extend your legs straight out in front of you and then return to the bent-knee position.

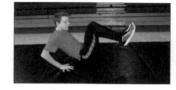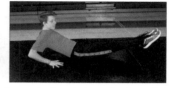

In-out abs: Intensity Level 2

Intensity Level 3

Sit on a cushioned surface with your arms held straight above your head. Keeping your knees bent, lift both legs until they are parallel to the ground. Extend your legs straight out in front of you and then return to the bent-knee position.

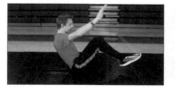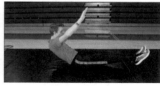

In-out abs: Intensity Level 3

FORWARD LUNGES

muscle focus: glutei maximi, hamstrings, and quadriceps

Intensity Level 1

Perform alternate forward lunges. Start with your feet together. Step 1 foot forward and bend your knee as low as you comfortably can. Do not exceed a 90-degree angle. Return to the starting position and then repeat the exercise with your other leg.

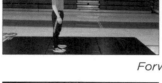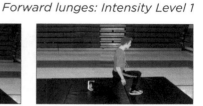

Forward lunges: Intensity Level 1

Intensity Level 2

Perform alternate forward lunges. Start with your feet together. Step 1 foot forward and bend your knee to a 90-degree angle. Return to the starting position and repeat the exercise with your other leg.

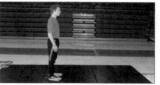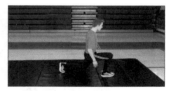

Forward lunges: Intensity Level 2

Intensity Level 3

Start with your feet together. Step your right foot forward and bend your knee to a 90-degree angle. Go back to the starting position. Continue lunging with your right foot until you have completed the repetitions. Next, lunge by stepping forward with your left foot until you complete the repetitions.

Forward lunges: Intensity Level 3

RIGHT-ANGLE PUSH-UPS

muscle focus: pectoralis majors, deltoids, triceps, biceps, and abdominal muscles

Intensity Level 1

Perform knee push-ups. Kneel on a cushioned surface with your back straight and your hands on the ground under your shoulders. Bend your elbows 90 degrees and then return to the straight-arm position, or plank position.

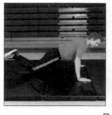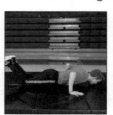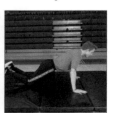

Right-Angle Push-ups: Intensity Level 1

Intensity Level 2

Lie on your stomach. Place your hands under your shoulders. Straighten your arms to lift up your body. Make sure that your back and legs are straight from head to toe. Lower your body by bending your elbows as far as you can without exceeding 90. Straighten your arms to lift your body back up to the plank position, keeping your back and legs straight.

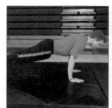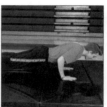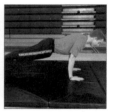

Right-Angle Push-ups: Intensity Level 2

Intensity Level 3

Lie on your stomach. Place your hands under your shoulders. Straighten your arms to lift up your body. Make sure that your back and legs are straight from head to toe. Lower your body by bending your elbows 90 degrees. Straighten your arms to lift your body back up to the plank position, keeping your back and legs straight.

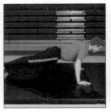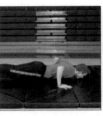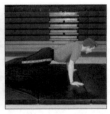

Right-Angle Push-ups: Intensity Level 3

ALTERNATE 6 INCHES

muscle focus: abdominal muscles

Intensity Level 1

Lie on your back on a cushioned surface. Pull 1 knee toward your chest. Extend your other leg straight out in front of you and parallel to the floor. Hold your extended leg 6 to 10 inches above the ground for 3 seconds. Switch legs.

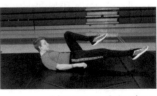

Alternate 6 inches: Intensity Level 1

Intensity Level 2

Lie on your back on a cushioned surface. Extend 1 leg up toward the ceiling with your knee bent. Extend your other leg straight out in front of you and parallel to the floor. Hold your extended leg 6 to 10 inches above the ground for 6 seconds. Switch legs.

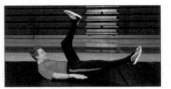

Alternate 6 inches: Intensity Level 2

Intensity Level 3

Lie on your back on a cushioned surface. Extend 1 leg straight up toward the ceiling. Extend your other leg straight out in front of you and parallel to the floor. Hold your extended leg 6 inches above the ground for 6 seconds. Switch legs.

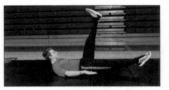

Alternate 6 inches: Intensity Level 3

SQUATS

muscle focus: glutei maximi, hamstrings, and quadriceps

Intensity Level 1

Stand with your legs shoulder-width apart and your hands on your hips. Lower your body by bending your knees and hips as low as you comfortably can. Do not lower your hips below knee level.

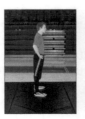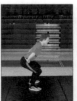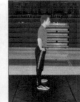

Squats: Intensity Level 1

Intensity Level 2

Stand with your legs shoulder-width apart and your arms extended out in front of you at shoulder height. With your legs apart, lower your body by bending your knees and hips until your hips are even with your knees.

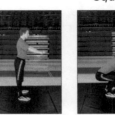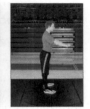

Squats: Intensity Level 2

Intensity Level 3

Perform ¼-squat jumps. Standing with your legs shoulder-width apart, lower your body by bending your knees and hips until your hips are even with your knees. Jump to the right, making a quarter turn and landing gently in a squat position. Continue until you are back to the starting position. Repeat the exercise to the left.

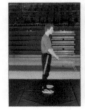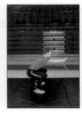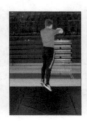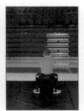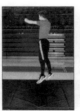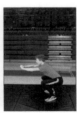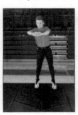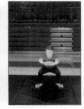

Squats: Intensity Level 3

TRICEPS PUSH-UPS (NARROW PUSH-UPS)

muscle focus: pectoralis majors, pectoralis minors, deltoids, triceps, biceps, and abdominal muscles

Intensity Level 1

Perform knee push-ups. Kneel on a cushioned surface with your back straight and your hands on the ground inside your shoulders. Bend your elbows 90 degrees and return to straight arms.

Intensity Level 2

Lie on your stomach. Place your hands on the floor close to your body at chest level. Lift your body up with your triceps until you return to the straight-arm position. Make sure that your back and legs are straight from head to toe. Lower your body by bending your elbows as far as you can without exceeding 90 degrees. Return to the straight-arm position.

Intensity Level 3

Lie on your stomach. Place your hands on the floor close to your body at chest level. Lift your body up with your triceps until you return to the straight-arm position. Make sure that your back and legs are straight from head to toe. Lower your body by bending your elbows 90 degrees. Return to the straight-arm position.

SIT-UPS

muscle focus: abdominal muscles

Intensity Level 1

Perform fitness curl-ups. Lie on a cushioned surface with your knees flexed and your feet about 12 inches from your buttocks. With your arms at your sides, slide your fingertips 3 to 4 inches forward along the ground, simultaneously lifting your head and shoulders off the ground. Slowly lower your head and shoulders back to the ground.

Intensity Level 2

Perform sit-ups. Lie on a cushioned surface with your knees flexed and your feet about 12 inches from your buttocks. A partner may hold your feet. Cross your arms, placing your hands on opposite shoulders and holding your elbows close to your chest. Raise your body until your elbows touch your thighs; then, lower your body until your shoulder blades touch the ground.

Intensity Level 3

Perform sit-ups. Lie on a cushioned surface with your knees flexed and your feet about 12 inches from your buttocks. Cross your arms, placing your hands on opposite shoulders and holding your elbows close to your chest. Raise your body until your elbows touch your thighs; then, lower your body until your shoulder blades touch the ground.

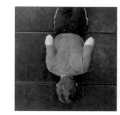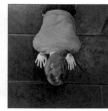

Triceps push-ups

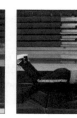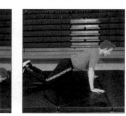

Triceps push-ups: Intensity Level 1

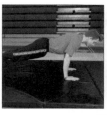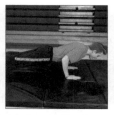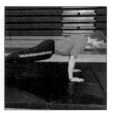

Right-Angle Push-ups: Intensity Level 2

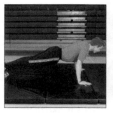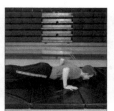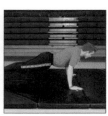

Right-Angle Push-ups: Intensity Level 3

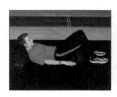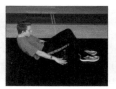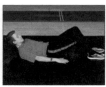

Sit-ups: Intensity Level 1

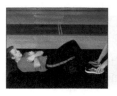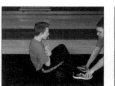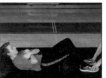

Sit-ups: Intensity Level 2

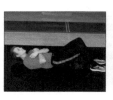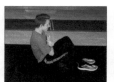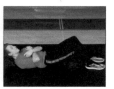

Sit-ups: Intensity Level 3

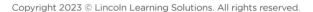

STEP-BACK LUNGES

muscle focus: glutei maximi, hamstrings, and quadriceps

Intensity Level 1

Perform alternate step-back lunges. Start by standing with your feet together and your hands on your hips. Step back with 1 foot and lower your knee as low as you comfortably can. Go back to the starting position and repeat this with your other leg.

Intensity Level 2

Perform alternate step-back lunges with high arms. Start by standing with your feet together and your arms extended straight above your head. Step back with 1 foot and lower your knee as far as you comfortably can. Return to the starting position and repeat this with your other leg.

Intensity Level 3

Start by standing with your feet together. Step back with your right foot and lower your knee as far as you comfortably can. Return to the starting position and continue lunging back with your right foot until you have completed the repetitions. Next, step back with your left foot until you complete the repetitions. Your hands may remain on your hips or remain extended.

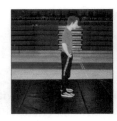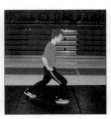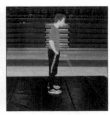

Step-back lunges: Intensity Level 1

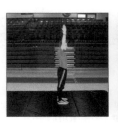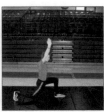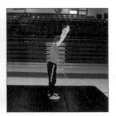

Step-back lunges: Intensity Level 2

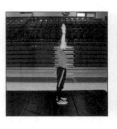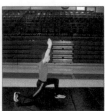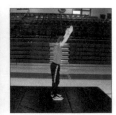

Step-back lunges: Intensity Level 3

WIDE PUSH-UPS

muscle focus: pectoralis majors, deltoids, triceps, biceps, and abdominal muscles

Intensity Level 1

Kneel on a cushioned surface with your back straight and your hands on the ground outside your shoulders. Bend your elbows 90 degrees. Return to the straight-arm position.

Intensity Level 2

Lie on your stomach. Place your hands outside your shoulders. Lift your body up to a straight-arm position. Make sure that your back and legs are straight from head to toe. Lower your body by bending your elbows as far as you can without exceeding 90 degrees. Return to the straight-arm position.

Intensity Level 3

Lie on your stomach. Place your hands outside your shoulders. Lift your body up to a straight-arm position. Make sure that your back and legs are straight from head to toe. Lower your body by bending your elbows 90 degrees. Return to the straight-arm position.

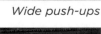

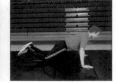

Wide push-ups

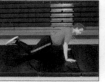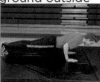

Wide push-ups: Intensity Level 1

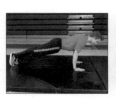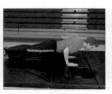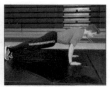

Wide push-ups: Intensity Level 2

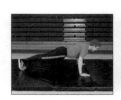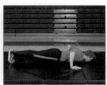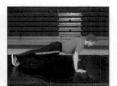

Wide push-ups: Intensity Level 3

Have a trusted adult or friend evaluate you for correct form for the previous exercises. Did you respond positively to the feedback?

Reciprocate and evaluate your friend. Were you able to provide feedback in a positive manner?

How to Use Your Body Weight in a Strength-Training Workout

- Warm up before your workout. Cool down after your workout.
- Choose the appropriate level of intensity for you.
- Perform each exercise 2 to 3 days per week.
- Begin with 1 set of 10 repetitions of each exercise. Increase sets and repetitions when the exercise becomes easy for you.
- Your goal should be to reach 3 sets of 15 repetitions of each exercise.

Write down an excuse that you have used to avoid strength training and how you overcame or will overcome that obstacle.

My Excuse for Not Exercising	What I Did to Overcome That Excuse

RESEARCH INTEGRATION

Research and participate in yoga, Pilates, or tai chi as an alternative way to improve strength and flexibility and to reduce stress. You can enroll in a class or follow a workout from a DVD or app.

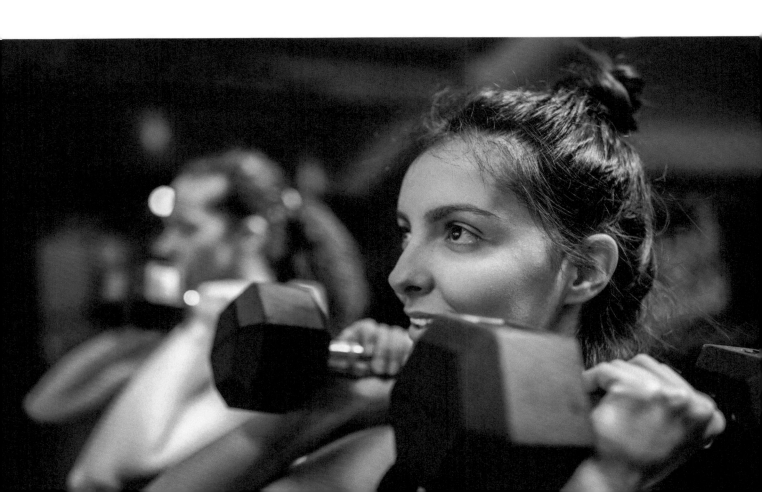

RESISTANCE EXERCISE: FITNESS BALL

Including a fitness ball (or exercise ball) in your exercise routine is a fun, efficient way to improve muscular strength, muscular endurance, flexibility, and balance. Your core muscles work to balance on an unstable ball while exercising a variety of muscle groups.

 CAUTION: Do not overinflate the ball.

FITNESS BALL EXERCISES

TIPS FOR USING A FITNESS BALL

- Exercises done on a firmer ball are more challenging.
- A beginner should start with a slightly-deflated ball.
- When you are seated on the ball, your feet should be flat on the floor.

Practice each of the following exercises, concentrating on proper form, prior to engaging in a workout.

BASIC ROLLOUTS

muscle focus: abdominal muscles

- Sit perfectly upright on the ball with your arms behind your head.
- Sit perfectly upright on the ball with your arms behind your head.
- Walk your feet out slowly.
- Holding your head still, tighten your abdominal muscles as you continue to walk your feet out. Keep your buttocks up as your feet leave the ball.
- Once the ball has reached your shoulders, walk your feet back to the starting position.
- Keep your body parallel to the ground during this exercise.

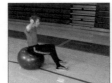
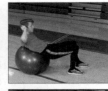
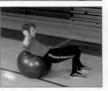
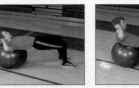
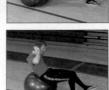
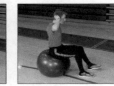

Basic rollouts

SIT-UPS

muscle focus: abdominal muscles

- Lie on your back on the ball. The middle of your back should be on the ball. Place your hands behind your head.
- Keep your elbows flat and in line with your head as you raise your upper body and back off the ball. You should end up almost in a sitting position.
- Lower your body slowly back to the starting position.

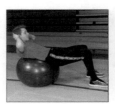
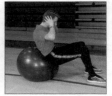

Sit-ups

PLANKS

muscle focus: abdominal muscles

- Place the ball on a flat surface on the ground. Place your forearms on the ball.

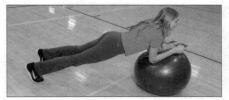

Planks

- Extend your legs straight out behind you and place them shoulder-width apart with your toes on the ground.
- Push yourself up on the ball so that your chest is not resting on your forearms. Only your forearms should be on the ball.
- Hold this position for 30 seconds.

LEG EXTENSIONS

muscle focus: quadriceps, hamstrings, and glutes

- Sit on the ball with both feet firmly on the ground.
- Lift your right leg so that your calf is parallel to the ground.
- Lower your right leg slowly back to the starting position.
- Lift your left leg so that your calf is parallel to the ground.
- Lower your left leg slowly back to the starting position.
- Continue to alternate legs until the exercise is complete.

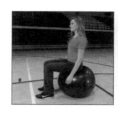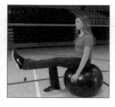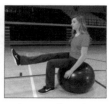

Leg extensions

LEG RAISES

muscle focus: abdominal muscles, quadriceps, hamstrings, and glutes

- Lie flat on your back on the ground, squeezing the middle of the ball tightly between your feet and ankles.
- From this position, keep your upper back and shoulders on the ground and slowly raise your legs about 6 inches off the ground.
- Bring the ball slowly down without resting it on the ground.

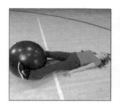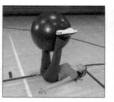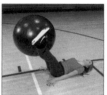

Leg raises

Have a trusted adult or friend evaluate you for correct form for the previous exercises. Did you respond positively to the feedback?

Reciprocate and evaluate your friend. Were you able to provide feedback in a positive manner?

The following is a suggested use of the fitness ball in a strength-building workout. Exercise to your level of fitness.

- Warm up and cool down.
- Perform each exercise 2 to 3 days per week.
- For the basic rollouts, sit-ups, planks, leg extensions, and leg raises, begin with 1 set of 10 repetitions. Increase sets and the number of repetitions when the current number is easy for you to complete. Hold each plank for 20 to 30 seconds.
- For the basic rollouts, sit-ups, planks, leg extensions, and leg raises, your goal should be to reach 3 sets of 10 to 15 repetitions. Your goal for each plank should be to hold it for 30 to 60 seconds.

RESEARCH INTEGRATION

Research the benefits of using an exercise ball as a replacement for a desk chair.

CROSS-TRAINING CARDIOVASCULAR AND STRENGTH CIRCUIT

For a combination cardiovascular and strength workout, you can do a cross-training circuit. This cross-training circuit alternates strength exercises with aerobic movements. Cross-training saves time by giving you 1 workout that has both strength and aerobic benefits. It is important for you to set your own goals based on your ability level and determine your intensity and duration based on your individual target heart rate zone.

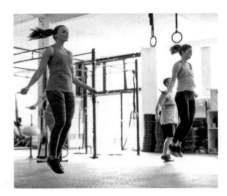

The purpose of this lesson is to encourage you to create and implement a cross-training circuit workout. The workout would be included in the recommended 60 minutes of daily physical activity and would count as both an aerobic and strength workout. **The Cardiovascular Endurance section of this manual includes the target heart rate zone formula and the Borg Rating of Perceived Exertion Scale to help you to determine if you are exercising for heart health.** You can also use available technology to monitor your pulse rate and workout intensity.

 CAUTION: Do not overinflate the ball.

CROSS-TRAINING CIRCUIT WORKOUT: CARDIOVASCULAR, STRENGTH, AND FLEXIBILITY

Review the following example and use the information to establish a workout regimen that fits into your schedule. Adhere to the FITT principle (frequency, intensity, time, and type of exercise). This workout requires a jump rope and a fitness ball. You should have a mat or cushioned surface for sit-ups and push-ups.

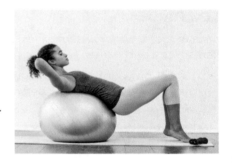

SAMPLE CROSS-TRAINING CIRCUIT WORKOUT

Build cardiovascular endurance, strength, and flexibility in a cross-training circuit workout using exercises from the appropriate sections of your PE Manual: Cardiovascular Endurance, Muscle Strength, Muscle Endurance, and Flexibility. Review the 7th-grade Aerobics, 8th-grade Jump Rope, 8th-grade Strength Training, and 8th-grade Fitness Ball sections in your PE Manual to practice correct forms for the skills.

Warm-up: Perform 5 to 10 minutes of light cardio to increase your heart rate, breathing rate, and body temperature. Do some dynamic stretches to increase flexibility.

Perform each exercise for 30 seconds. Rest and hydrate when necessary.

1. jumping jacks
2. sit-ups
3. high knees
4. fitness ball leg extensions
5. jump rope
6. right-angle push-ups
7. burpees
8. fitness ball plank
9. jog in place
10. squats
11. jump rope
12. triceps push-ups (narrow push-ups)
13. ¼-squat jumps
14. fitness ball sit-ups
15. knee tucks
16. forward lunges
17. jump rope
18. wide push-ups

Repeat for an 18-minute workout.

Cool-down: Walk slowly until your heart rate, breathing rate, and body temperature have returned to baseline. Do some static stretches to increase flexibility.

Use the cross-training information to create your personal circuit workout.

RATE YOUR ENJOYMENT OF A CROSS-TRAINING CIRCUIT

On a scale from 1 to 4, where 1 is not enjoyable and 4 is very enjoyable, rate this activity.

1	It was not enjoyable, and I will not participate again.
2	It was not enjoyable, but I will participate again for exercise.
3	It was enjoyable, and I will complete a cross-training circuit again.
4	It was very enjoyable, and I will create more cross-training routines outside of PE class.

Explain to a trusted adult or friend how you can make your cross-training workout more enjoyable.

🖥 RESEARCH INTEGRATION

Review the appropriate sections in your manual to practice the correct forms for basic locomotor skills before creating your movement sequence.

♥ HEALTH INTEGRATION

Use available technology to monitor your pulse rate and workout intensity. Apply the results to your overall fitness plan.

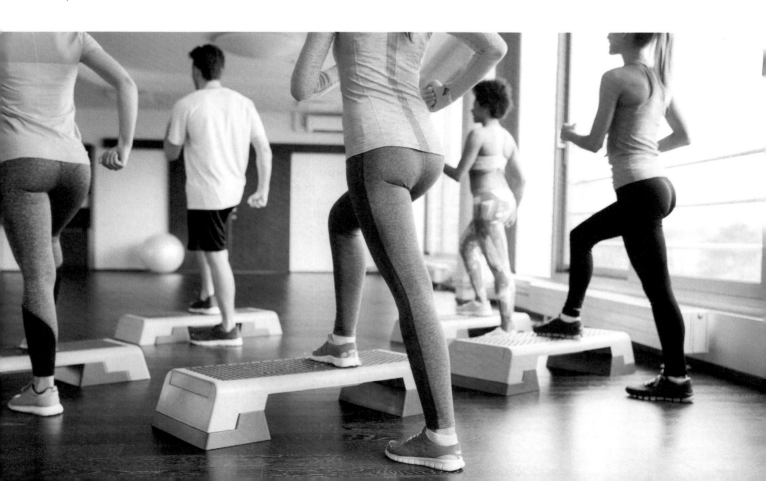

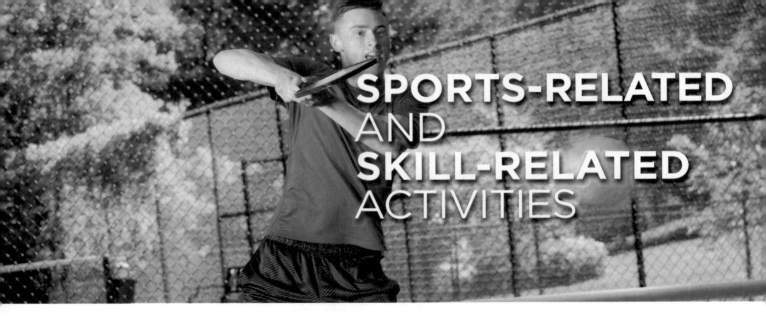

SPORTS-RELATED AND SKILL-RELATED ACTIVITIES

FITNESS TIP: Prior to beginning your physical education activities, read the following safety information that applies to every lesson, review the timeline, and review the assessment rubric.

SAFETY ALERT: Before you exercise, make sure that you are properly warmed up and have enough room to perform each activity. Wear proper equipment and follow activity-specific safety rules. Stay hydrated and take breaks as needed. Exercise only if you are healthy, and always exercise at your own pace. If an exercise starts to hurt, if you feel dizzy, or if you feel light-headed, stop the exercise completely and get help. Upon completion of any workout, cool down and stretch.

TIMELINE

Review all of the activity information before beginning. Use the scoring rubrics as assessment tools. You may ask a trusted adult or friend to observe your performance and provide feedback. Progress according to your skill level. The time that it takes you to complete a module will depend on your personal progress.

Practice and assess the first skill until competent.

Apply skills in a game situation.

Continue to progress until you have practiced and assessed each skill until competent.

ASSESSMENT RUBRIC

You will find a rubric assessment tool following some of the basic skills. Use this tool to evaluate and score your progress in learning the elements of a new skill.

SKILL	PROGRESSING	COMPETENT	PROFICIENT
skill 1	1 or 2 of the elements	3 or 4 out of 5 elements	all elements met

FLOOR HOCKEY

Floor hockey is played by 2 opposing teams each made up of 6 players on a rectangular court. A point is scored when the puck or hockey ball goes into a goal. It is a fast, energetic sport that does not permit physical contact with other players. Playing floor hockey helps you develop hand-eye coordination, balance, agility, and physical fitness. Many people choose to complete aerobic workouts by playing in fun pick-up games like floor hockey.

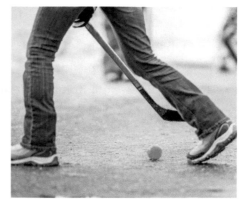

The purpose of this lesson is for you to participate in aerobic exercise and in skill-building activities. Game participation will depend upon the availability of a facility and players. When you are playing floor hockey, be sure to follow game rules, communicate with teammates in a positive and effective manner, and exhibit appropriate behavior with your team and the opposing team.

⚠️ **CAUTION: Keep 2 hands on the hockey stick. Keep the stick below waist level. Do not body check or otherwise contact anyone.**

FLOOR HOCKEY SKILLS

GRIP

- Place your dominant hand lower on the hockey stick and your non-dominant hand near the top of the stick. Now, switch hands so that your non-dominant hand is lower on the stick and your dominant hand is near the top of the stick. You may use the hand position that is most comfortable for you.

- Face your palms up like you are shaking hands with someone. Place your hands 6 to 8 inches apart on the stick. Bend your elbows and keep them loose. Let your arms hang loose and ready to play.

- Always keep the tip of the stick below your waist.

- Your bottom hand is the pivot, and your top hand is the control.

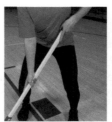
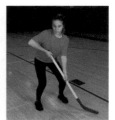
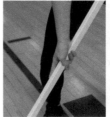
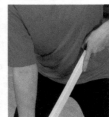

STICKHANDLING

- Stay in place and move the puck from side to side or from front to back.

SIDE TO SIDE

- Your feet should be slightly wider than shoulder-width apart.

- Move the puck from right to left using both sides of the stick to softly tap the puck.

- Keep the blade of the stick on the floor.

- The puck should remain slightly in front of your feet.

- Keep your head up.

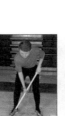
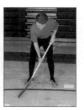
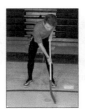
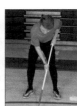

SKILL	PROGRESSING	COMPETENT	PROFICIENT
side to side	1 or 2 of the elements	3 or 4 out of 5 elements	all elements met

FRONT TO BACK

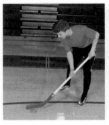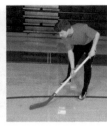

- Your feet should be staggered so that 1 is forward and 1 is back.
- Push the puck forward with the front of the blade (the side facing away from you) and then backward with the back of the blade using soft taps and not pushing the puck beyond your toes.
- Keep the blade on the floor.
- Transfer your weight from your front foot to your back foot.
- Keep your head up.
- Switch your feet so that the other foot is forward and repeat the exercise.

SKILL	PROGRESSING	COMPETENT	PROFICIENT
front to back	1 or 2 of the elements	3 or 4 out of 5 elements	all elements met

DRIBBLING ON THE MOVE

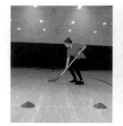

- The puck should stay in contact with the stick blade on 1 side only.
- Practice moving the puck on both the right and left sides of the stick.
- Move the puck forward with short taps or pushes.
- Tilt the stick blade slightly over the puck for better control.
- Keep the puck in the middle of the blade.
- Hold your head up as you move.
- To switch direction, move the puck in front of you rather than to the side. Use short taps while pushing the puck from side to side in the middle of the blade.

SKILL	PROGRESSING	COMPETENT	PROFICIENT
dribbling on the move	1, 2, or 3 of the elements	4 or 5 out of 6 elements	all elements met

SHOOTING THE PUCK

There are 2 types of shots: wrist shots and slap shots. Wrist shots are used for shorter distances and quick execution, while slap shots are used for moderate to long distances.

WRIST SHOT

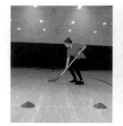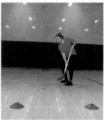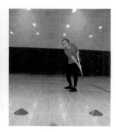

- Touch the puck with the stick blade before you shoot the puck.
- Look toward the target.
- When you are shooting, move your lower hand down the stick for better control.
- Follow through your shot with the stick ending no higher than your hips.

SKILL	PROGRESSING	COMPETENT	PROFICIENT
wrist shot	1 or 2 of the elements	3 out of 4 elements	all elements met

SLAP SHOT

- When you are approaching the puck, move your lower hand slightly down the stick for better control.

- Keep your eyes on the puck.

- Swing the stick behind you to about waist level and in line with the target.

- Swing the stick quickly forward and hit through the puck.

- Follow through your shot with the stick ending no higher than your hips. Finish with all your weight on your front foot.

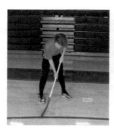
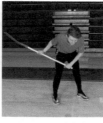
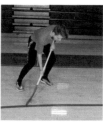
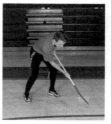
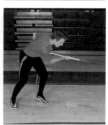

SKILL	PROGRESSING	COMPETENT	PROFICIENT
slap shot	1 or 2 of the elements	3 or 4 out of 5 elements	all elements met

PASSING AND RECEIVING THE PUCK

PASSING

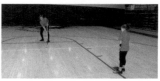

Keep the stick blade upright.

Use your lower hand to execute a smooth, sweeping motion.

Do not raise the stick above your waist during the backswing or forward swing.

Pass slightly ahead of your receiver on their stick side. This is called a lead pass.

Aim the puck to where the receiver will be able to intercept it.

SKILL	PROGRESSING	COMPETENT	PROFICIENT
passing	1 or 2 of the elements	3 or 4 out of 5 elements	all elements met

RECEIVING

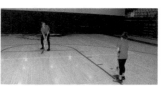

Track the puck with your eyes.

Move into position to receive the puck.

Intercept the puck by placing your stick blade over the puck to trap it.

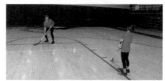

Cushion the pass by allowing the stick blade to give during impact (let the stick move slightly backward to keep control of the puck).

SKILL	PROGRESSING	COMPETENT	PROFICIENT
receiving	1 or 2 of the elements	3 out of 4 elements	all elements met

PRACTICE THE SKILLS

Practice each skill until you are competent.

- Shoot a stationary puck at a wall or other target. Use the wrist shot with forehand and backhand shooting.

- Dribble and shoot toward a target using a forehand and backhand wrist shot.

- Shoot a stationary puck at a wall or other target using the slap shot.

- Pass with a partner while both of you are stationary. Pass the puck quickly back and forth. Trap the puck with the blade of the stick and pass it immediately back to your partner.
- While standing still, pass the puck to your partner while your partner is on the move. Your partner should stop, trap the puck, and pass it back to you. Repeat this 5 times and switch roles.
- Pass the puck back and forth while you and your partner are moving forward. Try short passes and long passes.

OFFENSIVE AND DEFENSIVE SKILLS

Quick, fast, agile footwork is an essential component of a floor hockey game. Practice footwork skills to improve your offensive and defensive play.

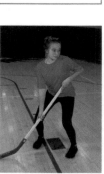

OFFENSIVE SKILLS

FAKE

The purpose of the fake is to lead your opponent in a different direction.

- Look in 1 direction, and then pass or move in another direction.
- Stay on the balls of your feet.
- Move quickly.

SKILL	PROGRESSING	COMPETENT	PROFICIENT
fake	1 of the elements	2 out of 3 elements	all elements

GIVE AND GO

The purpose of the give and go in a hockey game is to for you to pass the puck to a teammate and to quickly relocate so that you can receive a pass.

- Pass the puck to a teammate.
- Move quickly to relocate and support your offense.
- Indicate (call out) that you are ready and open to receive the puck.
- Receive the puck.

SKILL	PROGRESSING	COMPETENT	PROFICIENT
give and go	1 or 2 of the elements	3 out of 4 elements	all elements

DEFENSIVE SKILLS

READY POSITION FOR DEFENSE

The purpose of the ready position is to keep you on the balls of your feet and ready to react as appropriate.

- Bending your knees, stand with your feet shoulder-width apart.
- Keep your head up and your weight on the balls of your feet.
- Hold your hockey stick with both hands, letting the edge of the stick rest on the floor.

SKILL	PROGRESSING	COMPETENT	PROFICIENT
ready position	1 of the elements	2 out of 3 elements	all elements met

DEFENSIVE SLIDES

The purpose of defensive slides in floor hockey is to keep up with your opponent and to legally take the puck or legally disrupt the opponent's pass or shot.

- Place your weight on the balls of your feet.
- Slide to the side or diagonally backward with quick steps.
- Do not cross your feet.
- Keep your knees bent.
- Face your hips toward your opponent.
- Hold your stick with both hands in front of you and keep the tip of the blade near the floor.
- Anticipate and react quickly to your opponent's movements.

SKILL	PROGRESSING	COMPETENT	PROFICIENT
defensive slides	1, 2, or 3 of the elements	4, 5, or 6 out of 7 elements	all elements met

PRACTICE OFFENSIVE AND DEFENSIVE SKILLS

Practice each skill until you are competent.

- Practice the **give and go** with a partner and a defender. Pass the puck, quickly relocate, and then receive the pass, avoiding the defender.
- Practice the **fake** independently. Set up a cone as a decoy. Fake the pass toward the cone and then pass to your partner until you feel comfortable with the movement.
- Practice the **fake** with a partner defending you. Dribble, fake, and move in another direction to get around the defensive player. Do this until you feel comfortable with the fake.
- Practice the **defensive slide** with a partner. As your partner dribbles, defensive slide to try to prevent them from making a successful pass or shot. Do this until you feel comfortable with the defensive slide.

FACING OFF

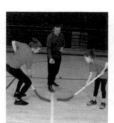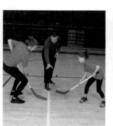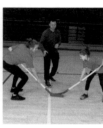

A face-off starts a hockey game. It is also used to restart the game after each point is scored.

- Stand facing your opponent in the center of the court, about a stick-length apart. Face the goal your team is trying to score in. Place the stick blades on the floor so they are almost touching. Slide your lower hand down the shaft of your stick for more power and control.
- The referee will drop the puck between you and your opponent. Once the puck hits the floor, try to gain control of the puck.

PLAYING THE GAME

- You should play in a large gym or on a rectangular court. Play begins in the center of the court. You may play off the walls, but tape off the goalie area for safety.
- Each goal that is scored is worth 1 point.
- A floor hockey team consists of 1 goalie, 2 defensive backs, and 3 forwards.
- A face-off between the 2 center forwards starts the game and restarts it after a goal is scored. After every goal, the center forward should switch with 1 of the other forwards.
- Play an even number of minutes for halves with a 2-minute halftime to switch sides of the court. If there are extra players, swap so that everyone gets a chance to play.

- A goalie may use their hands, stick, or feet to stop the puck inside their own goal area. They must release the puck within 3 seconds of catching it. A goalie cannot throw or shoot the puck toward their opponent's goal.
- Defensive players cannot cross the center line.
- Center forwards may play the entire floor.
- Wing forwards may play from their start position and go forward, staying out of the back-court area.
- If the puck gets trapped under bleachers or against a wall, a face-off takes place at the nearest X spot (the spot away from the bleachers or walls often marked with tape) or the game can be restarted close to where the puck was lost.
- If any of the fouls listed below are made, the puck will be given to the opposite team at the place where the foul occurred. The opposite team is then allowed a penalty shot, which means that the team gets a free shot where the foul was made. Defensive players must stay 15 feet away when the puck is put back into play.
    - touching the puck with your hands
    - swinging the stick above your shoulders
    - having a player other than the goalie inside the goalie box
    - having guards and forwards out of position
    - stepping on, holding, or lying on the puck
- If any of the personal fouls listed below are made, the player who made the foul will be given a 2-minute penalty.
    - tripping someone with a stick or foot
    - pushing or body checking
    - checking someone with a stick
    - using bad language

Insert hockey court from Getty images # 1008822910

Prior to playing a pick-up game, establish and review the game rules so that all participants understand them. If problems arise, while self-officiating, work as a group to solve them in a positive and effective manner. Appreciate different players' abilities. Consider the number of participants, the facility, the amount of equipment, and other variables to establish game rules for your personal situation. An example of a rule that you may want to implement is to switch positions after a certain period of time so that everyone can play both offense and defense.

Below are our game rules for safety and fairness.
1.
2.
3.
4.
5.

RATE YOUR ENJOYMENT OF FLOOR HOCKEY

On a scale from 1 to 4, where 1 is not enjoyable and 4 is very enjoyable, rate this activity.

1	It was not enjoyable, and I will not participate again.
2	It was not enjoyable, but I will participate again for exercise.
3	It was enjoyable, and I will play again.
4	It was very enjoyable, and I will initiate future games.

 RESEARCH INTEGRATION

Research the official rules and regulations of ice hockey and compare them to the rules for floor hockey presented in this lesson.

HEALTH INTEGRATION

Count your pulse during and after playing floor hockey to determine if you are exercising in your personal target heart rate zone. Predict and then compare the difference between your heart rate after playing in the goalie position and your heart rate after playing in a running position. Apply your results to your overall fitness plan.

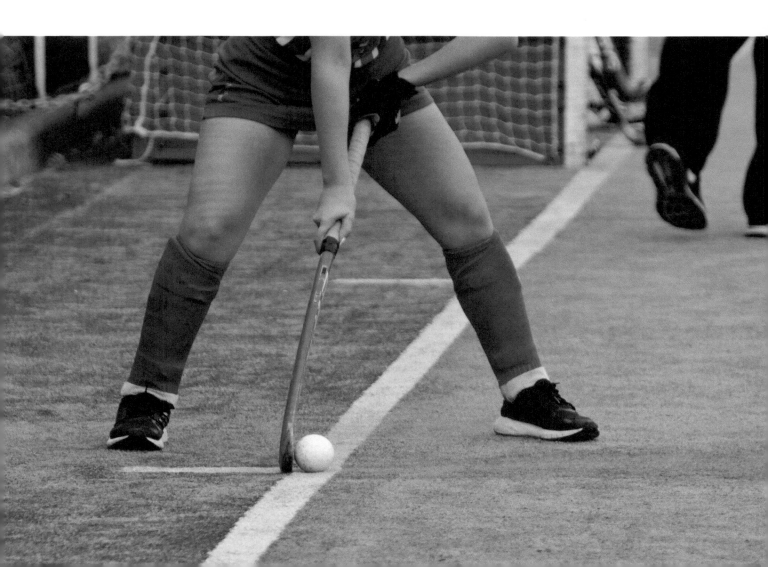

JUGGLING

Juggling improves focus and coordination, and it increases the range of motion in your arms and shoulders. Juggling requires intense concentration, which can help relieve stress because it requires your mind to stay focused on the task. Juggling is a workout that you can take almost anywhere and that requires little space. Juggling is unique and adds variety to your 60 minutes of daily activity and regular aerobic workouts.

The purpose of this lesson is for you to participate in juggling in and outside of PE class.

JUGGLING PROGRESSIONS

1-CUBE JUGGLE

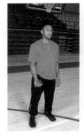 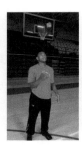 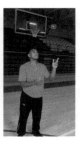

- Hold 1 juggling cube in your dominant hand.
- Throw the cube in an arc pattern from your dominant hand to your non-dominant hand. Do not throw the cube high; rather, throw it at eye level.
- Throw the cube at eye level in an arc pattern from your non-dominant hand back to your dominant hand.
- Continue tossing the cube from 1 hand to the other until it feels comfortable. Make sure that you throw in an arc pattern, not a circle.

SKILL	PROGRESSING	COMPETENT	PROFICIENT
1 cube juggling	1 or 2 of the elements	3 out of 4 elements	all elements met

2-CUBE JUGGLE

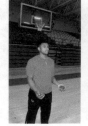 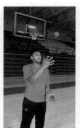 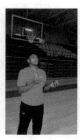 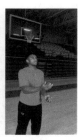

Do not toss the cubes at the same time. Wait for 1 cube to reach eye level before tossing the other cube. It may help to say to yourself, "Toss, toss, catch, catch."

- Hold a cube in each hand.
- Toss 1 cube in an arc pattern from your dominant hand to your non-dominant hand.
- After the cube tossed from your dominant hand has reached eye level, toss the cube in your non-dominant hand in an arc pattern to your dominant hand.
- Catch the cube tossed from your dominant hand with your non-dominant hand. Then, catch the cube tossed from your non-dominant hand with your dominant hand.

SKILL	PROGRESSING	COMPETENT	PROFICIENT
2-cube juggle	1 or 2 of the elements	3 out of 4 elements	all elements met

Challenge: Toss 2 cubes, beginning by tossing with your non-dominant hand first.

3-CUBE JUGGLE

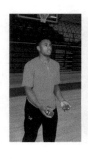 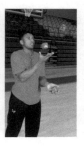

- Place 2 cubes in your dominant hand and 1 cube in your non-dominant hand.
- Toss the first cube from your dominant hand in an arc pattern to your non-dominant hand.
- After the cube tossed from your dominant hand has reached eye level, toss the cube in your non-dominant hand in an arc pattern to your dominant hand.

- Catch the first cube tossed from your dominant hand with your non-dominant hand.
- After the cube tossed from your non-dominant hand has reached eye level, toss the second cube in your dominant hand in an arc pattern to your non-dominant hand.
- Catch the cube tossed from your non-dominant hand with your dominant hand. Then, catch the second cube tossed from your dominant hand with your non-dominant hand.

SKILL	PROGRESSING	COMPETENT	PROFICIENT
3-cube juggle	1, 2, or 3 of the elements	4 or 5 out of 6 elements	all elements met

After you are proficient in juggling the cubes, start the exercises from the beginning and use the juggling balls.

RATE YOUR ENJOYMENT OF JUGGLING

On a scale from 1 to 4, where 1 is not enjoyable and 4 is very enjoyable, rate this activity.

1	It was not enjoyable, and I will not participate again.
2	It was not enjoyable, but I will participate again for exercise.
3	It was enjoyable, and I will juggle again.
4	It was very enjoyable, and I will include juggling in my regular orkout schedule.

RESEARCH INTEGRATION

1. Research the origin of juggling.
2. Research how to juggle with a partner.

HEALTH INTEGRATION

Count your heart rate during and after juggling to determine if you are exercising in your personal target heart rate zone. Apply the results to your overall fitness plan.

PICKLEBALL

Pickleball is a popular game that is enjoyed by players of all ages. Pickleball is a paddle sport that combines elements of badminton, tennis, and table tennis. It is played with a paddle, a pickleball ball, and a low net on a hard court. This striking activity helps you develop concentration, hand-eye coordination, footwork, and fitness.

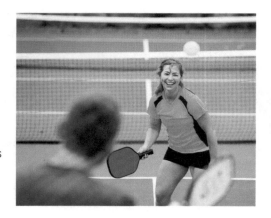

The purpose of this lesson is for you to participate in aerobic exercise and in skill-building activities. Game participation will depend upon the availability of a facility and players. When you are playing pickleball, be sure to follow game rules, communicate with teammates in a positive and effective manner, and exhibit appropriate behavior with your team and the opposing team.

⚠️ **CAUTION: Make sure that nobody is close to you before you swing the paddle. Do not walk into the path of another person who is swinging a paddle.**

PICKLEBALL SKILLS

STROKES

READY POSITION

- Wait for the ball, keeping your paddle in front of the middle of your chest. This way, you are ready to return the ball from wherever it goes.
- Bend your knees and stand with your feet shoulder-width apart.
- Keep your head up and your weight on the balls of your feet.
- Hold the paddle in your dominant hand.

HANDSHAKE GRIP

- Hold the paddle in your dominant hand away from your body and at waist height.
- Placing the head of the paddle vertical to the ground, point the handle toward your belly button.

UNDERHAND STROKE

- Hold the paddle so that the head is facing the ground and is positioned under the ball.
- Flick your wrist to hit the ball with the center of the paddle.
- Rotate your forearm so that it faces upward on contact.
- Follow through to your target.

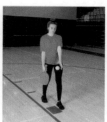
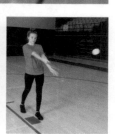

SKILL	PROGRESSING	COMPETENT	PROFICIENT
underhand stroke	1 or 2 of the elements	3 out of 4 elements	all elements met

OVERHAND STROKE

- Bend your elbow slightly and position the paddle under the ball.
- Flick your wrist to hit the ball with the center of the paddle.
- Extend your arm when you make contact.
- Follow through to your target.

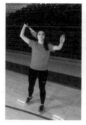 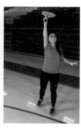 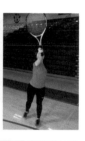

SKILL	PROGRESSING	COMPETENT	PROFICIENT
overhand stroke	1 or 2 of the elements	3 out of 4 elements	all elements met

FOREHAND STROKE

- The paddle should be on the same side of your body as your dominant hand.
- Face the palm of your hand forward.
- Extend your arm and flick your wrist to hit the ball.
- Point the face of the paddle up to get the ball over the net.
- Follow through to your target.

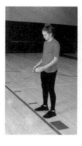 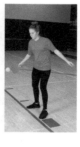 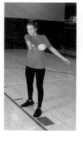 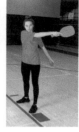

SKILL	PROGRESSING	COMPETENT	PROFICIENT
forehand stroke	1 or 2 of the elements	3 or 4 out of 5 elements	all elements met

BACKHAND STROKE

- Rotate the paddle and extend it across your body.
- Rotate your feet and shoulders in the same direction as the paddle.
- Face the back of your hand (your knuckles) forward.
- Flick your wrist as you hit the ball with the center of the paddle.
- Follow through to your target.

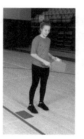 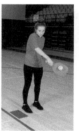 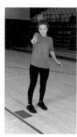

OPTION: 2-HANDED BACKHAND STROKE

- Place your non-dominant hand below your dominant hand.
- Rotate the paddle.
- Rotate your feet and shoulders in the same direction as the paddle.
- Flick your wrists as you hit the ball with the center of the paddle.
- Follow through to your target.

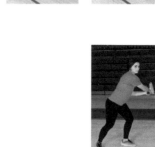

SKILL	PROGRESSING	COMPETENT	PROFICIENT
backhand stroke	1 or 2 of the elements	3 or 4 out of 5 elements	all elements met

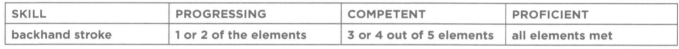

UNDERHAND SERVE

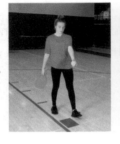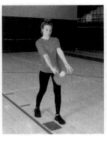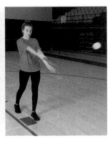

- Hold the paddle in your dominant hand. Hold the ball in your non-dominant hand.
- Hold the head of the paddle down toward the ground.
- Step forward with your non-dominant foot.
- Drop the ball slightly below your waist.
- Hit the ball with the center of the paddle. Flick your wrist as you make contact.
- Follow through to your target.
- Serve successfully 70 percent of the time.

SKILL	PROGRESSING	COMPETENT	PROFICIENT
underhand serve	1, 2, 3, or 4 of the elements	5 or 6 out of 7 elements	all elements met

PRACTICE THE STROKES

- Practice each stroke by hitting the ball against a wall with the paddle.
  - Allow the ball to bounce before striking it.
  - Volley the ball against the wall. This means that you should not allow the ball to bounce off the ground.
- Strike the ball toward the wall using various levels of force.
- Aim and strike the ball to the left of the target.
- Aim and strike the ball to the right of the target.
- Hit the ball back and forth with a partner. How many times can you hit it back and forth?

SHOTS

DINK SHOT

LOB

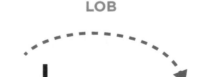

DRIVE

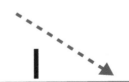

The most effective short-hand shots, or dinks, are those that bounce in front of the no-volley line (the area 7 feet from the net, where volleying is not allowed). Dinks should be short and low.

A lob is high and pushes your opponent to the rear of the court. This slows down the game to give you a chance to get ready for your opponent's shot.

A drive is a hard, fast hit that is difficult to return.

PRACTICE THE SHOTS

Practice the shots independently by bouncing or tossing the ball at the appropriate height for each shot. Practice with a net set up.

- Practice the dink shot forward and crosscourt.
- Practice the lob shot.
- Practice the drive shot.
- Describe a shot and then execute it. Do this for the 3 shots.
- Have a partner toss the ball for you. Practice each shot and then switch roles. Be supportive and encouraging to your partner.

PLAYING A GAME

- Pickleball is a singles game with 2 players or a doubles game with 4 players.

- Start by serving the ball underhand from the right side of the court. Serve diagonally to your opponent on the left. Stand behind the serving line when you start your serve.

  - If a point is scored, the server then serves from the left side of the court. Continue this side-to-side pattern until the serve is lost. In a doubles game, the other teammate then serves. Once the second teammate loses the serve, the opposing team serves.

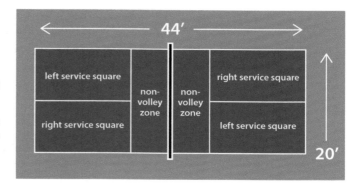

- The ball must land in the opponent's section of the court.

- Your opponent must let the ball bounce once before returning the serve.

- After each team hits the ball once, you may either let the ball bounce once or hit it. This starts the game.

- Points are only scored when a player is serving.

- Games are played to 11 points. A team must win by 2 points.

- Faults include the following.

  - hitting the ball out of bounds

  - serving faults

  - allowing the ball to bounce more than once

  - hitting the ball on the fly in the non-volley zone

  - hitting the ball to the wrong service court

PICKLEBALL OPTIONS

- Play at picnics and group outings.

- Make a net by tying jump ropes together and then tying the jump ropes to the tops of chairs. If there are 2 trees in your playing area, tie the jump ropes to the trees. You may also go to a park with a tennis court and set smaller boundaries on the tennis court.

DEMONSTRATE POSITIVE GAME BEHAVIOR

- Follow the rules.

- Call for a shot, when appropriate, to identify that you are going to hit it. This is for safety and game efficiency.

- Be supportive and encouraging to your teammate.

- Treat your opponents with respect.

SKILL	PROGRESSING	COMPETENT	PROFICIENT
game behavior	1 or 2 of the elements	3 out of 4 elements	all elements met

RATE YOUR ENJOYMENT OF PICKLEBALL

On a scale from 1 to 4, where 1 is not enjoyable and 4 is very enjoyable, rate this activity.

1	It was not enjoyable, and I will not participate again.
2	It was not enjoyable, but I will participate again for exercise.
3	It was enjoyable, and I will play again.
4	It was very enjoyable, and I will initiate future games.

 ## RESEARCH INTEGRATION

Research pickleball's country of origin and who invented the game.

♥ HEALTH INTEGRATION

Count your pulse during and after playing pickleball to determine if you are exercising in your personal target heart rate zone. Apply the results to your overall fitness plan. Many people choose to complete aerobic workouts by playing in casual games with friends.

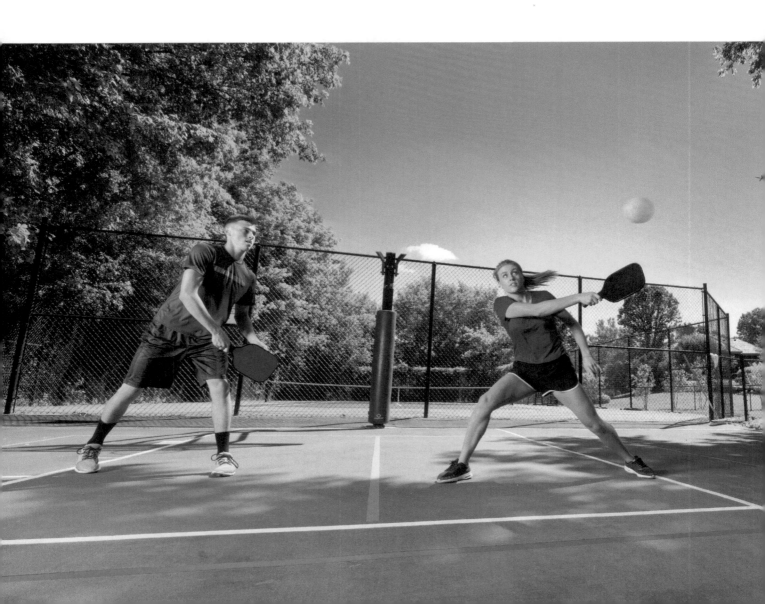

PLAYGROUND BALL GAME

SPEED BALL: INDOOR BASKETBALL VERSION

Speed ball is a game that is played by 2 teams of 7 players and is a combination of basketball, soccer, and team handball. It is played with a playground ball on a basketball court. There are 2 goals at each end of the court—a basketball hoop and a soccer goal placed beneath the hoop. The object of the game is to shoot the ball through the basketball hoop and kick or throw the ball into the soccer goal to score.

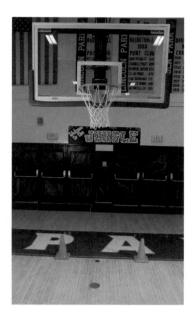

Playing the game utilizes and improves the skill-related components of agility, balance, coordination, speed, power, and reaction. Playing speed ball is an aerobic workout. The game also provides the opportunity to work as a team to develop offensive and defensive strategies as well as the ability to transition quickly between them.

The purpose of this lesson is for you to participate in aerobic exercise and in skill-building activities. Game participation will depend upon the availability of a facility and players. When you are playing speed ball, be sure to follow game rules, communicate with teammates in a positive and effective manner, and exhibit appropriate behavior with your team and the opposing team.

 CAUTION: Do not overinflate the ball.

SPEED BALL SKILLS

Speed ball utilizes skills from basketball, soccer, and team handball. Practicing skills from these 3 sports will enhance your ability to play each of those sports as well as lead to better performance in speed ball. You can find a full description of each of the 3 sports in the 7th-grade section of your PE Manual.

BASKETBALL SKILLS USED IN SPEED BALL: USE A PLAYGROUND BALL

HAND DRIBBLING

- Using your dominant hand, spread your fingers and push the ball down gently toward the ground with your finger pads. Do not slap the ball.

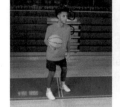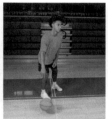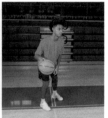

- Let the ball bounce on the ground and come back to your hand. Do not let the ball bounce higher than your waist.

- Flex your wrist and push the ball back to the ground with your finger pads. This is a continuous movement; do not catch the ball after every bounce.

- Dribble with your head up.

- Keep your eyes looking forward, not watching the ball.

- Repeat dribbling the ball with your non-dominant hand.

SKILL	PROGRESSING	COMPETENT	PROFICIENT
right-handed dribble	1 or 2 of the elements	3 or 4 out of 5 elements	all elements met
left-handed dribble	1 or 2 of the elements	3 or 4 out of 5 elements	all elements met

PRACTICE HAND DRIBBLING

- See how many times you can dribble the ball with your dominant hand without losing control of it.
- Push the ball down with different amounts of force to make it bounce at different levels.
- Try pushing the ball with a soft force so that it bounces at a low level.
- Try pushing the ball with a hard force so that it bounces at a high level.
- Dribble with your dominant hand.
- Dribble with your non-dominant hand.
- Dribble from 1 hand to the other.
- Dribble from 1 hand to the other while moving.
- Dribble while moving, increasing and decreasing your speed.
- Dribble while moving and change directions.

BASIC SHOOTING

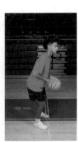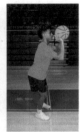
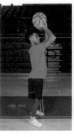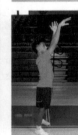

- Stand facing the hoop with your feet shoulder-width apart and your knees slightly bent.
- Place your dominant hand on the back of the ball and bend your wrist. Place your non-dominant hand on the side of the ball.
- Place the ball on the finger pads of your dominant hand.
- Use your non-dominant hand as your guide.
- Position your elbow so that it is behind the ball, not out to the side.
- Look at the target—the front of the rim.
- Push your dominant hand toward the target while straightening your legs to give you more power to shoot.
- Shoot the ball toward the target and follow through with your arm and wrist. Snap your wrist as the ball leaves your hand.
- Remember BEEF.
  - **Balance** the ball in your dominant hand.
  - Place your **elbow** behind the ball, not out to the side.
  - Keep your **eyes** on the target.
  - **Follow** through with a snap of your wrist.

SKILL	PROGRESSING	COMPETENT	PROFICIENT
BEEF elements	1 or 2 of the elements	3 out of 4 elements	all elements

PRACTICE SHOOTING

- Shoot from a variety of spots inside the 3-point line.

TEAM HANDBALL SKILLS USED IN SPEED BALL: USE A PLAYGROUND BALL

OVERHAND PASS

- Grip the ball with your hands.
- Step toward your target and transfer your weight to your front foot.
- Move your arms forward in the direction of your target.
- Snap your wrists.
- Aim and pass to your target by releasing the ball, using the appropriate force to reach your target.

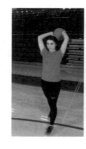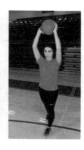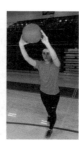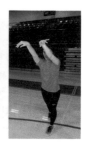

SKILL	PROGRESSING	COMPETENT	PROFICIENT
passing	1 or 2 of the elements	3 or 4 out of 5 elements	all elements met

RECEIVING

- Spread your fingers to catch the ball.
- Catch the ball firmly using only your hands.
- Gain control of the ball.
- Maintain your balance throughout the catch.
- Make the necessary pass or run with the ball after the catch.

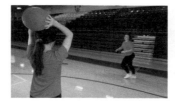

SKILL	PROGRESSING	COMPETENT	PROFICIENT
receiving	1 or 2 of the elements	3 or 4 out of 5 elements	all elements met

RECEIVING WHILE RUNNING

- Keep your eyes on the ball.
- Anticipate the throw. Change your speed and direction to accommodate the throw.
- Use speed and direction to create an opening.
- Catch the majority of throws.

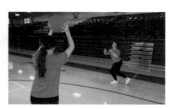

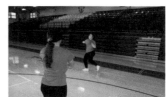

SKILL	PROGRESSING	COMPETENT	PROFICIENT
receiving while running	1 or 2 of the elements	3 out of 4 elements	all elements met

PRACTICE THROWING AND CATCHING

- Throw the ball against a wall and catch it.
- Throw and catch the ball with a partner.

SOCCER SKILLS USED IN SPEED BALL: USE A PLAYGROUND BALL

FOOT DRIBBLING

Use your peripheral vision, or your side vision, to watch the ball as you dribble it. Dribbling is a series of small, controlled touches that you complete in order to move with the ball in your possession. Dribble the ball with the insides and outsides of your feet as well as with the tops of your feet, where your shoelaces lay. Do not dribble the ball with your toes, otherwise, you risk losing control of the ball.

- Start with the ball positioned in front of you on the ground.

- Dribble forward, keeping the ball close—no more than 3 to 5 feet in front of you.

- Move the ball with the insides, outsides, and/or tops of both of your feet.

- Keep your head up.

- Match your speed to your skill.

- Change directions.

SKILL	PROGRESSING	COMPETENT	PROFICIENT
foot dribbling	1, 2, or 3 of the elements	4 or 5 out of 6 elements	all elements

PRACTICE FOOT DRIBBLING

- Practice dribbling by placing discs in various locations around your practice area. As you are dribbling, weave in and out of the discs.

PASSING

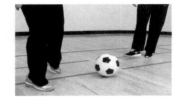

Players pass the ball to each other in order to keep the other team from gaining control of the ball and to progress the ball toward the other team's goal.

- Start with the ball on the ground, next to the inside of your dominant foot.

- Position the inside of your kicking foot behind the middle of the ball.

- Establish your non-kicking foot slightly behind you.

- Swing your kicking leg back, keeping it straight throughout your entire kick.

- Contact the middle of the ball with the inside of your foot. Follow through your kick with your foot and leg.

- Use appropriate force and direction to keep your pass on target.

SKILL	PROGRESSING	COMPETENT	PROFICIENT
passing	1, 2, or 3 of the elements	4 or 5 out of 6 elements	all elements

PRACTICE PASSING

- Set up 2 discs about 3 feet apart. Aim to pass the ball between the discs.

- Pass back and forth with a partner.

TRAPPING: OPTION 1

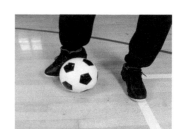

Trapping is a way of stopping the ball, receiving a pass, or gaining control of the ball.

- Start with the ball positioned in front of you on the ground.

- Place your dominant foot on top of the ball. To do this, lift your foot slightly off the ground, keeping your ankle locked and your toes up.

- Repeat this with your non-dominant foot.

SKILL	PROGRESSING	COMPETENT	PROFICIENT
trapping: option 1	1 of the elements	2 out of 3 elements	all elements

TRAPPING: OPTION 2

Trapping is also a way to stop the ball in order to quickly gain control and transition to your next move.

- When the ball comes toward you, turn the ankle of whichever foot you are trapping with so that your instep, or the inside of your foot, is facing forward.

- Cushion the ball with your foot as you stop it lightly, as if you were catching an egg.

- Repeat this with your other foot.

SKILL	PROGRESSING	COMPETENT	PROFICIENT
trapping: option 2	1 of the elements	2 out of 3 elements	all elements

SHOOTING ON GOAL

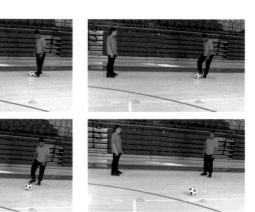

The purpose of shooting is to get the ball into your opponent's goal by striking it with your foot.

- Stand so that your dominant leg, or kicking leg, is pulled back behind you.

- Place your non-kicking foot alongside the ball, with your toes pointing at your goal.

- Bend the knee of your kicking leg by pulling your foot back. Then, in a single motion, swing your leg forward, straightening your leg and pointing your toes to kick the ball with the top of your foot. Kick the center of the ball with the laces of your shoe, pointing your toes down. You do not want to kick the ball with your toes.

- Follow through your kick, making sure that you finish with your toes pointing toward the goal.

SKILL	PROGRESSING	COMPETENT	PROFICIENT
shooting on goal	1 or 2 of the elements	3 out of 5 elements	all elements

PRACTICE TRAPPING AND SHOOTING ON GOAL

- Place 2 disc cones about 4 feet apart to use as your goal. Place them 10 to 20 feet away from you.

- Toss the ball slightly up in the air, trapping it with your foot and guiding it to the ground just in front of you.

- Dribble the ball toward the goal.

- When you get to about 5 feet away from the goal, shoot the ball through the discs.

OFFENSIVE AND DEFENSIVE SKILLS

OFFENSIVE SKILLS

OFFENSIVE READY POSITION

Being in the ready position allows you to move quickly in any direction. This position is used for both offense and defense.

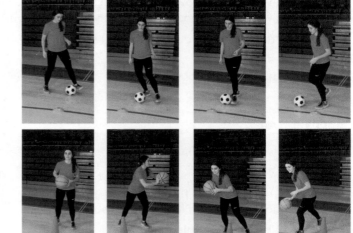

- With your elbows out, hold the ball with both hands to the dominant side of your chest.
- Bend your knees to keep your body low.
- Stand with your feet shoulder-width apart.
- Keep your head up and your weight on the balls of your feet.

SKILL	PROGRESSING	COMPETENT	PROFICIENT
offensive ready position	1 or 2 of the elements	3 out of 4 elements	all elements met

FAKE

SOCCER

BASKETBALL

- Look 1 direction, but pass or move in another direction.
- Stay on the balls of your feet.
- Move quickly.

SKILL	PROGRESSING	COMPETENT	PROFICIENT
fake	1 of the elements	2 out of 3 elements	all elements

GIVE AND GO

The purpose of the give and go is for you to pass the ball to a teammate and quickly relocate so that you can receive a pass.

SOCCER

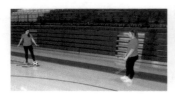 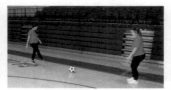 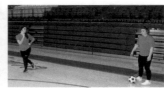 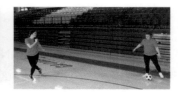

BASKETBALL

- Pass the ball to a teammate.
- Move quickly to relocate and support your offense.
- Indicate (call out) that you are ready and open to receive the ball.
- Catch the ball.

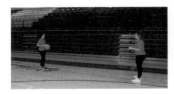 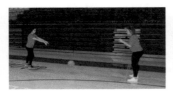 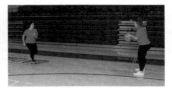 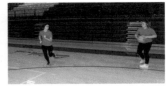

SKILL	PROGRESSING	COMPETENT	PROFICIENT
give and go	1 or 2 of the elements	3 out of 4 elements	all elements

PIVOT

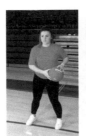 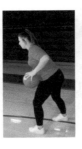 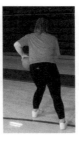 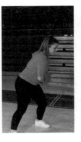 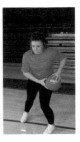

The purpose of the pivot in a speed ball game is for you to look around and decide to dribble, pass, or shoot.

- Plant 1 foot, which will be your pivot foot, in place on the ground.
- Place your weight on the balls of your feet.
- Slide your non-pivot foot and rotate your body 180 degrees.
- Repeat this exercise with your other foot.

SKILL	PROGRESSING	COMPETENT	PROFICIENT
pivot	1 of the elements	2 out of 3 elements	all elements

DEFENSIVE SKILLS

DEFENSIVE READY POSITION

Being in the ready position allows you to move quickly in any direction. This position is used for both offense and defense.

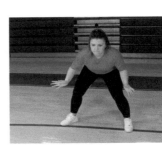

- Bend your knees to keep your body low.
- Stand with your feet shoulder-width apart.
- Keep your head up and your weight on the balls of your feet.
- Hold your arms extended out above waist height so that they are ready to receive the ball.
- React quickly.
- Anticipate direction.

SKILL	PROGRESSING	COMPETENT	PROFICIENT
defensive ready position	1, 2, or 3 of the elements	4 or 5 out of 6 elements	all elements met

DEFENSIVE SLIDES

The purpose of defensive slides in speed ball is to keep up with your opponent and to legally take the ball or legally disrupt the opponent's pass or shot.

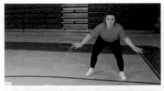
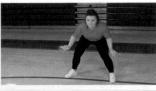
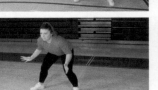
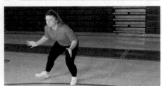

- Place your weight on the balls of your feet.
- Slide to the side with quick steps.
- Do not cross your feet.
- Keep your knees bent.
- Face your hips toward your opponent.
- Hold your hands up at chest level.
- Keep your eyes on your opponent's waistline.
- Stay with your opponent.
- Anticipate and react quickly to your opponent's movements.

SKILL	PROGRESSING	COMPETENT	PROFICIENT
defensive slides	1, 2, 3, 4, or 5 of the elements	6, 7, or 8 out of 9 elements	all elements met

PRACTICE OFFENSIVE AND DEFENSIVE SKILLS

- Practice the **pivot** by planting your right foot and rotating your left foot until you feel comfortable with the movement.
- Practice the **pivot** by planting your left foot and rotating your right foot until you feel comfortable with the movement.
- Practice the **give and go** with a partner and a defender. Pass the ball, quickly relocate, and then receive the pass, avoiding the defender.
- Practice the **fake** independently. Set up a cone as a decoy. Fake the pass toward the cone and then pass to your partner until you feel comfortable with the movement.
- Practice the **fake** with a partner defending you. Dribble, fake, and move in another direction to get around the defensive player. Do this until you feel comfortable with the fake.
- Practice the **defensive slide** with a partner. As your partner dribbles, defensive slide to try to prevent them from making a successful pass or shot. Do this until you feel comfortable with the defensive slide.

SPEED BALL GAME

OBJECT OF THE GAME

Speed ball is a combination of basketball, soccer, and team handball. A player is allowed 3 steps when they are in possession of the ball. They can take 3 steps then throw, hand dribble 3 steps then pass, or foot dribble 3 steps then pass. If the ball is on the floor, the ball is moved like in soccer; if the ball is in the players' hands, the ball is moved like in basketball. The players continue to move the ball until a goal is made, the ball is turned over to the other team, or a penalty occurs.

SPEED BALL SETUP

- It is recommended to have a trusted adult supervise the game.
- Play on a basketball court.
- Set up a soccer goal under each basketball hoop.
  - You can use nets or cones to mark off the goals.
- Use a playground ball to play the game.
- Establish 2 teams of 7 players each.
  - The number of players on each team can be adjusted according to the number of available players. This means that you have the option of playing a 3-on-3 game, a 4-on-4 game, and so on.

RULES OF THE GAME

- Establish the time of your game or the total points to reach in your game.
- Begin the game at mid-court with a jump ball. Have a neutral person toss the ball between 2 designated opposing players.
- In the event where there is nobody to toss the ball, perform a coin toss to decides which team has first possession of the ball.
- After a score, the opposing team throws the ball in.
- A player can hold onto the ball for 3 seconds before moving or passing.
- A player can take 3 steps before throwing the ball.
- Bounce passes are not allowed.
- A player is allowed 3 hand or foot dribbles before passing the ball.
- A turnover occurs when an incomplete pass or an interception is made.
- A dropped ball turns the game to soccer.
- A player can flip the ball from the floor from feet to hands (soccer to basketball).
- A player can be in possession of the ball for only 30 seconds.
  - No physical contact is allowed.
  - Defensive physical contact is a penalty that results in a basketball foul shot for the offensive player.
  - Offensive physical contact results in a turnover, or a change in possession of the ball between teams.

SCORING

1 point: Throw the ball into the goal from outside the 3-point line.
  - You cannot throw the ball into the goal from inside the 3-point line.

2 points: Soccer kick the ball into the goal from inside the 3-point line.
  - You cannot kick the ball into the goal from behind the 3-point line.

3 points: Shoot a basket from inside the 3-point line.
  - The 3-point line is the arc line.

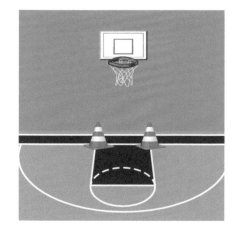

Prior to playing the game, establish and review the game rules so that all participants understand them. If problems arise, work as a group to solve them in a positive and effective manner. Appreciate different players' abilities. Provide game options and variations to fit your circumstances; for example, if you want to play a version of the game on an outdoor field, eliminate the hand dribble and basketball basket.

Below are our game rules for safety and fairness.
1.
2.
3.
4.
5.

RATE YOUR ENJOYMENT OF SPEED BALL

On a scale from 1 to 4, where 1 is not enjoyable and 4 is very enjoyable, rate this activity.

1	It was not enjoyable, and I will not participate again.
2	It was not enjoyable, but I will participate again for exercise.
3	It was enjoyable, and I will play again.
4	It was very enjoyable, and I will initiate future games.

RESEARCH INTEGRATION

1. Research the basic skills for speed ball in the 7th-grade sections for basketball, team handball, and soccer in your PE Manual.

2. Research the game of 4 square in the 7th-grade section of your PE Manual for another playground ball activity option.

HEALTH INTEGRATION

Count your pulse during and after playing speed ball to determine if you are exercising in your personal target heart rate zone. Apply the results to your overall fitness plan. Many people complete aerobic workouts by playing in team games like speed ball.

TENNIS

Tennis is a sport that is played by striking a ball with a racket over a net. It is played against a single opponent or as a doubles game. This striking activity helps you develop concentration, hand-eye coordination, and footwork. You may play tennis as a competitive sport or as an opportunity for social play.

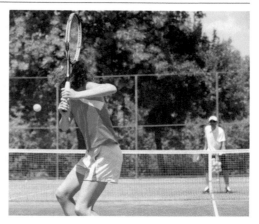

The purpose of this lesson is for you to participate in aerobic exercise and in skill-building activities. Game participation will depend upon the availability of a facility and players. When you are playing tennis, be sure to follow game rules, communicate with teammates in a positive and effective manner, and exhibit appropriate behavior with your team and the opposing team.

⚠ **CAUTION: Make sure that nobody is close to you before you swing the racket. Do not walk into the path of another person who is swinging a racket.**

RACKET SKILLS

READY POSITION

The ready position allows a player to move quickly in any direction.

- Bend your knees and stand with your feet shoulder-width apart.
- Keep your head up.
- Keep your weight on the balls of your feet.
- Hold the racket in your dominant hand.

SKILL	PROGRESSING	COMPETENT	PROFICIENT
ready position	1 or 2 of the elements	3 out of 4 elements	all elements met

HANDSHAKE GRIP

- Hold the racket in your dominant hand like you are about to shake someone's hand.
- Place your 4 fingers around the racket, and then wrap your thumb around the racket.
- Hold the racket so that the head is vertical to the ground. Make sure that the strings on the racket head are facing front and back.
- Point the handle toward your belly button.

SKILL	PROGRESSING	COMPETENT	PROFICIENT
handshake grip	1 or 2 of the elements	3 out of 4 elements	all elements met

FOREHAND STROKE

- Begin in the ready position.
- Pivot to bring the racket back on the same side of your body as your dominant hand.
- Face the palm of your hand forward.

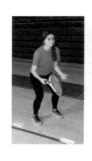 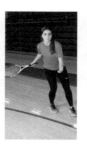 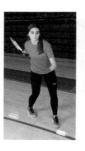 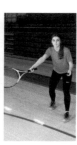

- Shift your weight from your back foot to your front foot while stepping forward and swinging the racket with your dominant hand.
- Extend your arm and flick your wrist to hit the ball, pointing the face of the racket up to get the ball over the net.
- Follow through to your target.

SKILL	PROGRESSING	COMPETENT	PROFICIENT
forehand stroke	1, 2, or 3 of the elements	4 or 5 out of 6 elements	all elements met

BACKHAND STROKE

- Begin in the ready position.
- Rotate the racket and extend it across your body.
- Rotate your feet and shoulders in the same direction as the racket.
- Face the back of your hand (the side that your knuckles are on) forward.
- Step forward with your non-dominant foot while swinging the racket.
- Flick your wrist when hitting the ball with the center of the racket.
- Follow through to your target.

SKILL	PROGRESSING	COMPETENT	PROFICIENT
backhand stroke	1, 2, 3, or 4 of the elements	5 or 6 out of 7 elements	all elements met

2-HANDED BACKHAND STROKE

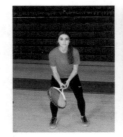 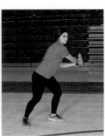 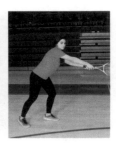

- Place your non-dominant hand below your dominant hand on the racket handle.
- Rotate the racket and extend it across your body.
- Rotate your feet and shoulders in the same direction as the racket.
- Flick your wrists when you are hitting the ball with the center of the racket.
- Follow through to your target.

OVERHAND STROKE

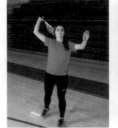 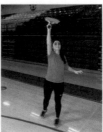 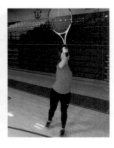

- Bend your elbow slightly and position the racket under the ball.
- Flick your wrist to hit the ball with the center of the racket.
- Extend your arm as you make contact.
- Follow through to your target.

SKILL	PROGRESSING	COMPETENT	PROFICIENT
overhand stroke	1 or 2 of the elements	3 out of 4 elements	all elements met

SERVES

Every game starts with a serve

PUNCH SERVE

Stand behind the service line at a 45-degree angle to the net. A punch serve is an excellent stroke to use as a beginner.

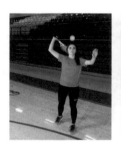

- If you are right-handed, place your left foot forward; if you are left-handed, place your right foot forward. Put your weight on your back foot.

- Hold the racket with a forehand grip in your dominant hand. Raise the racket over your head and slightly back.

- Hold the ball with your fingertips in your non-dominant hand.

- Toss the ball slightly in front of you and high above the racket. Look up at the ball.

- As the ball comes back down, hit it up and forward with the racket. Extend your arm and the racket while you are hitting the ball.

- Follow through to your target. Swing out, across, and down.

SKILL	PROGRESSING	COMPETENT	PROFICIENT
punch serve	1 or 2 of the elements	4 out of 6 elements	all elements met

OVERHAND SERVE

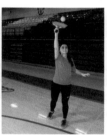
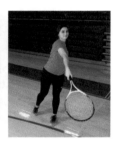

- Hold the racket with your dominant hand.

- Place your non-dominant foot toward the opposite post of the net and your dominant foot parallel to the court.

- Toss the ball into the air just above your head.

- Bring your dominant arm back with the head of the racket pointing toward the sky.

- Watch for the ball to begin to fall.

- Extend your arm up over your head and contact the ball with the head of the racket.

SKILL	PROGRESSING	COMPETENT	PROFICIENT
overhand serve	1, 2, or 3 of the elements	4 or 5 out of 6 elements	all elements met

PRACTICE

AGAINST A WALL

- Practice the various strokes and serves by hitting the ball against a wall with the racket. Catch the ball each time and repeat.

- Allow the ball to bounce before hitting it against the wall.

- Volley against the wall, aiming at and hitting certain spots.

WITH A PARTNER

You can use a jump rope to separate each side if a net is unavailable.

- Have a partner stand on 1 side of the net and toss the ball toward your forehand. Return with a proper forehand stroke.

- Have a partner stand on 1 side of the net and toss the ball toward your backhand. Return with a proper backhand stroke.

- Have a partner stand on 1 side of the net and toss the ball, mixing up forehand and backhand shots. Return with a proper forehand stroke or backhand stroke.

- Use the various strokes to hit the ball back and forth with a partner. Stand 15 feet away from your partner when you are volleying back and forth.

Have your partner evaluate you for correct form for the partner exercises. Did you respond positively to the feedback?

Reciprocate and evaluate your partner. Were you able to provide feedback in a positive manner?

GAME

OFFICIAL SINGLES GAME

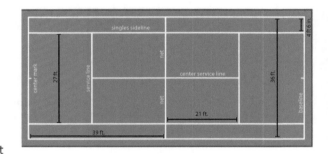

- You will need traditional tennis balls for this game.

- Start with an overhand serve from the right side of the court. Serve from behind the baseline to your opponent on the left.

- Get the ball into your opponent's service box. You have 2 tries to get the ball into the service box. If you hit the ball into your opponent's service box and your opponent cannot return it, you win that volley and get a point.

- Serve from the left side of the court next. When your score is an even number, serve from the right side of the court. When your score is an odd number, serve from the left side of the court.

- Continue serving the ball until the game is over. The receiver becomes the server during the next game.

- You may only hit the ball 1 time on each side.

- You score if your opponent does not have a successful serve, fails to return a serve, or hits the ball out of bounds.

- You lose a volley if you or the racket touch the net.

SCORING

- The server's score is always announced first.

- The point system is as follows.

  o no points or love = 0 points

  o 1 point = 15 points

  o 2 points = 30 points

  o 3 points = 40 points

  o 4 points = win

- To win a game, you must lead by at least 2 points.

- If the score is tied at 40 points (a deuce), you must earn 2 consecutive points (an advantage point) to win the game.

- You must win at least 6 games in a set. You must lead by 2 sets to win a match.

DEMONSTRATE POSITIVE GAME BEHAVIOR

- Follow the rules.
- There is to be no intentional hitting of an opposing player with the ball. You forfeit a point if you hit the opposing player with a ball.
- Be supportive and encouraging to your teammate.
- Treat your opponents with respect.

SKILL	PROGRESSING	COMPETENT	PROFICIENT
game behavior	1 or 2 of the elements	3 out of 4 elements	all elements met

RATE YOUR ENJOYMENT OF TENNIS

On a scale from 1 to 4, where 1 is not enjoyable and 4 is very enjoyable, rate this activity.

1	It was not enjoyable, and I will not participate again.
2	It was not enjoyable, but I will participate again for exercise.
3	It was enjoyable, and I will play again.
4	It was very enjoyable, and I will initiate future games.

RESEARCH INTEGRATION

1. Research proper tennis etiquette.
2. Attend a tennis game or watch a tennis game on television.

HEALTH INTEGRATION

Count your pulse to determine if you are exercising in your personal target heart rate zone. Count your pulse after practicing skills and after playing in a game. Apply the results to your overall fitness plan. Many people choose to complete aerobic workouts by playing in games with friends.

VOLLEYBALL

The official game of volleyball is played by 2 teams of 6 players on an indoor volleyball court. Another popular version of volleyball is beach volleyball, which is played by 2 teams of 2 to 6 players on a sand surface. The object of the game is to strike a ball over a net onto the ground so that the opposing team cannot return it.

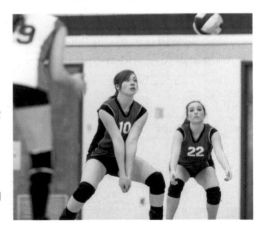

You may play volleyball as a competitive sport or as an opportunity for social play. Casual games of volleyball can be played by as few as 2 players and set up in a yard, park, beach, or gym.

The purpose of this lesson is for you to participate in aerobic exercise and in skill-building activities. When you play volleyball, be sure to follow the rules, communicate with teammates in a positive and effective manner, and exhibit appropriate behavior with your team and the opposing team.

 CAUTION: Do not overinflate the ball.

VOLLEYBALL SKILLS

The following striking skills will not only help to improve your volleyball game, but they may also enhance skills used in other sports and activities.

READY POSITION

The ready position will enable you to react quickly.

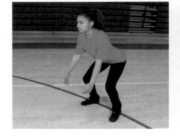 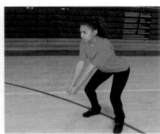

- Stand with your legs shoulder-width apart.
- Balance on the balls of your feet.
- Bend your knees slightly.
- Hold your shoulders rounded and slightly forward.
- Hold your arms in front of you and ready to react.

SKILL	PROGRESSING	COMPETENT	PROFICIENT
ready position	1 or 2 of the elements	3 or 4 out of 5 elements	all elements met

FOREARM GRIP

Try both of the following grips to decide which works better for you.

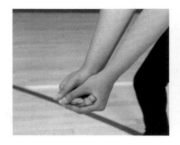 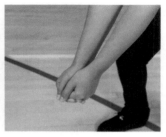

1. Right-handed players: Make a fist with your left hand, wrap the fingers of your right hand around your left hand, and line up your thumbs side by side on top. Left-handed players: Make a fist with your right hand, wrap the fingers of your left hand around your right hand, and line up your thumbs side by side on top.

2. Place 1 hand out flat with your palm up. Place the other hand underneath with the palm up. Curl your thumbs until they are next to each other, centered, and pointing down.

FOREARM PASS (BUMP)

- Stand in the ready position.
- Use the correct grip.
- Contact the ball with your forearm platform.
- Follow through toward your target.

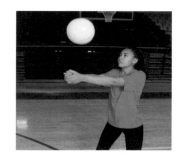

SKILL	PROGRESSING	COMPETENT	PROFICIENT
forearm pass	1 or 2 of the elements	3 out of 4 elements	all elements met

FOREARM PASS (BUMP) PRACTICE

- Forearm pass and catch: Toss the ball to yourself to begin. Pass it back up with your forearm platform, reaching toward your target and catching it. Do not allow your swing to be out of control.
- Forearm pass: Toss the ball to yourself to begin, then continue to pass it. How many times can you pass in a row?
- Wall forearm passes: Toss the ball to yourself to begin, then pass it against a wall. How many times can you pass in a row?
- Partner wall forearm passes: Take turns passing against a wall with a partner.
- Partner toss, forearm pass, and catch: Toss the ball to your partner. Your partner passes it back to you. You catch it. Switch roles.
- Partner forearm passes: How many times can you pass back and forth with a partner?

OVERHAND PASS (SET)

- Stand in the ready position.
- Hold your hands level with your forehead with your elbows bent. Form the size and shape of the ball with your fingers and thumbs.
- Contact the ball with your finger pads, not tips.
- Use a soft touch near your forehead and extend your elbows to push the ball up into the air.

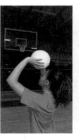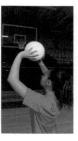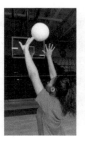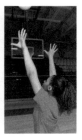

SKILL	PROGRESSING	COMPETENT	PROFICIENT
overhand pass	1 or 2 of the elements	3 out of 4 elements	all elements met

OVERHAND PASS (SET) PRACTICE

- Set and catch: Toss the ball to yourself to begin, set it back up with your finger pads, and catch it.
- Set: Toss the ball to yourself to begin, then continue to set it. How many times can you set in a row?
- Wall sets: Toss the ball to yourself to begin, then set it against a wall. How many times can you set in a row?
- Partner wall sets: Take turns setting against a wall with a partner.
- Partner toss, set, and catch: Toss the ball to your partner. Your partner sets it back to you. You catch it. Switch roles.
- Partner sets: How many times can you set back and forth with a partner?

UNDERHAND SERVE

- Put your non-dominant foot forward.
- Hold the ball on the palm of your non-dominant hand. Position that arm across your body at waist height.
- Make a fist with your striking hand.
- Bring your striking arm back and then forward, striking the ball with the heel of your hand.
- Shift your weight to your front foot.
- Serve successfully 70 percent of the time.

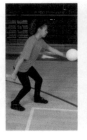 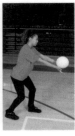 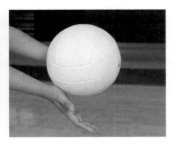

SKILL	PROGRESSING	COMPETENT	PROFICIENT
underhand serve	1 or 2 of the elements	4 or 5 out of 6 elements	all elements met

UNDERHAND SERVE PRACTICE

- Wall serves: Practice serving toward a wall.
- Partner serves: Serve to a partner and volley back and forth using the set and bump skills.

CHALLENGING VOLLEYBALL SKILLS

The following advanced skills are for students who have mastered the basic skills. The challenge level is recommended if you want to further explore the volleyball activity.

OVERHAND SERVE

- Put your non-dominant foot forward.
- Turn the non-dominant side of your body slightly toward the net or target.
- Hold the ball in your non-dominant hand.
- Bend your striking arm with your hand cupped near your ear.

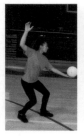 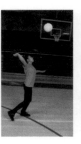 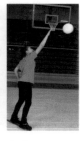 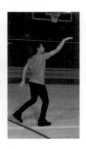

- Contact: Toss the ball 2 to 3 feet in the air, placing your weight on your back foot. Shift your weight to your front foot as you strike the ball approximately 12 inches above your head.
- Follow through in the direction of the ball.

SKILL	PROGRESSING	COMPETENT	PROFICIENT
overhand serve	1 or 2 of the elements	3, 4, or 5 out of 6 elements	all elements met

OVERHAND SERVE PRACTICE

- Wall serves: Practice serving toward a wall.
- Partner serves: Serve to a partner and volley back and forth using the set and bump skills.

OVERHAND HITTING (SPIKE)

1 player: Follow the overhand serve techniques.

2 players: A teammate hits the ball up high near the net.

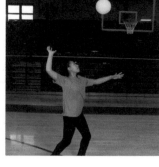

- As a hitter, approach from behind using a 4-step approach.
- Place your dominant foot forward.
- Step forward with your non-dominant foot, then quick step with your dominant then non-dominant foot. For example, if you are right-handed, you would start with your right foot forward, step left, then right, then left.
- Begin with your arms at waist height in front of your body. Swing them backward then forward until both of your arms are reaching high with your dominant arm slightly forward.
- Strike the ball with the fleshy part of your dominant hand.
- Follow through, facing the direction in which you want the ball to go.

SKILL	PROGRESSING	COMPETENT	PROFICIENT
overhand hit (spike)	1 or 2 of the elements	3, 4, or 5 out of 6 elements	all elements met

EXTENSION

If you have an available outdoor wall or garage door and permission from your parent or guardian, you can place a horizontal line of tape or chalk mark 7 feet 4½ inches from the ground to represent the height of a net. Begin approximately 10 feet back and practice the underhand and overhand serves. When you are successful, move back farther. Continue this until you are able to serve from 30 feet back, which is the official serving distance.

VOLLEYBALL GAMES

REGULATION VOLLEYBALL GAME

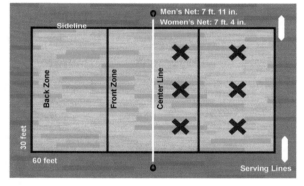

- There are 6 people on a team: 3 front row players and 3 back row players.
- Players rotate in order to reach the serving position.
- The players from the same team all rotate 1 position clockwise when it is their team's turn to serve.
- The serving position is behind the end line. Most players will serve from the right end line; however, for left-handed servers, you may serve from anywhere behind the end line.
- The objective is to serve the ball across the net into the opponent's court within the boundaries. The ball can hit the net on the way over and still be playable.
- Each team is allowed 3 hits, but no player can hit the ball twice in a row.
- A player may not make contact with any part of the net.
- A ball contacting the net is considered playable.

SCORING

- The serve starts the game.
- When the serving team wins the rally, a point is scored.
- If the rally is won by the non-serving team, that team gets a point and a chance to serve.
- The first team to score 25 points and be ahead by at least 2 points wins the game.
- A match consists of either winning 2 out of 3 games or 3 out of 5 games.

ALTERNATIVE: A COOPERATIVE SCORING GAME

- You will need at least 2 players.
- Toss a coin to see which side serves first.
- There will be 1 person or team on each side of the net. You may use a jump rope or disc cones to separate each side if a net is unavailable.
- Rally back and forth.
- Count each time the ball goes over the net except for the serve.
- There are unlimited hits per side, but a point is scored only when it goes over the net.
- Continue until the ball is not in play.
- Indicate the score.
- Rotate sides and players for each serve.
- Count again and try to beat your previous score.

DEMONSTRATE POSITIVE GAME BEHAVIOR

- Follow the rules.
- Call out when you are attempting to strike the ball to avoid collisions.
- Be supportive and encouraging to your teammates.
- Treat your opponents with respect.

SKILL	PROGRESSING	COMPETENT	PROFICIENT
game behavior	1 or 2 of the elements	3 out of 4 elements	all elements met

RATE YOUR ENJOYMENT OF VOLLEYBALL

On a scale from 1 to 4, where 1 is not enjoyable and 4 is very enjoyable, rate this activity.

1	It was not enjoyable, and I will not participate again.
2	It was not enjoyable, but I will participate again for exercise.
3	It was enjoyable, and I will play again.
4	It was very enjoyable, and I will initiate future games.

RESEARCH INTEGRATION

1. Research who invented the game of volleyball, including the rules and regulations.
2. Attend a volleyball game or watch a volleyball game on television and compare the skills you have practiced for the game of volleyball with the skills the players use.

HEALTH INTEGRATION

Count your pulse to determine if you are exercising in your personal target heart rate zone. Count your pulse after practicing skills and after playing in a game. Apply the results to your overall fitness plan.

GRADE 9
PE EQUIPMENT KIT

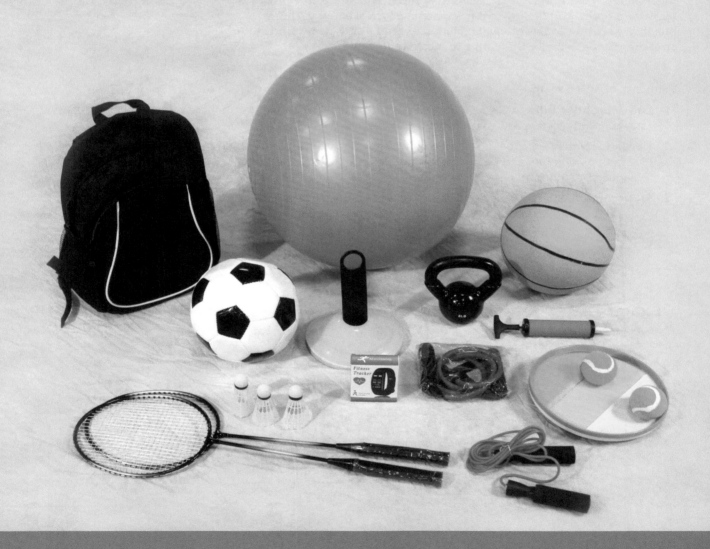

WARM-UP AND COOL-DOWN

⚠ **CAUTION: Stretching should not be painful; ease up if stretching hurts. See the Flexibility section of your PE Manual for more information.**

WARM-UP

The purpose of a warm-up is to gradually increase your heart rate, breathing rate, and body temperature. A good warm-up prior to exercise increases circulation and blood flow to your muscles. When your muscles are warmed up, their performance (for example, strength and speed) is enhanced, and the risk of injury is decreased.

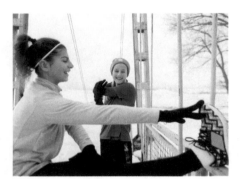

Stretching your muscles helps to minimize the risk of injury by making the muscle fibers pliable.

Before beginning any workout, you should always warm up. Getting your heart and muscles prepared for exercise is important. There are numerous ways to get your body ready to participate in physical activity. **The Flexibility section of this manual includes a variety of dynamic and static stretches for each major body part to increase flexibility.**

Elements of a Warm-Up

1. **Low-intensity cardio**: Walk, slow jog, or slow swim for 5 to 10 minutes to increase your heart rate, breathing rate, and body temperature before your workout.

2. **Dynamic stretch**: Perform a repeated motion—such as kicks, high knees, lunges, or arm circles—that will loosen up your joints and prepare your muscles for the exercise that you are about to do. Perform each dynamic stretch for at least 30 seconds.

3. **Static stretch**: Stretch your muscles slowly and hold each stretch for 20 to 30 seconds without bouncing in order to lengthen your muscles and increase your flexibility. Some important areas to stretch as a part of your warm-up are your neck, sides, shoulders, triceps, back, hamstrings, quadriceps, and groin.

Example 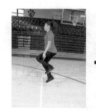 **+** 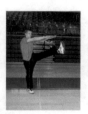 **+** 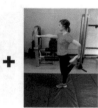 **= EFFECTIVE WARM-UP**

PERSONAL WARM-UP ACTIVITY

1. Select an exercise activity to participate in.

2. Design your personal warm-up plan for the activity that you selected. Any dynamic and static stretches that you choose to complete should be specific to the exercise activity that you chose.

3. Have a trusted adult or friend assess your stretches to make sure that you are using proper form.

4. Explain how the warm-up will decrease your risk of injury for this activity. _____

Procedure	Enter your personal warm-up regimen below.
1. **Low-intensity cardiovascular exercise:** Exercise for 5 to 10 minutes.	
2. **Dynamic stretches:** Perform dynamic stretches specifically for the selected activity.	
3. **Static stretches:** Perform static stretches specifically for the selected activity.	

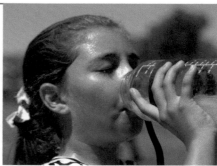

COOL-DOWN

After you have finished your workout, exercise, or activity, it is imperative that your body returns to its normal state. You want to avoid stopping immediately and sitting down **unless you are in pain, dizzy, or injured**. Be sure to slow your heart rate and breathing rate back to or slightly above their resting rates. There are several ways to do this. You can simply walk or slow down your exercise for a few minutes, or you can find your own way to slow your body back down. You also may want to incorporate static stretches to increase flexibility and to avoid your muscles tightening. **The Flexibility section of your PE Manual includes a variety of static stretches for each major body part.** Always keep hydrated by drinking water before, during, and after exercise.

Elements of a Cool-Down

1. **Slow down**: Walk or gradually slow down your exercise—such as returning to a slow swim if you are swimming—until your heart rate, breathing rate, and body temperature are back to normal.

2. **Static stretch**: Stretch your muscles slowly and hold each stretch for 20 to 30 seconds without bouncing in order to lengthen your muscles and increase flexibility. Some important areas to stretch as part of your cool-down are your neck, sides, shoulders, triceps, back, hamstrings, quadriceps, and groin.

WALK + STATIC STRETCHES = EFFECTIVE COOL-DOWN

Design your personal cool-down plan. You can perform the same cool-down each time you finish a physical activity or you can change each time in order to reflect the exercise activity, such as by slowing your pedaling if you are biking.

Procedure	Enter your personal cool-down regimen below.
1. **Slow down:** Perform this slowed activity for 5 to 10 minutes.	
2. **Static stretches:** Perform several lower-body and upper-body stretches.	

AEROBIC EXERCISE AND PROPER NUTRITION

Aerobic exercise is important for strengthening the heart and for reducing stress. Frequency, intensity, and time are essential to efficient aerobic exercise. **Any** exercise done in your target heart rate zone and performed for 20 to 60 minutes 3 to 5 days per week is aerobic exercise.

Proper nutrition is important for a healthy body and for keeping the arteries of the heart clear. Eating proper portions from the grain group, the fruit group, the vegetable group, the dairy group, and the protein group is essential to proper nutrition. Limit high-fat and sugary foods. You are more likely to commit to healthful eating if you plan and keep track of your nutrition.

Combining regular aerobic exercise with proper nutrition contributes to cardiovascular health as well as overall health.

The purpose of this lesson is to encourage you to develop a fitness portfolio, choreograph an aerobic exercise routine, participate in aerobic workouts, and plan for proper nutrition. **The Cardiovascular Endurance section of this manual includes the target heart rate zone formula and the Borg Rating of Perceived Exertion Scale to help you to determine if you are exercising for heart health.** You can also use available technology to monitor your pulse rate and intensity.

When beginning any exercise program, begin with workouts for your fitness level and then build accordingly. You want to feel refreshed after your exercise session, not exhausted. Use your pulse rate to monitor aerobic workouts.

 CAUTION: Wear proper equipment and follow activity-specific safety rules.

AEROBIC EXERCISE AND PROPER NUTRITION

Develop a fitness portfolio and make a commitment to aerobic exercise. Your fitness portfolio should include the following.

- endurance walk/run fitness score
- goals for improvement
- 4-week exercise plan (See below.)

TYPES OF AEROBIC EXERCISE

Sports: Examples include soccer, basketball, volleyball, swimming, hockey, lacrosse, tennis, badminton, pickleball, handball, gymnastics, dance, martial arts, wrestling, track and field, and so on.

Outdoor pursuits: Examples include walking, jogging, biking, canoeing, kayaking, golfing, fly fishing, hiking, rock climbing, horseback riding, skiing, and so on.

Fitness gyms: Find a gym that is convenient for you to attend where you can complete circuit exercises, use aerobic machines, take classes, and more.

Stationary exercise equipment: Examples include using a jump rope, treadmill, elliptical trainer, bike, mini trampoline, and so on.

Exercise apps or videos: Use a workout tutorial on an app, website, video, or other digital source.

Your own sequence workouts: You can also design your own workout sequences by following the steps below.

- Create your personal aerobic workout routines by blending activities that involve basic locomotor skills such as jogging in place, jumping jacks, high knees, and so on.
- Design the intensity and duration of the exercise according to your level of fitness.
- Perform your personal routine for some or all your aerobic workouts.

Choreograph a personal aerobic workout routine by blending basic locomotor skills. This is a workout that can be done at home for convenience. The suggested time for each skill is from 20 to 60 seconds with a 30-second rest every 4 to 5 minutes. Repeat for a 20- to 60-minute workout. Most important, exercise at your level of fitness and rest accordingly. Use the following skills to choreograph your routine, or use skills of your choice.

- Jogging in place: Run slowly in place.
- Jumping jacks: Stand with your feet apart with arms up, then feet together with arms at your sides.
- High knees: Alternate lifting your knees to waist height.
- Burpees: Jump vertically, then bend your knees and transition to a push-up position.
- Side slides: Step to the right. Bring the other foot over in a step-together motion. Repeat left.
- Squat jumps: Jump and land softly into a squat (hips even with knees).
- March in place: Alternate lifting knees to waist height.
- Carioca: Step to the side with 1 foot and cross with your other foot in a step-cross-step-cross movement. Alternate the step-cross movement with a cross behind the lead foot and a cross in front of the lead foot.
- Front kicks: Alternate lifting your legs forward.

EXTENSION: Work with a friend to create aerobic routines. Evaluate each other's level of fitness and schedule (school/work) to create and plan personalized workouts.

Plan your exercise. The following is an example of how to schedule and track aerobic exercise for 1 week. Plan for 4 weeks.

WARM UP BEFORE EACH WORKOUT.

Week 1	Exercise	Time of Day	Exercise Time (min.)	Heart Rate (bpm)
Mon.	jump rope	morning	20	160
Tues.				
Wed.	my routine	morning	30	155
Thurs.	volleyball	evening	60	145
Fri.				
Sat.	tennis	evening	45	140
Sun.				

COOL DOWN AFTER EACH WORKOUT.

Plan your nutrition. Keep track of the food you eat each day for 1 week. Include food from the grain group, the fruit group, the vegetable group, the dairy group, and the protein group each day. Drink water daily. Limit high-fat and sugary foods. Exercise burns calories, so it is important to get food from all of the food groups. Plan for and eat healthful snacks. Review what you eat each day, discuss your diet with a trusted adult, and adjust so that you are getting a well-rounded, healthful diet. Be aware of false diet claims and rely on your doctor for advice.

 CAUTION: Do not consume foods to which you are allergic.

EXAMPLE

Day 1	Time	Servings	Total Servings
Grain	breakfast	2	6
	lunch	2	
	dinner	2	
Fruit	breakfast	1	4
	lunch	2	
	dinner	1	
Vegetable	breakfast	O	5
	lunch	2	
	dinner	3	
Dairy	breakfast	2	4
	lunch	1	
	dinner	1	
Protein	breakfast	O	3
	lunch	1	
	dinner	2	
Snacks	granola bar	1	2
	apple	1	

 RESEARCH INTEGRATION

1. Research proper nutrition, focusing on food groups and portion servings.
2. Research proper nutrition in relation to exercise and your body. Consider the daily calories necessary to consume to meet your workout duration and intensity; how you should fit in snacks before, during, and after vigorous exercise; and the importance of staying hydrated.

♥ HEALTH INTEGRATION

Use available technology to monitor your pulse rate and workout intensity. Apply the results to your overall fitness plan.

DANCE

Dancing is an exercise option for aerobic workout, for competition, or just for fun. You can dance on your own or with others. Dancing is expressing yourself through repeated patterns of movement which are usually set to music. Some forms of dance include creative, tap, ballet, hip-hop, modern, folk, square, jazz, line, Latin, ballroom, and social.

Social dance is dancing with a partner or a group in a social situation for enjoyment. Social dancing is common at events like weddings and parties. Dancing freestyle with a partner or following a choreographed line dance are some examples of social dancing.

The purpose of this lesson is for you to perform basic locomotor movements using common dance concepts in rhythmic patterns to create your own line dance for aerobic exercise.

SOCIAL DANCE

CREATE YOUR PERSONAL DANCE ROUTINE

COMMON CONCEPTS OF DANCE TO USE FOR YOUR PERSONAL DANCE

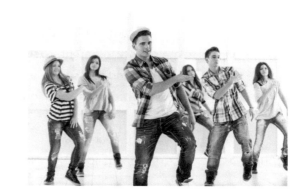

- The concept of space includes the following.
  - high, medium, or low **levels**
  - forward, backward, right, or left **direction**
  - curved, zigzag, straight, circle, or square **pathways**
- The concept of time includes the following.
  - slow, medium, or fast **speeds**
  - a pattern for **rhythm**
- The concept of force includes the following.
  - applying light, moderate, or strong **weights**

CREATE A LINE DANCE

Create a dance that can be done individually for an aerobic workout but that can also be done with a partner or small group for a social experience.

Start with the dance steps described below. Start moving to the right. When you jump, turn, and clap, turn to the right as you step and land. Continue this pattern until you complete the square. Next, complete the routine by adding your own dance steps. Set the dance to music.

1. Combine the sidestep and step-hop for a double step (step together then step-hop and clap).

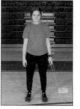 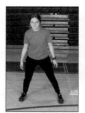 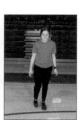
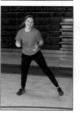 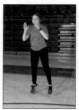 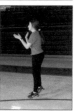

- Step to the right with your right foot.
- Bring your left foot in to meet your right foot.
- Step out to the right side with your right foot.
- Bring your left foot in, simultaneously jumping and clapping.
- Step to the right with your right foot.
- Bring your left foot in to meet your right foot.
- Step out to the right side with your right foot.
- Bring your left foot in and simultaneously **jump, turn, and clap**.
- Repeat these steps until you complete a square pattern.

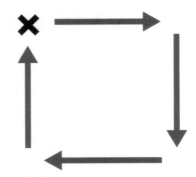

2. Next, add your own dance steps to complete the dance. Create the steps, write a description of each step, and practice the steps.

- Choose locomotor skills to blend (slides, cariocas, turns, and so on).
- Use your arms to accompany the footwork, for example: step, cross, step, clap.
- Perform the skills at different levels.
- Move at medium and fast speeds.
- Use light, moderate, and strong force to move your body.
- Create a pattern.
- Use an 8 count for each move.

Option: Dance with friends outside of PE class for a social experience.

RATE YOUR ENJOYMENT OF SOCIAL LINE DANCING

On a scale from 1 to 4, where 1 is not enjoyable and 4 is very enjoyable, rate this activity.

1	It was not enjoyable, and I will not participate again.
2	It was not enjoyable, but I will participate again for exercise.
3	It was enjoyable, and I will dance again.
4	It was very enjoyable, and I will create more dances.

RESEARCH INTEGRATION

1. Research the historical and cultural role of dance in a society. Discuss your research with a friend or trusted adult.
2. Research and compare the 2 dance types folk and ballroom.
3. Join a dance from the USB if provided in your PE program.

HEALTH INTEGRATION

Count your pulse to determine if you are exercising in your personal target heart rate zone. Apply the results to your overall fitness plan. Many people choose to get their aerobic workouts through dance.

JUMP ROPE

A jump rope is an inexpensive piece of exercise equipment. It can be used indoors, outdoors, and in a small space. A jump rope promotes adherence to participation in physical activity by eliminating cost and space barriers.

The purpose of this lesson is for you to use jumping rope to improve your cardiovascular fitness and foot speed.

JUMP ROPE BASICS

FITTING THE JUMP ROPE TO YOUR HEIGHT

- Place a jump rope handle in each hand.
- Stand on the middle of the rope with 1 foot.
- Move the handles straight up, making sure that the rope is straight and pulled tight.
- The tops of the handles should reach close to your shoulders.

Fitting The Jump Rope To Your Height

ELEMENTS OF JUMP ROPE

- Keep your eyes forward.
- When you are turning the rope, keep your elbows near your sides, maintaining a 45-degree angle and making 2-inch circles with your wrists.
- Leave just enough space for the rope to pass under your feet when you jump.
- Stay on the balls of your feet.
- Land softly, keeping your knees slightly bent.

BASIC SKILLS

BASIC JUMP

- Pick up the rope. Holding a handle in each hand, rest the rope behind your feet. Stand on the balls of your feet. This is the ready position.
- Your hands should be just above the height of your waist.
- Swing the rope up and over your head.
- Jump over the rope when it approaches your toes.
- Continue as long as you can without stopping.

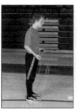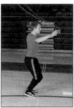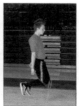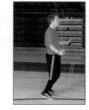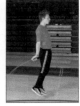

Basic jump

BACKWARD JUMP

- Begin with the rope in front of your feet.
- Swing the rope up and over your head.
- Jump over the rope when it approaches your feet.

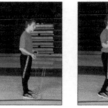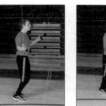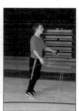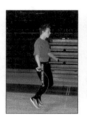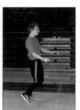

Backward jump

ALTERNATE-FOOT JUMP

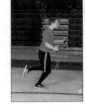
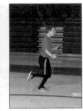

- Pick up the rope. Holding a handle in each hand, rest the rope behind your feet. Stand on the balls of your feet. This is the ready position. Note that 1 foot will be lifted off the ground during each turn of the rope before the other foot jumps.

- Turn the rope from behind you up over your head. When the rope reaches your toes, jump over it with your right foot.

- Turn the rope again from behind you up over your head. When the rope reaches your toes this time, jump over it with your left foot.

Alternate-foot jump

- Continue turning the rope and alternating feet as if you were running in place. Try it jumping backward.

Practice the basic jump rope skills until competent. Next, design a jump rope routine using basic jump rope skills that will improve footwork speed.

SAMPLE OF A WORKOUT TO IMPROVE FOOTWORK SPEED	
• basic jump 1 minute at a medium pace	• rest 30 seconds
• basic jump 30 seconds at a fast pace	• alternate-foot jump 1 minute at a medium pace
• rest 30 seconds	• alternate-foot jump 30 seconds at a fast pace
• backward jump 1 minute at a medium pace	• rest 30 seconds
• backward jump 30 seconds at a fast pace	• repeat as needed

DESIGN YOUR PERSONAL FOOTWORK SPEED ROUTINE

CHALLENGE SKILLS

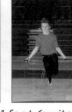

The following challenges are for students who have mastered the basic jump rope skills. The challenge level is recommended to learn advanced skills and add a variety of skills to your workout.

HOP ON 1 FOOT

- Perform the basic jump on your right foot.

- Perform the basic jump on your left foot.

Hop on 1 foot (switch)

SKIER

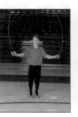
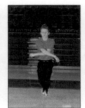

- With both feet together, hop side to side while turning the rope.

Skier

CROSSOVERS

- After the rope moves over your head, cross the rope in front of you, jump, and uncross the rope.

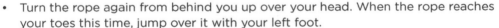

Crossovers

FRONT KICKS

- Kick 1 foot forward as the rope passes under your feet with a skip-step in between.
- Alternate kicks.

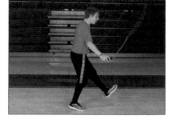

Front kicks

SIDE KICKS

- Kick 1 foot and then the other out to the side with a skip-step in between.

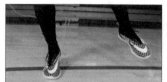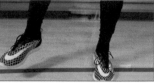

Side kicks

CRISSCROSS FEET

- Cross and uncross your feet while jumping.

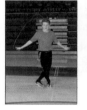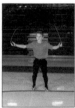

Practice the challenge jump rope skills until competent. Next, design your personal aerobic jump rope routine by blending the basic jump rope skills and the challenge skills. Set your routine to music.

Crisscross feet

BLENDING: Perform 1 jump rope skill and transition smoothly to another jump rope skill without stopping between moves.

SAMPLE OF A CARDIOVASCULAR CONDITIONING WORKOUT

- blend basic jump/crossovers/basic jump **2 minutes**
- march or jog in place **30 seconds**
- blend backward jump/hop on 1 foot/backward jump **2 minutes**
- march or jog in place **30 seconds**
- blend alternate-foot jump/basic jump/crisscross feet **2 minutes**
- walk or jog in place **30 seconds**
- blend skier/front kicks/side kicks **2 minutes**
- march or jog in place **30 seconds**
- repeat for a 20-minute workout

DESIGN YOUR PERSONAL CARDIOVASCULAR JUMP ROPE ROUTINE. SET IT TO MUSIC.

 HEALTH INTEGRATION

Count your pulse during and after jumping rope to determine if you are exercising in your personal target heart rate zone for health benefits. Apply the results to your overall fitness plan.

FITNESS BALL

Including a fitness ball (or exercise ball) in your exercise routine is a fun, efficient way to improve muscular strength, muscular endurance, flexibility, and balance. Your core muscles work to balance on an unstable ball while exercising a variety of muscle groups.

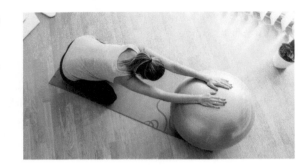

 CAUTION: Do not overinflate the ball.

FITNESS BALL STRENGTH-BUILDING EXERCISES

TIPS FOR USING A FITNESS BALL

- Exercises done on a firmer ball are more challenging.
- A beginner should start with a slightly-deflated ball.
- When you are seated on the ball, your feet should be flat on the floor.

Practice each of the following exercises, concentrating on proper form, prior to engaging in a workout.

SQUATS

muscle focus: quadriceps, hamstrings, and glutes

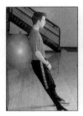 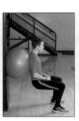 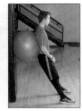

Squats

- Place the fitness ball against your lower back, between you and the wall.
- Holding the ball against the wall, place your feet shoulder-width apart and slightly out in front of you. Your body should be at an angle.
- Slide your body down into a seated position (the fitness ball should now be against your upper back), making sure your knees do not go past your toes.
- Stand back up to the starting position. The fitness ball should still be between you and the wall against your lower back.

BACK EXTENSIONS

muscle focus: erector spinae (iliocostales, longissimi, and spinales)

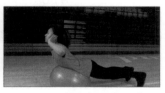

Back extensions

- Place the fitness ball on the floor.
- Place your abdomen on the ball. Your legs should be extended behind you and about shoulder-width apart for balance.
- Place your hands behind your head on your neck (like when doing a crunch).
- Lift your upper body so that you are hyperextending your back.
- Come back down to the starting position.

CRUNCHES

muscle focus: recti abdominis and oblique abdominal muscles

- Place the fitness ball on the floor.
- Place yourself on the fitness ball so that your lower back is on the ball. You do not want your shoulders on the ball.
- Your feet should be shoulder-width apart for balance.
- Place your hands behind your head on your neck.
- Bend your torso upward, performing a crunch.
- Come back down to the starting position, making sure your abdomen is still tight. Do not extend back the whole way as that would release the tension in your abdomen.

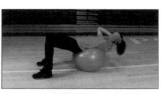
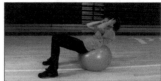

Crunches

TWISTS

muscle focus: abdominal muscles and erector spinae

- Place the fitness ball on the floor.
- Sit on the fitness ball so that your knees are at 90-degree angles.
- Your feet should be together on the floor.
- In a single motion, swing your legs to the right as you swing your arms to the left.
- Then, simultaneously swing your legs to the left as you swing your arms to the right.
- Move in 1 motion back and forth from side to side.
- Remember to twist opposite legs and arms.

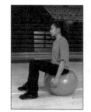
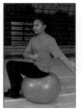
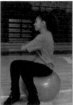

Twists

HAMSTRING CURLS

muscle focus: abdominal muscles, erector spinae, hamstrings, and glutes

- Place the fitness ball on the floor.
- Lie down with your hands slightly out to your sides.
- Put your lower calves and ankles on the ball. Your feet should be together, and your glutes should be lifted off the ground.
- Bring your knees in toward your chest, moving the ball toward your glutes. The bottoms of your feet should be resting on the ball.
- Straighten your legs to return to the starting position.

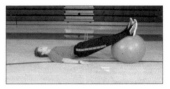
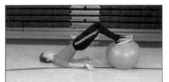
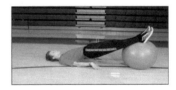

Hamstring curls

LEG EXTENSIONS

muscle focus: quadriceps, hamstrings, and glutes

- Sit on the ball with both feet firmly on the ground.
- Lift your right leg so your calf is parallel to the ground.
- Lower your right leg slowly back to the starting position.
- Lift your left leg so your calf is parallel to the ground.
- Lower your left leg slowly back to the starting position.
- Alternate legs.

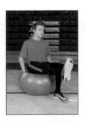
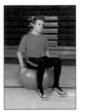
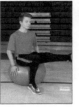
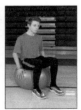

Leg extensions

Have a trusted adult or friend evaluate you for correct form for the previous exercises. Did you respond positively to the feedback?

Reciprocate and evaluate your friend. Were you able to provide feedback in a positive manner?

The following is a suggested use of the fitness ball in a strength-building workout. Exercise to your level of fitness.

Warm up and cool down.

- Perform each exercise 2 to 3 days per week.
- Begin with 1 set of 10 repetitions. Increase sets and the number of repetitions when the current number is too easy.
- Your goal should be to reach 3 sets of 10 to 15 repetitions.

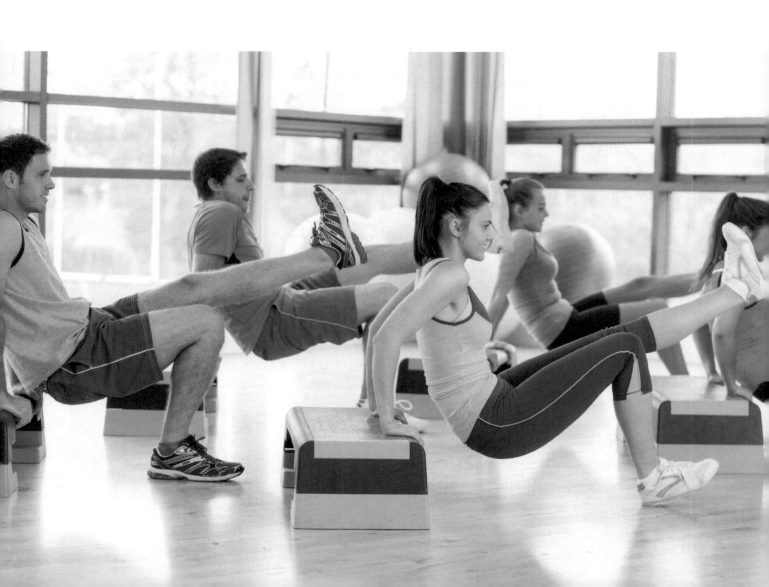 **RESEARCH INTEGRATION**

Research flexibility exercises that are performed with an exercise ball.

RESISTANCE BANDS

Resistance bands are elastic bands with or without handles that are used to improve flexibility, muscular strength, muscular endurance, and body composition. When you are using resistance bands, start with the lightest resistance and gradually increase to a higher resistance as you get stronger.

The purpose of this lesson is to encourage you to use resistance bands for strength training.

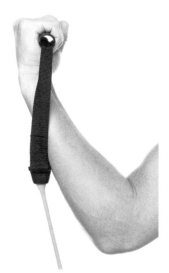

FITNESS TIP: When using resistance bands, you should make sure that the band is secured in a way that the length is appropriate to give resistance for the entire exercise. Wrap the band around your hands if you need an increased resistance level.

CAUTION: Check the resistance bands for damage or wear before exercising. When exercising, secure the band before adding any resistance.

RESISTANCE BANDS STRENGTH-BUILDING EXERCISES
BENEFITS OF STRENGTH TRAINING WITH RESISTANCE BANDS

- is an effective overall strength workout that does not require weights
- offers a variety of resistance adjustments for beginner through advanced levels
- requires inexpensive pieces of equipment
- requires equipment that is easy to carry with you when you are traveling

Practice each of the following exercises, concentrating on proper form, prior to engaging in a workout.

SQUATS

muscle focus: quadriceps, hamstrings, and glutei maximi

- Stand on the middle of the band with your feet shoulder-width apart.
- Hold an end of the band in each hand. Bend your elbows and place your hands by your ears.
- Bend your legs as if you were sitting in a chair. Bend until your legs are at 90-degree angles. Do not let your knees go past your toes.
- Stand back up to the starting position. Do not lock your knees.

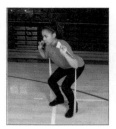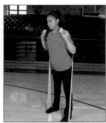

Squats

LEG EXTENSIONS

muscle focus: quadriceps, hamstrings, and glutei maximi

- Lay with your back flat on the ground and with your right knee bent to your chest.
- Wrap your band around the bottom of your right foot, holding an end in each hand.
- Keep your left leg flat on the ground.
- Hold the band firmly in your hands and push your right leg straight out without fully straightening your knee.
- Bring your leg slowly back to the starting position.
- After completing the set, switch to your left leg.

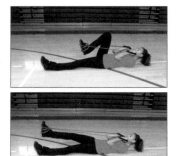

Leg extensions

CHEST PRESSES

muscle focus: pectoralis majors, anterior deltoids, and triceps

- Sit on the exercise ball and place the band behind your back.
- Place your hands in front of your shoulders in the loops of the band. You may need to hold closer to the middle of the band if it is too long for you.
- Push your arms straight out in front of you while holding onto the loops of the resistance band.
- Lower your arms slowly back toward your body, but do not go so far that your arms reach a resting position.

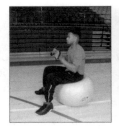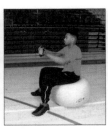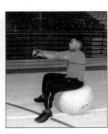

Chest presses

TRICEPS EXTENSIONS

muscle focus: triceps and biceps

- Sit on the exercise ball with the middle of the band under you. You should be sitting on the band.
- Hold the right handle in your right hand and the left handle in your left hand.
- Place both hands over your head with your elbows bent.
- Extend both hands above your head, straightening your elbows.

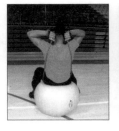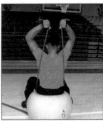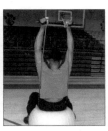

Tricep extensions

BICEP HAMMER CURLS

muscle focus: biceps and triceps

- Stand on the middle of the exercise band with your feet shoulder-width apart.
- Hold both ends of the resistance band with your palms facing in toward your body.
- Bend at your elbows, and slowly bring each hand toward the respective shoulder while keeping your elbows by your sides and your palms toward your body.
- Return your arms slowly back to the starting position without fully straightening your elbows.

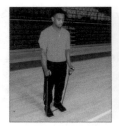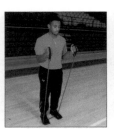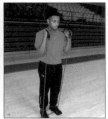

Biceps hammer curls

LATERAL RAISES

muscle focus: deltoids

- Place an end of the resistance band under your right foot and hold the other end in your right hand.
- Keep your arm straight at your side and make sure that the tension of the resistance band is at a good level. If the resistance is not enough, wrap the band around your hand until the resistance is comfortable.
- Keep your arm straight and raise it out to your side so that it is parallel with the floor.
- Bring your arm slowly back down to your side. Make sure you are keeping your arm straight during the entire exercise.

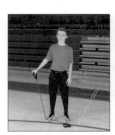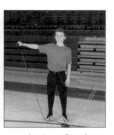

Lateral raises

SEATED ROWS

muscle focus: erector spinae, trapezii, rhomboids, and latissimi dorsi

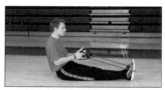
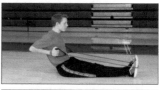
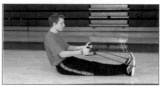

- Sit on the ground. Your feet and legs should be straight out in front of you.
- Place the middle of the band around the bottom of both feet. The resistance band should be across the instep of both feet. Hold an end in each hand.
- Start with your arms straight out in front of you. Make sure there is good tension with the resistance band.
- Make sure your forearms and wrists are rotated so that your thumbs are on top of the grip. Your palms should be facing each other.
- Keep your back upright. In a single motion, bend your elbows back and pinch your shoulder blades together. Do not bring your elbows so far back that they are almost touching; bring them back so that they are slightly behind you.
- Bring your arms slowly straight in front of you, back to the starting position.

Seated rows

CALF RAISES

muscle focus: gastrocnemii and solei

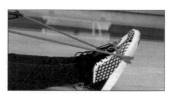
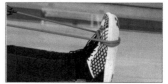

- Sit on the ground. Your feet and legs should be straight out in front of you.
- Place the middle of the resistance band around the bottom of both feet. The band should be across the balls of your feet (closer to the toes, but not on the toes). Hold an end in each hand.
- Flex your feet and point your toes away from your leg.
- Bring your toes slowly up toward your leg.

Calf raises

Have a trusted adult or friend evaluate you for correct form for the previous exercises. Did you respond positively to the feedback?

Reciprocate and evaluate your friend. Were you able to provide feedback in a positive manner?

The following is a suggested use of resistance bands in a strength-building workout. Exercise to your level of fitness.

- Warm up before your workout. Cool down after your workout.
- Perform each resistance band exercise 2 to 3 days per week. Do not exercise the same muscle group on consecutive days.
- Begin with 1 set of 10 repetitions for each exercise. Increase sets and the number of repetitions when the current number is too easy.
- Your goal should be to reach 3 sets of 10 to 15 repetitions.

Wrap the band to increase resistance as necessary.

🖥 RESEARCH INTEGRATION

Research the importance of proper form and technique to exercise efficiency and safety.

KETTLEBELLS

A kettlebell is a weighted ball with a handle. Using a kettlebell is a great way to get a combination strength and aerobic workout. Performing exercises with kettlebells requires your whole body to work hard, which results in more calories being burned.

The purpose of this lesson is to encourage you to use kettlebells to improve your muscular endurance and muscular strength.

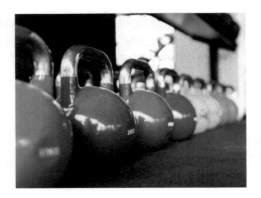

FITNESS TIP: Have a certified trainer plan for you and supervise you when you are working with any type of weights.

⚠ CAUTION: Make sure that no one is close to you before you swing a kettlebell. Do not walk into the path of another person who is swinging a kettlebell. Keep all kettlebell movements controlled to avoid injury.

KETTLEBELL STRENGTH-BUILDING EXERCISES
BENEFITS OF STRENGTH TRAINING WITH KETTLEBELLS

- requires only 1 piece of equipment
- can be done almost anywhere
- is time effective, allowing you to get an overall workout in a short time
- combines cardio and strength training
- requires you to use your core and other major muscle groups
- boosts metabolism and burns fat even after the workout is over
- improves focus and coordination

Practice each of the following exercises, concentrating on proper form, prior to engaging in a workout.

SWINGS

muscle focus: quadriceps, hamstrings, abdominal muscles, glutes, latissimi dorsi, and deltoids

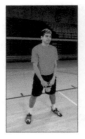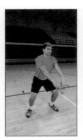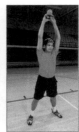

Swings

- Hold the kettlebell handle with both hands. Relax your arms in front of you.
- Place your feet shoulder-width apart.
- In a single motion, bend your knees (make sure your knees do not go past your toes) and bend at the hips to bring the kettlebell between your legs behind you.
- In another single motion, straighten your legs and hips as the kettlebell swings up to chest height.
- Always keep your arms straight.

SQUATTING SHOULDER PRESSES

muscle focus: quadriceps, hamstrings, deltoids, and triceps

- Hold the kettlebell by the handle with your right hand. Place your left hand on top of your right hand.
- Hold the kettlebell at chest height in front of the center of your chest.

- Stand with your feet shoulder-width apart.
- Bend your knees and lower your glutes toward the ground so that you are in a squatting position. Make sure that your knees do not go over your toes.
- In a single motion, straighten your knees and hips as you lift the kettlebell with your right arm up straight up in the air. Release your left hand.
- Rotate your shoulder and wrist so that the fingers of your fist face forward.
- Come back down into the squatting position while bringing the kettlebell back down to your chest where you started.
- After completing the repetitions with your right hand, switch to your left hand.

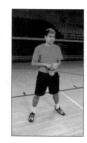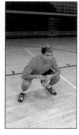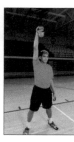

Squatting shoulder presses

LUNGE TWIST

muscle focus: abdominal muscles, erector spinae, hamstrings, and glutes

- Hold the kettlebell by the handle with your right hand. Place your left hand on top of your right hand.
- Hold the kettlebell at chest height in front of the center of your chest.
- Stand with your feet shoulder-width apart.

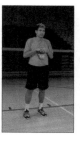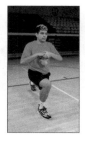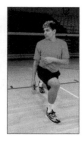

Lunge Twist

- In a single motion, step forward with your right foot. Bend your right knee so that it is over top of your toes but not past them. Your left knee should bend so that it is almost touching the ground and your heel is off the ground. This is a lunge position.
- In another single motion, bring the kettlebell from your chest down to the side of your right thigh while twisting your torso to the right.
- Come back up to the starting position.
- After completing the repetitions to the right, switch to perform repetitions to the left.

SIDE LUNGES WITH BICEPS CURLS

muscle focus: quadriceps, hamstrings, glutei maximi, adductors, hip flexors, and biceps

- Stand with your feet together.
- Hold the kettlebell with your right hand, holding your arm down at your side.
- With your left leg, step out to the side, keeping your right leg straight. Keep your left foot and ankle in line with your thigh. Bend your left knee, making sure that your knee does not go past your toes. This position is a side lunge.

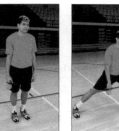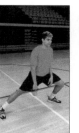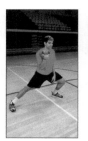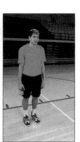

Side lunges with biceps curls

- Hang your arms so that the kettlebell is between your legs.
- While lunging to the left, bring the kettlebell up to chest height, bending at your elbow and keeping your wrist straight.
- Lower the kettlebell back down. Bring your left leg back to the starting position.
- After completing the repetitions lunging to the left, switch to the other side.

TRICEPS LIFTS

muscle focus: triceps

- Stand with your feet shoulder-width apart.
- Start by holding the kettlebell with your right hand. Lift the kettlebell straight above your head.
- Bend your right arm until the kettlebell rests near the back of your shoulder.
- Lift the kettlebell straight up above your head.
- Return to the starting position.
- After completing the repetitions on the right, switch to the other side.

ROWS

muscle focus: back muscles, latissimi dorsi

- Stand with your feet shoulder-width apart and your knees slightly bent.
- Hold the kettlebell with your right hand, holding your right arm down at your side.
- Bend slightly forward at the waist
- Bend your elbow to lift the kettlebell to chest height.
- Return to the starting position.
- After completing the repetitions with your right hand, switch to the other side.

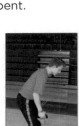
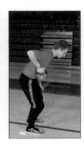
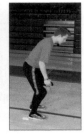

Triceps lifts

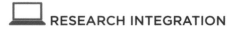

Rows

Have a trusted adult or friend evaluate you for correct form for the previous exercises. Did you respond positively to the feedback?

Reciprocate and evaluate your friend. Were you able to provide feedback in a positive manner?

The following is a suggested use of kettlebells in a combination strength-building and aerobic workout. Exercise to your level of fitness.

- Warm up before your workout. Cool down after your workout.
- Perform each kettlebell exercise 2 to 3 days per week. Do not exercise the same muscle group on consecutive days.
- Begin with 15 seconds per exercise per side. Increase to 30 seconds per exercise per side when the current time is too easy.
- Your goal should be to reach 3 sets of 30 seconds per exercise per side.

 RESEARCH INTEGRATION

Research kettlebell workouts.

♥ HEALTH INTEGRATION

Count your pulse to determine if you are exercising in your personal target heart rate zone. Apply the results to your overall fitness plan.

STRENGTH-TRAINING PROGRAM: USING WHAT YOU HAVE LEARNED

Skeletal muscles that are not used and not exercised become weak. Strength training, or resistance training, builds muscular strength and endurance. Applying tension to a muscle builds its strength. Fibers that make up your muscles break down during the exercise phase. After your workout, when your muscles are resting, the muscle fibers repair and strengthen. It is recommended that you allow 24 hours between strength training the same muscle group to allow the muscle fibers to repair and strengthen.

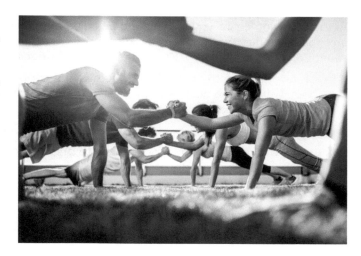

The purpose of this lesson is to encourage you to design your personal strength-training program and to perform exercises 2 to 3 days per week to obtain health benefits. A certified trainer should help you set up a balanced, effective strength-training program.

 CAUTION: Have a certified trainer plan for you and supervise you when you are working with weights.

STRENGTH-TRAINING PROGRAM

There are a variety of exercises from which to choose. Do strength exercises for the muscles of your upper body, lower body, and core. Opposing muscles (antagonistic muscles), such as biceps and triceps, should be equally trained because they work together. Choose the intensity of the exercise to fit your fitness level. For example, if you are struggling doing a right-angle push-up, switch to a knee push-up. Limit excuses and make a commitment to exercise!

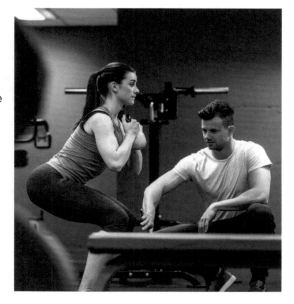

STRENGTH-TRAINING EXERCISE IDEAS

Weightlifting machines: You can use large stationary machines like those typically found in gyms.

Free weights: You can use free-weight equipment such as dumbbells, barbells, medicine balls, kettlebells, resistance bands, and weighted ropes to perform strength-training exercises.

Pilates or yoga: Pilates and yoga sessions are excellent workouts for muscle lengthening and muscle strengthening.

Personal workouts: You can use your own body weight as a source of resistance and create your own strength-training workouts. Create a personal workout by blending basic strength-building exercises such as sit-ups, push-ups, pull-ups, planks, and so on, and design the intensity and duration of each exercise according to your level of fitness. Include upper-body, lower-body, and core exercises in your workout. Perform your personal routine for some or all your strength-training workouts.

MUSCULAR STRENGTH AND MUSCULAR ENDURANCE SAMPLE WORKOUT

The following workout regimen is strictly an example of how to use the FITT principle to increase muscular strength and muscular endurance. The exercises are described in the Flexibility section, Muscular Endurance section, and PE Equipment Kit section of your PE Manual.

In the following chart, you will find a block plan for a weekly schedule based on increasing your muscular strength and muscular endurance. The chart includes the days of the week, muscle groups, exercises, sets and repetitions (for example, 3 · 10 = 3 sets of 10 repetitions), and the type of equipment used.

There is a column on the chart for you to design your personal workout. You can use fitness equipment or your own body weight. The plan you design should be for your fitness level. Personalized exercise plans work for all fitness levels and body types.

- Have a certified trainer plan and supervise you when you are working with weights.
- Before working out, warm up properly to prepare your body. The warm-up should increase your heart rate, breathing rate, and body temperature.
- Never begin vigorous exercise with cold muscles.
- Cool down after working out to allow your body to return to its baseline.

Warm-up: Complete 3 sets of this warm-up before exercising.

Exercise	Duration
• basic jump rope	• 1 minute
• high knees	• 30 seconds
• forward arm circles	• 30 seconds
• backward arm circles	• 30 seconds
• rear kicks	• 30 seconds

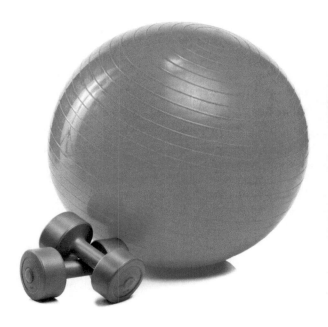

Day	Muscle Group	Exercise Sample	Sets/ Reps	Equipment	Personal Workout for Each Muscle Group
Mon. Wed.	chest shoulders	chest presses	3 · 10	resistance band/ fitness ball	
		lateral raises	3 · 15	resistance band	
		squatting shoulder presses	3 · 10 right 3 · 10 left	kettlebell	
		swings	3 · 10	kettlebell	
		wide-arm push-ups	3 · 15	body weight	
Mon. Wed.	biceps triceps	triceps extensions	3 · 15	resistance band/ fitness ball	
		biceps hammer curls	3 · 15	resistance band	
		triceps lifts	3 · 10 right 3 · 10 left	kettlebell	
		side lunges with bicep curls	3 · 10 right 3 · 10 left	kettlebell	
		triceps push-ups (narrow push-ups)	3 · 10	body weight	
Tue. Thur.	legs	leg extensions	3 · 15	fitness ball	
		hamstring curls	3 · 15	fitness ball	
		leg extensions	3 · 15	resistance band	
		calf raises	3 · 15	resistance band	
		swings	3 · 10	kettlebell	
		lunges	3 · 10	body weight	
Tue. Thur.	back	back extensions	3 · 15	fitness ball	
		seated rows	3 · 15	resistance band	
		rows	3 · 10	kettlebell	
		pull-ups	3 · 10	body weight	
Mon. Wed. Fri.	core	crunches	3 · 15	fitness ball	
		twists	3 · 15	fitness ball	
		lunge twists	3 · 10	kettlebell	
		planks	3 · 30 seconds	body weight	

Cool-down: Complete this cool-down after exercising.

Exercise	Duration
• hamstring stretch	• 30 seconds
• quadriceps stretch	• 30 seconds
• shoulder/triceps stretch	• 30 seconds
• side stretch	• 30 seconds
• lower back/hip stretch	• 30 seconds
• groin stretch	• 30 seconds

List at least 1 response to each of the following questions about strength training.

Question	Response
What positive emotional response did you experience by participating in strength training?	
What type of strength training do you enjoy the most?	
How would the previously mentioned activity lead to good physical and mental health?	

🖥 RESEARCH INTEGRATION

Research and describe isometric, concentric, and eccentric contractions in a squat.

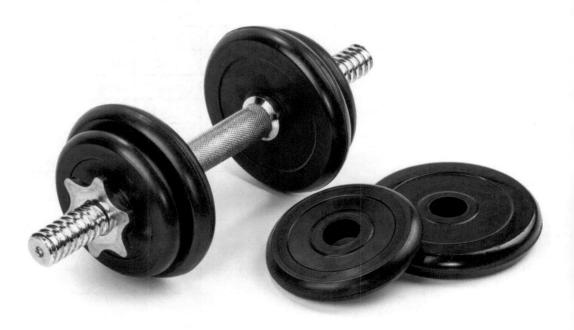

CROSS-TRAINING CARDIOVASCULAR AND STRENGTH CIRCUIT: USING WHAT YOU HAVE LEARNED

For a combination cardiovascular and strength-building workout, you can do a cross-training circuit. This cross-training circuit alternates strength exercises with aerobic movements. Cross-training saves time by giving you a single workout that has both strength and aerobic benefits. It is important for you to set your own goals based on your ability level and determine your intensity and duration based on your individual target heart rate zone.

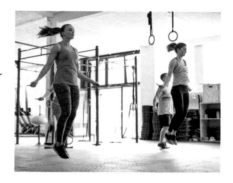

The purpose of this lesson is to encourage you to create and implement a cross-training circuit workout. The workout would be included in the recommended 60 minutes of daily physical activity and would count as both an aerobic and a strength workout. **The Cardiovascular Endurance section of this manual includes the target heart rate zone formula and the Borg Rating of Perceived Exertion Scale to help you to determine if you are exercising for heart health.** You can also use available technology to monitor your pulse rate and intensity.

 CAUTION: Do not overinflate the ball.

CROSS-TRAINING CIRCUIT WORKOUT: CARDIOVASCULAR AND STRENGTH

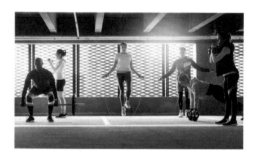

Review the following example and use the information to establish a workout regimen that fits into your schedule. Adhere to the FITT principle (frequency, intensity, time, and type of exercise). This workout requires a jump rope, fitness ball, resistance bands, and kettlebell. You should have a mat or cushioned surface for sit-ups and push-ups.

SAMPLE CROSS-TRAINING CIRCUIT WORKOUT

Build cardiovascular endurance, strength, and flexibility in a cross-training circuit workout using exercises from the appropriate sections of your PE Manual: Cardiovascular Endurance, Muscle Strength, Muscle Endurance, and Flexibility. Review the Aerobic Exercise and Proper Nutrition, Jump Rope, Fitness Ball, Resistance Bands, and Kettlebells sections in your PE Manual to practice correct forms for the skills.

Warm-up: Perform 5 to 10 minutes of light cardio to increase your heart rate, breathing rate, and body temperature. Do some dynamic stretches to increase flexibility.

Perform each exercise for 30 seconds. Rest and hydrate when necessary. Set the workout to music.

1. jumping jacks
2. sit-ups
3. high knees
4. kettlebell swings
5. jump rope
6. resistance band biceps hammer curls
7. rear kicks
8. fitness ball back extensions
9. jog in place
10. right-angle push-ups
11. jump rope
12. kettlebell squatting right shoulder presses
13. ¼-squat jumps
14. kettlebell squatting left shoulder presses
15. march in place
16. resistance band seated rows
17. jump rope
18. fitness ball crunches
19. burpees
20. kettlebell lunge twists (alternate sides)

Repeat for a 20-minute workout.

Cool-down: Walk slowly until your heart rate, breathing rate, and body temperature have returned to baseline. Do some static stretches to increase flexibility.

CREATE A PERSONAL WORKOUT

Use the cross-training information to create a personal circuit workout you would enjoy.

CREATE A PERSONAL WORKOUT FOR A PERSON WITH A JOB

Objective: to overcome exercise barriers you may face when you are finished with school and ready for a career

Create a cross-training workout for a family member who works full time. A job is often a barrier to exercise, and many people have trouble fitting exercise into their schedules. Try to help your family member find the time to exercise.

- Make sure the family member has a doctor's approval to exercise.
- Interview the family member to evaluate the level of fitness and plan accordingly.
- Use exercises and equipment that the family member prefers. A beginner may need to march in place and use the resistance bands only.
- Review the family member's daily and weekly schedules to find at least 3 available times for regular exercise.
- Establish an exercise plan that may work for your family member.

RESEARCH INTEGRATION

Research good health and its connection to positive job performance.

HEALTH INTEGRATION

Use available technology to monitor your pulse rate and intensity. Apply the results to your overall fitness plan.

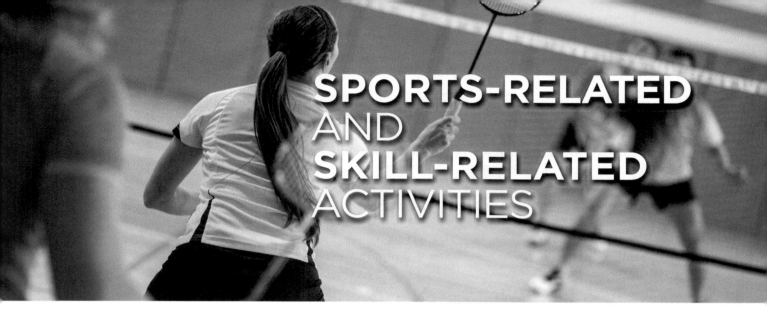

SPORTS-RELATED AND SKILL-RELATED ACTIVITIES

FITNESS TIP: Prior to beginning your physical education activities, read the following safety information that applies to every lesson, review the timeline, and review the assessment rubric.

SAFETY ALERT: Before you exercise, make sure that you are properly warmed up and have enough room to perform each activity. Wear proper equipment and follow activity-specific safety rules. Stay hydrated and take breaks as needed. Exercise only if you are healthy, and always exercise at your own pace. If an exercise starts to hurt, if you feel dizzy, or if you feel light-headed, stop the exercise completely and get help. Upon completion of any workout, cool down and stretch.

TIMELINE

Review all of the activity information before beginning. Use the scoring rubrics as assessment tools. You may ask a trusted adult or friend to observe your performance and provide feedback. Progress according to your skill level. The time that it takes you to complete a module will depend on your personal progress.

Practice and assess the first skill until competent.

Continue to progress until you have practiced and assessed each skill until competent.

Apply skills in a game situation.

ASSESSMENT RUBRIC

You will find a rubric assessment tool following some of the basic skills. Use this tool to evaluate and score your progress in learning the elements of a new skill.

SKILL	PROGRESSING	COMPETENT	PROFICIENT
skill 1	1 or 2 of the elements	3 or 4 out of 5 elements	all elements met

BADMINTON

Badminton is a sport that is played by striking a shuttlecock, or birdie, with a racket over a net. This striking activity helps you develop concentration, hand-eye coordination, and footwork. You may play badminton as a competitive sport or as an opportunity for social play.

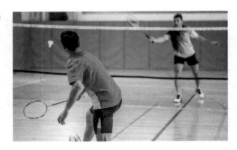

Badminton is considered a lifetime sport because it is not hard to learn and not physically hard on the body. The equipment is easy to set up. You can find badminton games in your local area or set up your own league.

The purpose of this lesson is for you to practice badminton skills and encourage participation in games for a lifetime of physical activity.

⚠ **CAUTION: Make sure that nobody is close to you before you swing your racket. Do not walk into the path of another person who is swinging a racket.**

BADMINTON STROKES

READY POSITION

- Bending your knees, stand with your feet shoulder-width apart.
- Keep your head up and your weight on the balls of your feet.
- Hold the racket in your dominant hand.
- React quickly.
- Anticipate direction.

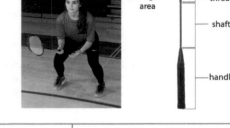

SKILL	PROGRESSING	COMPETENT	PROFICIENT
ready position	1 or 2 of the elements	3 or 4 out of 5 elements	all elements met

HANDSHAKE GRIP (V GRIP)

- Hold the handle of the racket in your dominant hand in a handshake grip.
- Form a V with your thumb and forefinger.
- Point the racket away from your body at waist height.
- Placing the head of the racket vertical to the ground, point the handle toward your belly button.
- Support the throat of racket lightly with your non-dominant hand.

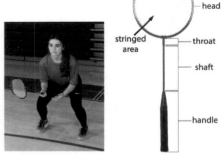

SKILL	PROGRESSING	COMPETENT	PROFICIENT
handshake grip	1 or 2 of the elements	3 or 4 out of 5 elements	all elements met

UNDERHAND STROKE

- Hold the racket so that the head is facing the ground and is under the birdie.
- Step forward with your non-dominant foot.
- Flick your wrist to hit the birdie with the center of the racket.
- Rotate your forearm so that it faces upward on contact.
- Follow through to your target.

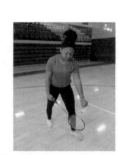

SKILL	PROGRESSING	COMPETENT	PROFICIENT
underhand stroke	1 or 2 of the elements	3 or 4 out of 5 elements	all elements met

OVERHAND STROKE

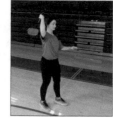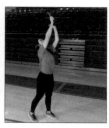

- Bend your elbow so that your racket is in a back-scratching position.
- Reach up and position the racket under the birdie.
- Flick your wrist to hit the birdie with the center of the racket. Extend your arm when you make contact.
- Follow through to your target.

SKILL	PROGRESSING	COMPETENT	PROFICIENT
overhand stroke	1 or 2 of the elements	3 out of 4 elements	all elements met

FOREHAND STROKE

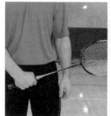

- The racket should be on the same side of your body as your dominant hand.
- Face the palm of your hand forward.
- Rotate your hips in the direction that you are hitting.
- Extend your arm and flick your wrist to hit the birdie.
- Point the face of the racket up to get the birdie over the net.
- Follow through to your target.

SKILL	PROGRESSING	COMPETENT	PROFICIENT
forehand stroke	1, 2, or 3 of the elements	4 or 5 out of 6 elements	all elements met

BACKHAND STROKE

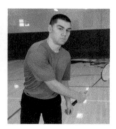

Create a 5-step or 6-step rubric for the backstroke using the following information. Keep in mind that the concept of rotation is important to the backstroke.

Rotate the racket and extend it across your body. Rotate your feet and shoulders in the same direction as the racket. Rotate your hips in the same direction as you are swinging the racket. The back of your hand (your knuckles) faces forward. Flick your wrist as you hit the shuttlecock with the center of the racket. Complete the stroke by following through your swing.

UNDERHAND SERVE

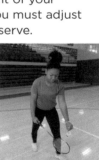

You may perform a low or high underhand serve. The low serve sends the shuttlecock to the front of your opponent's court. The high serve sends the shuttlecock to the back of your opponent's court. You must adjust the power of the shot and the arc—light and low for the low serve or hard and high for the long serve.

- Hold the racket in your dominant hand with the head of the racket pointed down toward the ground.
- Hold the birdie by the feathers in your non-dominant hand.
- Step forward with your non-dominant foot.
- Drop the birdie slightly below your waist.
- Hit the birdie with the center of the racket. Flick your wrist when you make contact.
- Follow through to your target.

SKILL	PROGRESSING	COMPETENT	PROFICIENT
underhand serve	1, 2, or 3 of the elements	4 or 5 out of 6 elements	all elements met

PRACTICE THE STROKES

Practice independently by holding the birdie by the feathers in your non-dominant hand. Hold the racket appropriately for the stroke. Drop the birdie and make contact with the racket.

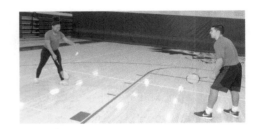

- First, practice each stroke without using the birdie.

- Then, practice each stroke using the birdie.

- Practice the underhand stroke by holding the head of the racket down toward the floor. Drop the birdie and make contact with the racket slightly below your waist. Flick your wrist and make contact with the birdie. How many times you can hit the birdie in a row?

- Strike the birdie toward a target using the various strokes.

- Strike the birdie toward a target using different levels of force.

- Aim and strike the birdie to the left of a target.

- Aim and strike the birdie to the right of a target.

- Practice with a partner. Hit the birdie back and forth with a partner. How many times can you hit it back and forth?

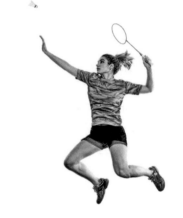

BADMINTON SHOTS

CLEAR SHOT

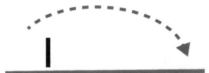

The overhead and underhand defensive clear shots arc or lob the birdie high and push your opponent to the rear of the court. This slows down the game to give you a chance to get ready for your opponent's shot.

DROP SHOT

The overhand drop shot keeps the pace of the game the same. It is sent at a steep angle, forcing your opponent to rush forward.

SMASH SHOT

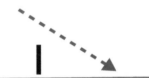

The overhand smash shot is a powerful hit at a severe angle. You need to contact the birdie high, which may even require you to jump to hit the birdie. This shot is often used to end a game.

PRACTICE THE SHOTS

Practice the shots independently by tossing the birdie at the appropriate height for each shot. Practice with a set-up net.

- Practice the clear shot with both the underhand and overhand strokes.

- Practice the drop shot.

- Practice the smash shot.

- Practice with a partner. Have a partner toss the birdie for you. Practice each shot and then switch roles. Be supportive and encouraging to your partner.

- Strike the shuttlecock to your partner using different levels of speed. Make each strike for accuracy using the necessary speed for success. Discuss with your partner the speed you needed to use for each shot to achieve accuracy.

BADMINTON GAME

- Badminton is usually a singles game with 2 players or a doubles game with 4 players.
- Start with an underhand serve from the right side of the court. Serve from behind the end line to your opponent on the left.
- If you hit the birdie onto your opponent's side and your opponent cannot return it, you win the rally—which is the series of consecutive strokes back and forth until a point is earned—and get a point.
- Now, serve from the left side of the court.
- When your score is an even number, serve behind the right end line. When your score is an odd number, serve behind the left end line.
- In a doubles game, the same player on a team serves throughout a rally, alternating serving sides until losing the rally. The opponent then serves until the rally is lost. Partners alternate turns serving.
- You may only hit the birdie 1 time on each side.
- You lose a rally if you or your racket touch the net.
- You lose a rally if you hit the birdie into the net, hit it out of bounds, or miss it when you swing.

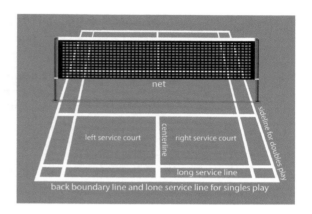

DEMONSTRATE POSITIVE GAME BEHAVIOR

- Follow the game rules.
- Call for the shot, when appropriate, to identify that you are going to hit the shot. This is for safety and game efficiency.
- Be supportive and encouraging to your teammate.
- Treat your opponents with respect.

SKILL	PROGRESSING	COMPETENT	PROFICIENT
game behavior	1 or 2 of the elements	3 or 4 out of 5 elements	all elements met

HOW TO SCORE

- You score a point when you hit the birdie over the net and onto your opponent's side before your opponent can return it. You also score a point when your opponent hits the birdie either into the net or out of bounds.
- A match consists of 3 games of 21 points.
- If you win a rally, you score 1 point.
- If the score is tied at 20 points, the first team to score 2 points wins the game.
- If the score is tied at 29 points, the first team to score its 30th point wins the game.
- The winning team serves first in the next game.

RATE YOUR ENJOYMENT OF BADMINTON

On a scale from 1 to 4, where 1 is not enjoyable and 4 is very enjoyable, rate this activity.

1	It was not enjoyable, and I will not participate again.
2	It was not enjoyable, but I will participate again for exercise.
3	It was enjoyable, and I will play again.
4	It was very enjoyable, and I will initiate future games.

RESEARCH INTEGRATION

Research the historical and cultural role of badminton in society.

HEALTH INTEGRATION

Count your pulse during and after playing badminton to determine if you are exercising in your personal target heart rate zone. Apply the results to your overall fitness plan. Keep in mind that many people choose to complete aerobic workouts by playing in casual games with friends.

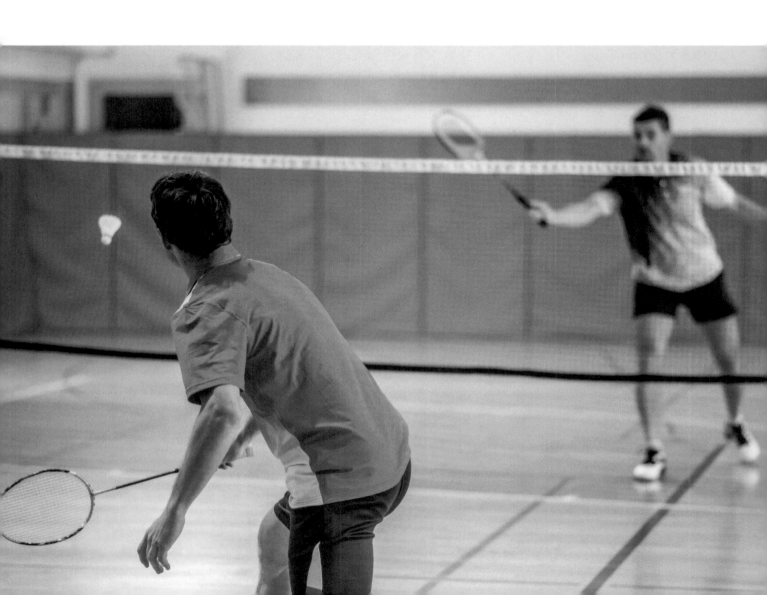

BASKETBALL

Basketball is an official team sport played from the elementary level through the professional level. Playing the official game requires a high level of skill and fitness. Recreational or intramural basketball is for players who enjoy the game but do not want to play in an official capacity. Former high school basketball players who do not play official college basketball often play college intramural basketball along with other basketball enthusiasts.

Basketball is usually not considered a lifetime sport due to the physicality of the game, however there are adult leagues that provide the opportunity to play a slowed, less physical version of the game. Playing basketball at any level is a great way to complete a moderate to intense aerobic workout.

The official game of basketball is played by 2 opposing teams that are each made up of 5 players. The players play on a basketball court. Points are scored when the ball goes through a basketball hoop. There are also other basketball games and activities that you can enjoy, such as independent shooting and dribbling challenges, shooting games, and half-court games of 1-on-1, 2-on-2, and 3-on-3 versions of the official game.

The purpose of this lesson is for you to participate in aerobic exercise and in skill-building activities. Game participation will depend upon the availability of a facility and players. Any time you play a game of basketball, be sure to follow game rules, communicate with teammates in a positive and effective manner, and exhibit appropriate behavior with your team and the opposing team.

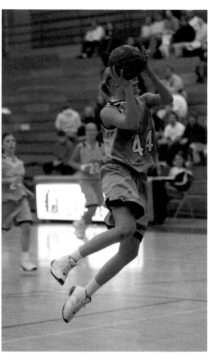

 CAUTION: Do not overinflate the basketball.

DRIBBLING SKILLS
Learning to dribble efficiently with both your right hand and left hand is necessary for playing a game of basketball.

BASIC STATIONARY DRIBBLING

- Using your dominant hand, spread your fingers and push the ball down gently toward the ground with your finger pads. Do not slap the ball.
- Let the ball bounce on the ground and come back to your hand. Do not let the ball bounce higher than your waist.
- Flex your wrist and push the ball back to the ground with your finger pads. This is a continuous movement; do not catch the ball after every bounce.
- Dribble with your head up.
- Keep your eyes looking forward, not watching the ball.
- Repeat dribbling the ball with your non-dominant hand.

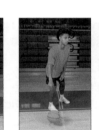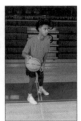

Basic stationary dribbling

SKILL	PROGRESSING	COMPETENT	PROFICIENT
right-handed dribble	1 or 2 of the elements	3 or 4 out of 5 elements	all elements met
left-handed dribble	1 or 2 of the elements	3 or 4 out of 5 elements	all elements met

STATIONARY DRIBBLING

- See how many times you can dribble the ball with your dominant hand without losing control of the ball.
- Push the ball down with different amounts of force to make it bounce at different levels.
- Try pushing the ball with a soft force so that it bounces at a low level.
- Try pushing the ball with a hard force so that it bounces at a high level.
- Dribble with your dominant hand.
- Dribble with your non-dominant hand.
- Dribble the ball from 1 hand to the other.

CREATE A PRACTICE PLAN TO IMPROVE DRIBBLING WHILE MOVING

- Include practice for both hands.
- Include concepts of speed and direction

CROSSOVER DRIBBLING

- Set up disc cones about 2 feet apart in a zigzag pattern.
- Start at the first cone and dribble the basketball to the next cone using the hand with which you are most comfortable.
- Reach the second cone and do a crossover (switch hands) in order to move on to the next cone.
- Complete a crossover at each cone until you have reached the last cone.
- Turn around and do the same thing back to the first cone.
- Continue this until you feel comfortable with dribbling and crossing over.

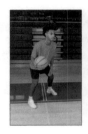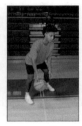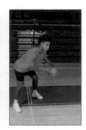

Crossover dribbling

CHALLENGE SKILLS

The following challenge skills are for those who are proficient in basic stationary dribbling. The challenge drills reinforce dribbling effectively with both the right hand and left hand. Practice as appropriate to your needs.

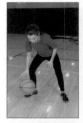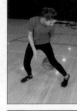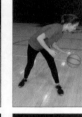
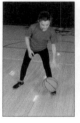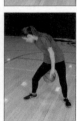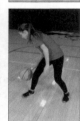

FIGURE-8 DRIBBLE

- Stand with your legs wide and your knees bent.
- Dribble the ball through your legs and around your ankles in a figure-8 pattern.
- Alternate hands while dribbling.
- Reverse directions for an advanced challenge.

Figure-8 dribble

FRONT 2, BACK 2 DRIBBLE

- Stand with your legs shoulder-width apart and your knees bent.
- Dribble twice in front of your body. Alternate hands while dribbling, but do not put both hands on the ball at the same time.
- Switch hands behind you, and dribble twice behind your body. This is a 1, 2, 3, 4 count.
- Move while making quarter turns for an advanced challenge.

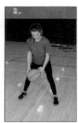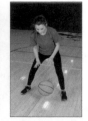
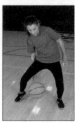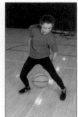

Front, back 2 dribble

2-BALL DRIBBLE

- Dribble 2 balls at the same time.
- Keep the balls at the same height.

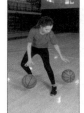

2-ball dribble

2-BALL HIGH-LOW DRIBBLE

- Dribble a ball with each hand.
- Dribble the ball on the right high while simultaneously dribbling the ball on the left low.
- Dribble the ball on the right low while simultaneously dribbling the ball on the left high.

2-ball high-low dribble

2-BALL FIGURE-8 DRIBBLE

- Dribble 1 ball between your legs while circling the other ball around 1 of your legs.
- When the ball that is circling your leg reaches the middle point between your legs, switch it with the ball between your legs.

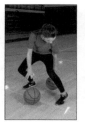 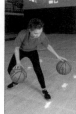

Check off the challenge skills that you have mastered.

_____FIGURE-8 DRIBBLE

_____FRONT 2, BACK 2 DRIBBLE

_____2-BALL DRIBBLE

_____2-BALL HIGH-LOW DRIBBLE

_____2-BALL FIGURE-8 DRIBBLE

2-ball figure-8 dribble

PASSING SKILLS

There are 2 common passes that are used in the game of basketball. The bounce pass and chest pass are used to move the ball to your teammates. You can practice these passes with a partner or against a wall.

BOUNCE PASS AND CATCH

BOUNCE PASS

- Stand facing the target.
- Hold the ball with both hands at chest level and your elbows out.
- Step toward the target.
- Extend both arms toward the target. The ball should bounce on the floor between you and the target before it reaches the target.

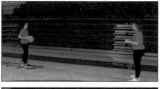

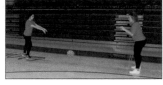

Bounce pass

CATCH

- When you are catching, watch the ball all the way until it reaches your hands.
- Move your hands toward the ball.
- Give with the ball (pull the ball slightly toward you) as it hits your hands to make a soft catch.

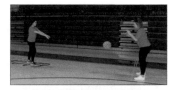

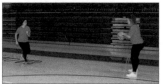

Catch

SKILL	PROGRESSING	COMPETENT	PROFICIENT
bounce pass	1 or 2 of the elements	3 out of 4 elements	all elements met
bounce-pass catch	1 of the elements	2 out of 3 elements	all elements met

CHEST PASS AND CATCH

CHEST PASS

- Stand facing the target.
- Hold the ball with both hands at chest level and your elbows out.
- Step toward the target.
- Extend both arms toward the target. The ball should not bounce on the floor.

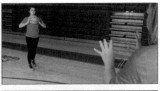
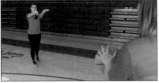
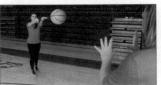

Chest pass

CATCH

- When you are catching, watch the ball all the way until it reaches your hands.
- Move your hands toward the ball.
- Give with the ball (pull the ball slightly toward you) as it hits your hands to make a soft catch.

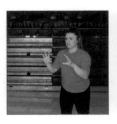
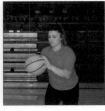
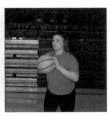

Catch

SKILL	PROGRESSING	COMPETENT	PROFICIENT
chest pass	1 or 2 of the elements	3 out of 4 elements	all elements met
chest-pass catch	1 of the elements	2 out of 3 elements	all elements met

PRACTICE PASSING WITH A PARTNER

- How many bounce passes can you and your partner do in a row?
- How many chest passes can you and your partner do in a row?
- Bounce pass to your partner. Your partner will send a chest pass back. Switch roles.
- Bounce pass as you and your partner move down the court.
- Chest pass as you and your partner move down the court.

BASIC SHOOTING SKILLS

BASIC SHOOTING

- Stand facing the hoop with your feet shoulder-width apart and your knees slightly bent.
- Place your dominant hand on the back of the basketball and bend your wrist. Place your non-dominant hand on the side of the ball.
- Place the ball on the finger pads of your dominant hand.
- Use your non-dominant hand as your guide.
- Position your elbow so that it is behind the ball, not out to the side.
- Look at the target—the front of the rim.
- Push your dominant hand toward the target while straightening your legs to give you more power to shoot.
- Shoot the ball toward the target and follow through with your arm and wrist. Snap your wrist as the ball leaves your hand.

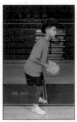
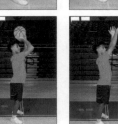

Basic shooting skills

- Remember BEEF.
  - ○ **Balance** the ball in your dominant hand.
  - ○ Place your **elbow** behind the ball, not out to the side.
  - ○ Keep your **eyes** on the target.
  - ○ **Follow** through with a snap of your wrist.

SKILL	PROGRESSING	COMPETENT	PROFICIENT
BEEF elements	1 or 2 of the elements	3 out of 4 elements	all elements

PRACTICE SHOOTING

- Practice some shooting drills after you become comfortable shooting the basketball.
- Pick different spots on the court, both closer and farther away from the hoop.
- Map out a pattern in your mind as to what spots you will go to first, second, third, and so on.
- Practice shooting from each spot.
- Start on 1 side of the hoop and move around to the other side.
- Work back around to the starting position.

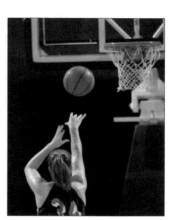

SHOOTING GAME

- You will need 2 or more players.
- The goal of the game is to be the first player to spell S-P-O-R-T.
- Determine who will go first and the order of the rest of the players.
- The first person chooses a spot to shoot from.
- If the player shoots and makes the basket, the player gets a letter and goes to the back of the line to wait for their next turn.
- The rest of the players must shoot from the first player's spot and make the basket to get a letter.
- The first player keeps the role of choosing a spot until they miss a shot.
- If the first player misses, they do not get a letter and they go to the back of the line.
- The second player in line selects a spot to shoot from and the above procedure is repeated.
- Continue to play until a player gets all of the letters to spell S-P-O-R-T.

OFFENSIVE AND DEFENSIVE SKILLS

Agile footwork is an essential component of basketball. Practice footwork skills to improve your offensive and defensive play.

OFFENSIVE SKILLS

Practice each of the following skills, concentrating on proper form, prior to using them in a game or other competition.

OFFENSIVE READY POSITION

The ready position allows a player to move quickly in any direction. It is used for both offense and defense.

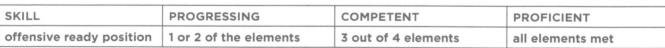

- With your elbows out, hold the ball with both hands to the dominant side of your chest.
- Bend your knees to keep your body low.
- Stand with your feet shoulder-width apart.
- Keep your head up and your weight on the balls of your feet.

SKILL	PROGRESSING	COMPETENT	PROFICIENT
offensive ready position	1 or 2 of the elements	3 out of 4 elements	all elements met

PIVOT

The purpose of the pivot in a basketball game is for you to look around and decide to dribble, pass, or shoot.

- Plant 1 foot, which will be your pivot foot, in place on the ground.
- Place your weight on the balls of your feet.
- Slide your non-pivot foot and rotate your body 180 degrees.
- Repeat this exercise with your other foot.

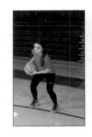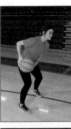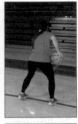
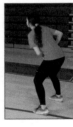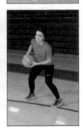

SKILL	PROGRESSING	COMPETENT	PROFICIENT
pivot	1 of the elements	2 out of 3 elements	all elements

FAKE

- Look in 1 direction, and then pass or move in another direction.
- Stay on the balls of your feet.
- Move quickly.

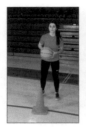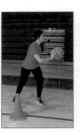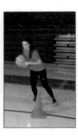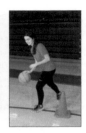

SKILL	PROGRESSING	COMPETENT	PROFICIENT
fake	1 of the elements	2 out of 3 elements	all elements

GIVE AND GO

The purpose of the give and go in a basketball game is to for you to pass the ball to a teammate and to quickly relocate so that you can receive a pass.

- Pass the ball to a teammate.
- Move quickly to relocate and support your offense.
- Indicate (call out) that you are ready and open to receive the ball.
- Catch the ball.

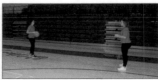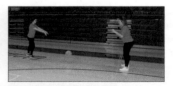
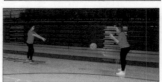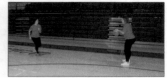
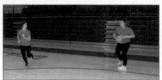

SKILL	PROGRESSING	COMPETENT	PROFICIENT
give and go	1 or 2 of the elements	3 out of 4 elements	all elements

DEFENSIVE SKILLS

Practice each of the following skills, concentrating on proper form, prior to using them in a game or other competition.

DEFENSIVE SLIDES

The purpose of defensive slides in basketball is to keep up with your opponent and to legally take the ball or legally disrupt the opponent's pass or shot.

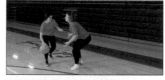
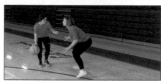
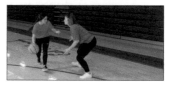

- Place your weight on the balls of your feet.
- Slide to the side with quick steps.
- Do not cross your feet.
- Keep your knees bent.
- Face your hips toward your opponent.
- Hold your hands up at chest level.
- Keep your eyes on your opponent's waistline.
- Stay with your opponent.
- Anticipate and react quickly to your opponent's movements.

SKILL	PROGRESSING	COMPETENT	PROFICIENT
defensive slides	1, 2, 3, 4, or 5 of the elements	6, 7, or 8 out of 9 elements	all elements met

PRACTICE OFFENSIVE AND DEFENSIVE SKILLS

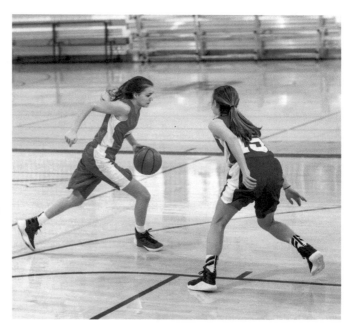

- Practice the **pivot** by planting your right foot and rotating your left foot until you feel comfortable with the movement.
- Practice the **pivot** by planting your left foot and rotating your right foot until you feel comfortable with the movement.
- Practice the **give and go** with a partner and a defender. Pass the ball, quickly relocate, and then receive the pass, avoiding the defender.
- Practice the **fake** independently. Set up a cone as a decoy. Fake the pass toward the cone and then pass to your partner until you feel comfortable with the movement.
- Practice the **fake** with a partner defending you. Dribble, fake, and move in another direction to get around the defensive player. Do this until you feel comfortable with the fake.
- Practice the **defensive slide** with a partner. As your partner dribbles, defensive slide to try to prevent them from making a successful pass or shot. Do this until you feel comfortable with the defensive slide.

BASKETBALL GAMES

OFFICIAL GAME

ABOUT THE GAME

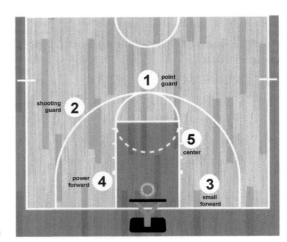

- The game is played by 2 opposing teams of 5 players each. Each team has a point guard, a shooting guard, a small forward, a power forward, and a center.
- The game is played on a basketball court 92 feet long and 50 feet wide.
- A 10-foot-high basketball hoop with a net is at each end of the court.
- The object of the game is to move the ball down the court by passing or dribbling and to score by shooting the ball through the opposing team's hoop.
- A high school game is divided into 8-minute quarters of play time with a rest period after 2 quarters of play.
- The team with the most points is the winning team.

PLAYING THE GAME

- The game begins with a jump ball at mid-court. A referee tosses the ball between 2 opposing players.
- The team that possesses the ball is on offense, and the other team is on defense.
- The player with the ball must dribble, pass, or shoot.
- When they are moving with the ball, the player must dribble. When the player stops dribbling, they cannot take any more steps.
- If a player walks without dribbling, the ball is turned over to the opposing team.
- The players on defense try to intercept, or take away, the ball.

DEMONSTRATE POSITIVE GAME BEHAVIOR

- Follow the rules of the game.
- Do not commit a foul or make illegal physical contact against an opposing player.
  - A foul against a non-shooting player results in a turnover, which is a change in possession of the ball between teams.
  - A foul against a shooting player results in the team getting free shots—2 shots for a foul on a player shooting a 2-point shot and 3 shots for a player shooting a 3-point shot.
  - A player who commits 5 fouls is removed from the game.
- Be supportive and encouraging to your teammates.
- Treat your opponents with respect.

SKILL	PROGRESSING	COMPETENT	PROFICIENT
game behavior	1 or 2 of the elements	3 out of 4 elements	all elements met

HOW TO SCORE

- An arc line, referred to as a 3-point line, is marked on the basketball court.
  - A player who makes a basket from behind the 3-point line is awarded 3 points.
  - A player who makes a basket from inside the 3-point line is awarded 2 points.
- Foul shots are worth 1 point each.

DESIGN AND COACH/REFEREE YOUR OWN GAME

Playing a basketball game like 1-on-1 or 2-on-2 allows you to practice your basketball skills and get an aerobic workout when you only have a few players. Use the following information to break down the barrier of not having enough players for an official game and to create a solution.

- Determine if you will play a half-court or full-court game.
- Determine the boundaries.
- Determine who will start with the ball.
- Determine where you will begin.
- Determine what happens after a team scores. Does the opposing team get the ball? Where does the team take it out?
- Establish scoring rules for your game. These can be the same as the official rules.
- Determine who will referee. You can alternate roles for fairness.

Prior to playing your game, establish and review the rules so that everyone understands them. If problems arise, work to solve them in a positive and effective manner. Appreciate different players' abilities. An example of a rule that you may want to decide upon is the boundaries.

Below are our game rules for safety and fairness.
1.
2.
3.
4.
5.

RESEARCH INTEGRATION

1. Research how to do a layup shot.
2. Research local facilities to learn where recreational basketball is played in your community.

HEALTH INTEGRATION

Count your pulse during and after playing basketball to determine if you are exercising in your personal target heart rate zone. Apply the results to your overall fitness plan. Many people choose to complete aerobic workouts by playing in fast-paced games like basketball.

SOCCER

Soccer is a sport that is popular around the globe. The object of the game is to use your feet to dribble, pass, and kick a ball in order to score goals by getting the ball into your opponent's net. Playing soccer is a great way to improve footwork, interact with others, have fun, and complete an aerobic workout.

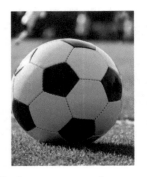

Playing official, competitive soccer requires high skill and fitness levels; however, people of all skill levels enjoy playing casual games of soccer. In most communities, there are soccer leagues for everyone from preschoolers to adults. Students who practice soccer skills are more likely to join a game and exercise outside of PE class. Playing recreational soccer at your age now and into college and your career can help to reduce stress, increase the opportunity to socialize, and count as exercise for good health.

The purpose of this lesson is for you to participate in soccer activities. You will practice skills, learn game rules, be encouraged to communicate with teammates in a positive and effective manner, and be reminded to exhibit appropriate behavior with your team and the opposing team.

 CAUTION: Wear appropriate safety equipment. Do not overinflate the ball.

SOCCER SKILLS

DRIBBLING

Use your peripheral vision, or your side vision, to watch the ball as you dribble it. Dribbling is a series of small, controlled touches that you complete in order to move with the ball in your possession. Dribble the ball with the insides and outsides of your feet as well as with the tops of your feet, where your shoelaces lay. Do not dribble the ball with your toes, otherwise, you risk losing control of the ball.

- Start with the ball positioned in front of you on the ground.
- Dribble forward, keeping the ball close—no more than 3 to 5 feet in front of you.
- Move the ball with the insides, outsides, and/or tops of both of your feet.
- Keep your head up.
- Match your speed to your skill.
- Change directions.

SKILL	PROGRESSING	COMPETENT	PROFICIENT
dribbling	1, 2, or 3 of the elements	4 or 5 out of 6 elements	all elements

PASSING

Passing the ball is an important part of soccer. Players pass the ball to each other in order to keep the other team from gaining control of the ball and to progress the ball up the field toward the other team's goal.

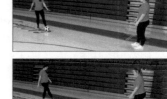
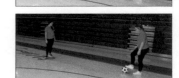

- Start with the soccer ball on the ground, next to the inside of your dominant foot.
- Position the inside of your kicking foot behind the middle of the soccer ball.
- Establish your non-kicking foot slightly behind you.
- Swing your kicking leg back, keeping it straight throughout your entire kick.
- Contact the middle of the ball with the inside of your foot. Follow through your kick with your foot and leg.
- Use appropriate force and direction to keep your pass on target.

SKILL	PROGRESSING	COMPETENT	PROFICIENT
passing	1, 2, or 3 of the elements	4 or 5 out of 6 elements	all elements

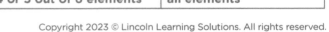

TRAPPING: OPTION 1

Trapping is a way of stopping the ball, receiving a pass, or gaining control of the ball.

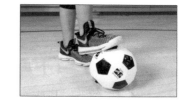

- Start with the ball positioned in front of you on the ground.

- Place your dominant foot on top of the ball. To do this, lift your foot slightly off the ground, keeping your ankle locked and your toes up.

- Repeat this with your non-dominant foot.

SKILL	PROGRESSING	COMPETENT	PROFICIENT
trapping: option 1	1 of the elements	2 out of 3 elements	all elements

TRAPPING: OPTION 2

Trapping is also a way to stop the ball in order to quickly gain control and transition to your next move.

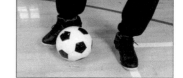

- When the soccer ball comes toward you, turn the ankle of whichever foot you are trapping with so that your instep, or the inside of your foot, is facing forward.

- Cushion the ball with your foot as you stop it lightly, as if you were catching an egg.

- Repeat this with your other foot.

SKILL	PROGRESSING	COMPETENT	PROFICIENT
trapping: option 2	1 of the elements	2 out of 3 elements	all elements

SHOOTING

The purpose of shooting is to get the soccer ball into your opponent's goal by striking it with your foot.

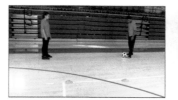
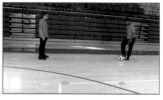
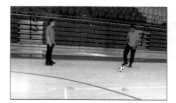
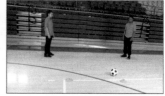

- Place 2 discs about 4 feet apart and 5 feet in front of you. Place the soccer ball on the ground in front of you.

- Stand so that your dominant leg, or kicking leg, is pulled back behind you.

- Place your non-kicking foot alongside the soccer ball, with your toes pointing at the goal that you made.

- Bend the knee of your kicking leg by pulling your foot back. Then, in a single motion, swing your leg forward, straightening your leg and pointing your toes to kick the soccer ball with the top of your foot. Kick the center of the soccer ball with the laces of your shoe, pointing your toes down. You do not want to kick the soccer ball with your toes.

- Follow through your kick, making sure that you finish with your toes pointing toward the goal.

SKILL	PROGRESSING	COMPETENT	PROFICIENT
shooting	1 or 2 of the elements	3 or 4 out of 5 elements	all elements

DEVELOP A PRACTICE PLAN

After you master the basic soccer skills, put them all together in practice drills to refine them. Use cones to set up dribbling pathways and a goal. Keep the following strategies in mind.

- When you are dribbling the soccer ball, keep it close to you.

- When you are passing the ball, kick with the instep of your foot.

- When you are trapping the ball, cushion it as if you were catching an egg.

- When you are shooting the soccer ball, point your toes down and kick the middle of the ball with the top of your foot. Your non-kicking foot should be next to the ball, pointing toward the target. When you follow through, make sure that your kicking toes end up pointing toward the target as well.

Skill	Practice Drill
Example: inside foot dribble	Example: Set up 3 cones 3 feet apart and dribble around them, increasing your speed when able.
inside foot dribble	
outside foot dribble	
front (laces) foot dribble	
trap	
pass	
shoot on goal	

EXTENSION: Coach another person through your personal practice drills.

ADVANCED BALL MANIPULATION SKILLS

The following advanced skills are for those who have mastered the basic skills. The challenge skills are recommended for those who want to improve their footwork.

TOE TAPS

With the ball stationary on the ground, hop onto your right foot and tap the top of the ball with the toes of your left foot. Then, hop onto your left foot and tap the top of the ball with the toes of your right foot. Continue this pattern. How fast can you go?

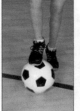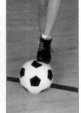

Toe taps

SIDE TO SIDE

With the ball between your feet, move the ball from side to side with the insteps of your feet while taking small hops.

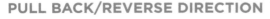

Side to side

PULL BACK/REVERSE DIRECTION

Place your foot on top of the ball. Pull your foot back so that the ball rolls along the bottom of your foot from back to front. This will pull the ball back so that you can make a quick turn to dribble or pass in the opposite direction.

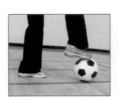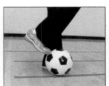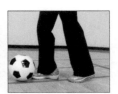

Pull back/Reverse direction

BACKSPIN/CATCH

Position your toes on the top of the ball to start. In a single motion, roll your toes backward and down along the ball to roll the ball back onto your toes.

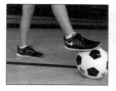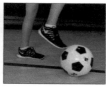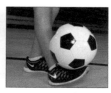

Backspin/Catch

SCISSORS

Swing 1 foot around the ball. Then, swing your other foot around the ball in the opposite direction. Try again, switching the directions that you swing your feet.

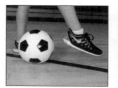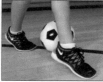

Scissors

KNEE JUGGLE

Drop the ball onto your knee, softly bouncing it back up. Use the same knee or your other knee to bounce the ball. See how many times you can bounce the ball on your knees to keep it from hitting the ground.

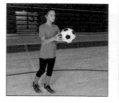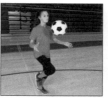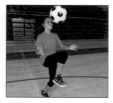

Knee juggle

INSIDE FOOT JUGGLE

Hold up 1 of your feet, bending at the knee to angle the instep of your foot up. Drop the ball and bounce it back up with the instep of your foot. Use the same foot or the instep of your other foot to bounce the ball back up again before it hits the ground. How many times can you juggle the ball with the insides of your feet before it touches the ground?

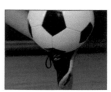

Inside food juggle

OUTSIDE FOOT JUGGLE

Drop the ball softly. Use the outside of 1 of your feet, angling your ankle down, to kick the ball back up. Repeat this with 1 or both of your feet. How long can you juggle the ball without it hitting the ground?

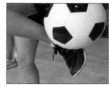

Outside food juggle

TOE JUGGLE

Drop the ball slightly in front of you. Gently kick the ball back up with the top part of your foot. Continue this with 1 or both of your feet to juggle the ball without letting it hit the ground for as long as you can.

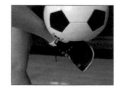

Toe juggle

COMBINATION JUGGLE

Use a combination of your knees and the insides, outsides, and tops of your feet to keep the ball up for as long as you can.

EXTENSION: After mastering the advanced ball manipulation skills, blend them for an aerobic workout. Perform each skill for 1 minute for a 10-minute workout. Monitor your pulse rate to make sure that you are exercising in your target range.

OFFENSIVE AND DEFENSIVE SKILLS

Quick, fast, agile footwork is an essential component of a soccer game. Practice footwork skills to improve offensive and defensive play.

OFFENSIVE SKILLS

FAKE

- Look 1 direction, but pass or move the ball in another direction.
- Stay on the balls of your feet.
- Move quickly.

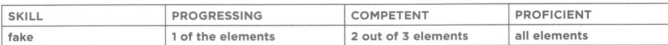

SKILL	PROGRESSING	COMPETENT	PROFICIENT
fake	1 of the elements	2 out of 3 elements	all elements

GIVE AND GO

The purpose of the give and go in a soccer game is for you to pass the ball to a teammate and quickly relocate so that you can receive a pass.

Pass the ball to a teammate.

Move quickly to relocate and support your offense.

Indicate (call out) that you are ready and open to receive the ball.

Receive the ball.

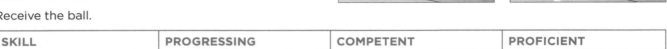

SKILL	PROGRESSING	COMPETENT	PROFICIENT
give and go	1 or 2 of the elements	3 out of 4 elements	all elements

THROW IN

The only time that a player other than a goalie can use their hands to touch the ball in a game is to perform a throw-in. A throw-in occurs when the ball goes out of bounds on either of the long sides of the field. The team that sends the ball out of bounds loses possession of the ball. The other team gains control of the ball and throws it in from the point where it went out of bounds.

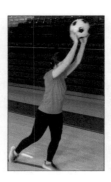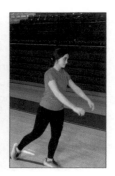

- Hold the ball in front of your body with both hands.
- Lift the ball over and behind your head.
- Step forward and throw the ball to a teammate. You cannot be the first person to touch the ball after you throw it in; or, you cannot throw-in to yourself.
- Follow through toward your target.
- Both of your feet must remain on the ground when you complete a throw-in. You can drag your back foot, but you cannot hop.

SKILL	PROGRESSING	COMPETENT	PROFICIENT
throw-in	1 or 2 of the elements	3 or 4 out of 5 elements	all elements

DEFENSIVE SKILLS

DEFENSIVE READY POSITION

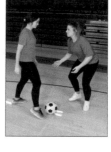

The ready position allows a player to move quickly in any direction. It is used for both offense and defense.

- Bend your knees to keep your body low.
- Stand with your feet shoulder-width apart.
- Keep your head up and your weight on the balls of your feet.
- Hold your arms extended out above waist height.
- Be ready to move and react quickly.
- Anticipate direction.

SKILL	PROGRESSING	COMPETENT	PROFICIENT
defensive ready position	1, 2, or 3 of the elements	4 or 5 out of 6 elements	all elements met

DEFENSIVE SLIDES

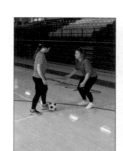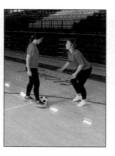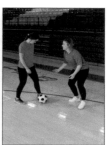

The purpose of the defensive slides in soccer is to keep up with your opponent and to legally take the ball or legally disrupt the opponent's pass or shot.

- Place your weight on the balls of your feet.
- Slide to the side with quick steps.
- Do not cross your feet.
- Keep your knees bent.
- Square your hips so that they face your opponent.
- Hold your hands up at chest level.
- Keep your eyes on your opponent's waistline.
- Stay with your opponent.
- Anticipate and react quickly to your opponent's movements.

SKILL	PROGRESSING	COMPETENT	PROFICIENT
defensive slides	1, 2, 3, 4, or 5 of the elements	6, 7, or 8 out of 9 elements	all elements met

PRACTICING OFFENSIVE AND DEFENSIVE SKILLS

- Practice the **give and go** with a partner and a defender. Pass the ball, quickly relocate, and then receive the pass, avoiding the defender.
- Practice the **fake** independently. Set up a cone as a decoy. Fake the pass toward the cone, and then pass to your partner. Practice until you feel comfortable with the movement.
- Practice the **fake** with a partner defending you. Dribble, fake, and then move in another direction to get around the defensive player. Practice until you feel comfortable with the fake.
- Practice the **defensive slides** with a partner. As your partner dribbles, defensive slide to try to prevent the player from making a successful pass or shot. Practice until you feel comfortable with the defensive slide.

SOCCER GAMES

SOCCER TENNIS

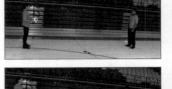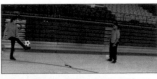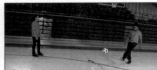

- You need 2 or 4 players to play this game.
- With discs, mark off an area that is 10 feet by 10 feet.
- Place jump ropes across the center of that area to represent a net that divides the area in half.
- If 2 people are playing, 1 person should be on either side of the net. If 4 people are playing, 2 people should be on either side of the net.
- Try to get the ball over the net. You can bounce the ball with your feet once before kicking it over the net.
- Points are awarded if you kick the ball over the net and the other team cannot return it.
- Play until a team scores 21 points.

SOCCER GAME

ABOUT THE GAME

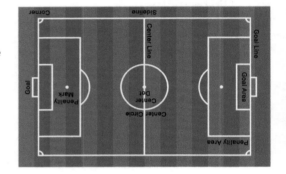

- To begin, 2 opposing teams of 11 players each including a goalie are established.
- All players must wear shin guards, socks that cover their shin guards, and appropriate cleats.
- The game is played on a rectangular grass or turf field.
- A goal is located at each end of the field.
- The object of the game is to move the ball down the field by passing or dribbling with your feet and to score by getting the ball into your opponent's goal.
- A game is divided into 45-minute halves.
- A goal is worth 1 point.
- The team with the most points at the end of the second half wins.

PLAYING THE GAME

- The game begins with a coin toss made by a referee at midfield.
- The team that possesses the ball is on offense and the other team is on defense.
- The first player to touch the ball at kickoff can only touch the ball once. They must kick the ball or pass it to another player who can dribble, pass, or kick the ball.
- No players except for the goalies or a player who is performing a throw-in can touch the ball with their hands. The entire arm counts as a hand in soccer, which means that a player cannot touch the ball anywhere from their fingertips to their upper arm.
- It is legal to use any body part other than a hand to contact the ball.
- If a player illegally uses their hands, which is referred to as a handball, the ball is turned over to the opposing team.
- The players on defense try to intercept, or take away, the ball from the offensive team to gain possession of the ball.

DEMONSTRATE POSITIVE GAME BEHAVIOR

- Follow all game rules.
- Do not conduct any fouls against another player (do not make illegal physical contact) and do not exhibit any unsportsmanlike behavior.
  - Fouls and unsportsmanlike behavior can result in a free kick for the other team, a yellow card warning for the offending player, or a red card ejection from the game for the offending player.
- Be supportive and encouraging to your teammates.
- Treat your opponents with respect.

SKILL	PROGRESSING	COMPETENT	PROFICIENT
game behavior	1 or 2 of the elements	3 out of 4 elements	all elements met

DESIGN AND COACH/REFEREE YOUR OWN GAME

Review the official game rules of soccer and think about how you can adjust them for casual games of 3-on-3, 4-on-4, and so on. Use the following information to break down the barrier of not having enough players for an official game and to create a solution.

- Determine the number of players.
- Determine the boundaries.
- Determine who starts with the ball.
- Establish safety rules.
- Establish scoring guidelines for your game. These can be the same as the official rules.
- Determine who will referee. You can alternate roles for fairness.

Prior to playing your game, establish and review the rules so that everyone understands them. If problems arise, work to solve them in a positive and effective manner. Appreciate different players' abilities. An example of a rule that you may want to decide upon is the boundaries.

Below are our game rules for safety and fairness.
1.
2.
3.
4.
5.

RATE YOUR ENJOYMENT OF THE SOCCER ACTIVITY THAT YOU ENJOYED MOST

On a scale from 1 to 4, where 1 is not enjoyable and 4 is very enjoyable, rate this activity.

1	It was not enjoyable, and I will not participate again.
2	It was not enjoyable, but I will participate again for exercise.
3	It was enjoyable, and I will play again.
4	It was very enjoyable, and I will initiate future games.

RESEARCH INTEGRATION

Research local facilities to find where soccer is played in your community for your age group.

HEALTH INTEGRATION

1. Count your pulse to determine if you are exercising in your personal target heart rate zone. Count your pulse after practicing skills and after playing in a game. Predict and then compare the difference between your heart rate after playing in the goalie position and your heart rate after playing in a running position. Apply the results to your overall fitness plan. Many people choose to complete aerobic workouts by playing in fast-paced games like soccer.

2. Discuss the protective gear worn by a soccer player and why they wear this gear.

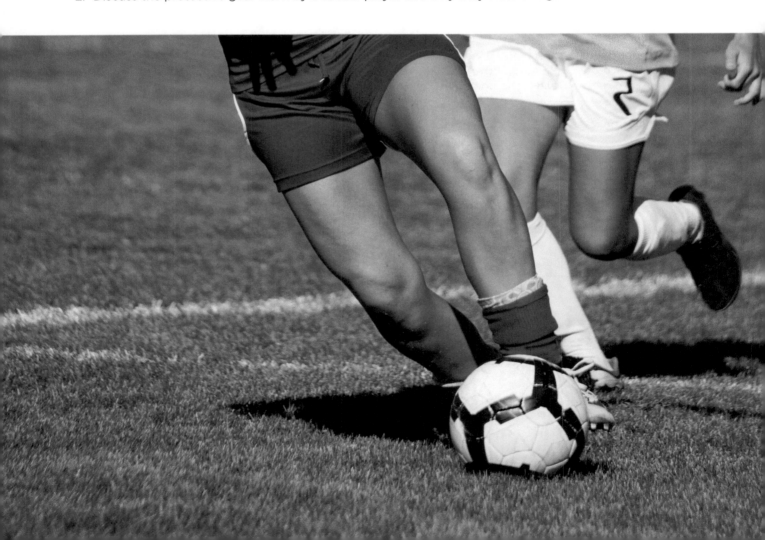

VELCRO® CATCH SET

Throwing and catching with the Velcro® catch set refines throwing, tracking, and catching skills while improving fitness. This activity also provides the opportunity for social interaction and enjoyment. It can be played in a yard, in a park, on a beach, and more.

The purpose of using the Velcro® catch set is to improve the necessary skills for throwing and catching and to provide another opportunity for exercise.

THROWING AND CATCHING SKILLS

UNDERHAND THROW

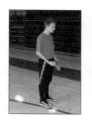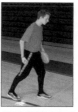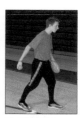
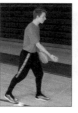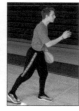

- Place the ball in your dominant hand.
- Face the direction in which you want the ball to go.
- Step with the foot opposite your throwing hand in the direction you want the ball to go. For example, if you are throwing with your right hand, step toward the target with your left foot.
- Swing your arm under and way back.
- Swing your arm forward, releasing the ball in front of you.
- Follow through toward the target with your throwing hand.

SKILL	PROGRESSING	COMPETENT	PROFICIENT
underhand throw	1 or 2 of the elements	3 or 4 out of 5 elements	all elements met

OVERHAND THROW

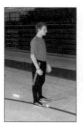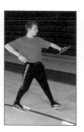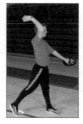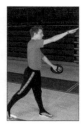

- Stand with the ball in your dominant hand.
- Turn to the side, pointing the shoulder of your non-throwing side in the direction you want the ball to go. For example, if you are throwing with your left hand, point your right shoulder toward the target.
- Bring your throwing arm up and way back behind your ear.
- Step with your opposite foot in the direction you want the ball to go. For example, if you are throwing with your left hand, step toward the target with your right foot.
- Follow through by letting your throwing arm come across the opposite side of your body.

SKILL	PROGRESSING	COMPETENT	PROFICIENT
overhand throw	1 or 2 of the elements	3 or 4 out of 5 elements	all elements met

CATCH

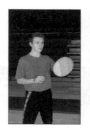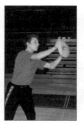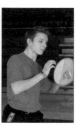

- Watch the ball all the way until it reaches your hands.
- As the ball comes toward you, reach your arms toward it.
- Give with the ball (pull the ball slightly toward you) as it hits your hands to make a soft catch.
- Bend your elbows slightly when catching the ball.

SKILL	PROGRESSING	COMPETENT	PROFICIENT
catch	1 or 2 of the elements	3 out of 4 elements	all elements met

VELCRO® CATCH SET SKILLS

UNDERHAND THROW TO YOURSELF

- Place the Velcro® pad on your non-dominant hand. Place the strap around your hand to secure the pad.
- Standing with your feet shoulder-width apart, hold the ball in your dominant hand.
- Use an underhand throw to toss the ball up in the air and then catch it with the Velcro® pad.

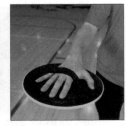
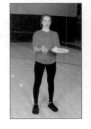
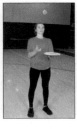
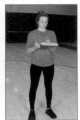

PRACTICE THE UNDERHAND THROW TO YOURSELF

- Continue to practice throwing the ball underhand and catching it, increasing the height of the ball as you improve.

PARTNER ACTIVITIES

Remember that to accurately throw to your partner, you will need to adjust direction and speed for every throw. You may be competent in the mechanics of a throw, but success also depends on accuracy.

UNDERHAND THROW WITH A PARTNER

- You and your partner should each wear a Velcro® pad on your non-dominant hand.
- Stand 10 feet away from your partner. Face each other.
- Using your dominant hand, throw the ball underhand to your partner so that your partner can catch it with their Velcro® pad.
- Increase your distance as you improve.

OVERHAND THROW WITH A PARTNER

- You and your partner should each wear a Velcro® pad on your non-dominant hand.
- Stand 10 feet away from your partner. Face each other.
- Using your dominant hand, throw the ball overhand to your partner so that your partner can catch it with their Velcro® pad.
- Increase your distance as you improve.

PARTNER CHALLENGE

- How many consecutive times can you throw and catch with your partner?
- Stand beside your partner and let them run ahead of you. Throw the ball to your partner. Then, run ahead of them and catch the ball. Continue to run, throw, and catch with your partner.

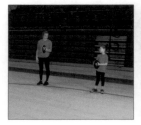
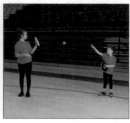
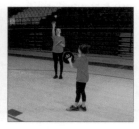
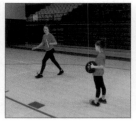
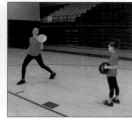

RATE YOUR ENJOYMENT OF THE VELCRO CATCH ACTIVITY THAT YOU ENJOYED MOST

On a scale from 1 to 4, where 1 is not enjoyable and 4 is very enjoyable, rate this activity.

1	It was not enjoyable, and I will not participate again.
2	It was not enjoyable, but I will participate again for exercise.
3	It was enjoyable, and I will play again.
4	It was very enjoyable, and I will initiate future games.

 RESEARCH INTEGRATION

Research and discuss the historical and cultural role of active games in a society.

♥ HEALTH INTEGRATION

Count your pulse to determine if you are exercising in your personal target heart rate zone. Many people choose to complete aerobic workouts by playing in casual games or activities with friends.

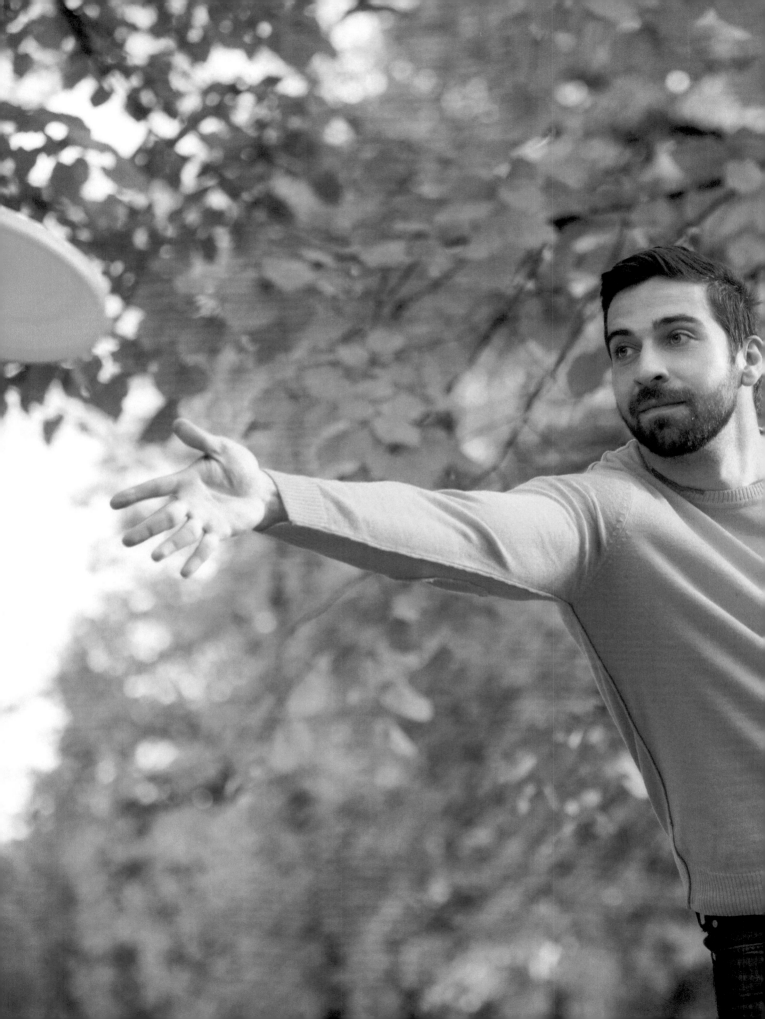

GRADE 10
PE EQUIPMENT KIT

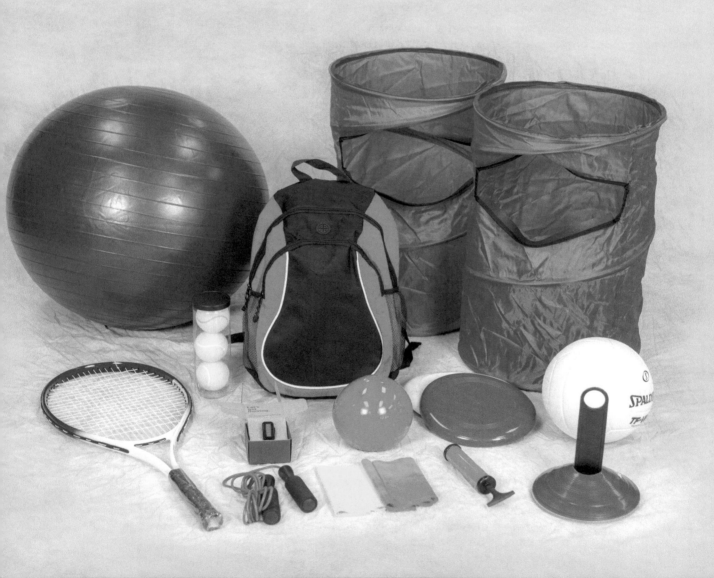

WARM-UP AND COOL-DOWN

⚠️ **CAUTION: Stretching should not be painful; ease up if stretching hurts. See the Flexibility section of your PE Manual for more information.**

WARM-UP

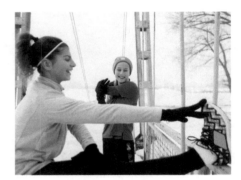

The purpose of a warm-up is to gradually increase heart rate, breathing rate, body temperature, and muscle temperature. Warming up prior to exercising increases circulation and blood flow to your muscles. When your muscles are warmed up, their performance—such as in the areas of strength and speed—is enhanced and risk of injury is decreased.

Stretching your muscles helps to minimize risk of injury by making the muscle fibers pliable, which means easy to bend or move.

Before you begin any workout, you should always warm up. Getting your heart and muscles prepared for exercise is important. There are numerous ways to get your body ready to participate in physical activity. **The Flexibility section of your PE Manual includes a variety of dynamic and static stretches for each major body part that will help you increase your flexibility.**

Elements of a Warm-Up

1. **Low-intensity cardio**: Walk, slow jog, or slow swim for 5 to 10 minutes to increase your heart rate, breathing rate, and body temperature before your workout.

2. **Dynamic stretch**: Perform a repeated motion—such as kicks, high knees, lunges, or arm circles—that will loosen up your joints and prepare your muscles for the exercise that you are about to do. Perform each dynamic stretch for at least 30 seconds.

3. **Static stretch**: Stretch your muscles slowly and hold each stretch for 20 to 30 seconds without bouncing in order to lengthen your muscles and increase your flexibility. Some important areas to stretch as a part of your warm-up are your neck, sides, shoulders, triceps, back, hamstrings, quadriceps, and groin.

Example 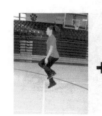 **+** 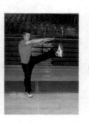 **+** 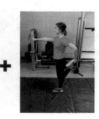 **= EFFECTIVE WARM-UP**

PERSONAL WARM-UP ACTIVITY

1. Select an exercise activity to participate in.

2. Design your personal warm-up plan for the activity that you selected. Any dynamic and static stretches that you choose to complete should be specific to the exercise activity that you chose.

3. Have a trusted adult or friend assess your stretches to make sure that you are using proper form.

4. Explain how the warm-up will decrease your risk of injury for this activity. _____

Procedure	Enter your personal warm-up regimen below.
1. **Low-intensity cardiovascular exercise:** Exercise for 5 to 10 minutes.	
2. **Dynamic stretches:** Perform dynamic stretches specifically for the selected activity.	
3. **Static stretches:** Perform static stretches specifically for the selected activity.	

COOL-DOWN

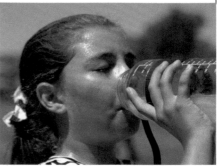

When you have finished your workout, exercise, or activity, it is imperative that your body returns to its normal state. You want to avoid stopping immediately and sitting down, **unless you are in pain, dizzy, or injured**. Be sure to slow your heart rate and breathing rate back to or slightly above their resting rates. There are several ways to do this. You could simply walk for a few minutes or slow down your exercise or find your own way to slow your body back down. You also may want to incorporate static stretches to increase flexibility and avoid your muscles tightening. **The Flexibility section of this manual includes a variety of static stretches for each major body part.** Always stay hydrated by drinking water before, during, and after exercise.

Elements of a Cool-Down

1. **Slow down**: Walk or gradually slow down your exercise—such as returning to a slow swim if you are swimming—until your heart rate, breathing rate, and body temperature are back to normal.

2. **Static stretch**: Stretch your muscles slowly and hold each stretch for 20 to 30 seconds without bouncing in order to lengthen your muscles and increase flexibility. Some important areas to stretch as part of your cool-down are your neck, sides, shoulders, triceps, back, hamstrings, quadriceps, and groin.

WALK + STATIC STRETCHES = EFFECTIVE COOL-DOWN

Design your personal cool-down plan. You can perform the same cool-down each time you finish a physical activity or you can change each time in order to reflect the exercise activity, such as by slowing your pedaling if you are biking.

Procedure	Enter your personal cool-down regimen below.
1. **Slow down:** Perform this slowed activity for 5 to 10 minutes.	
2. **Static stretches:** Perform several lower-body and upper-body stretches.	

AEROBIC EXERCISE AND PROPER NUTRITION

Aerobic exercise is important for strengthening the heart and for reducing stress. Frequency, intensity, and time are essential to efficient aerobic exercise. **Any** exercise done in your target heart rate zone and performed for 20 to 60 minutes 3 to 5 days per week is aerobic exercise.

You are more likely to commit to regular exercise if you plan a program that works for you. The equipment and facility should be affordable, and the location should be safe and convenient. Your exercise plan needs to accommodate your fitness level. Be prepared to adjust your workout plan if your schedule changes.

Proper nutrition is important for a healthy body and for keeping the arteries of the heart clear. Eating proper portions from the grain group, the fruit group, the vegetable group, the dairy group, and the protein group is essential to proper nutrition. Limit high-fat and sugary foods. You are more likely to commit to healthful eating if you plan and keep track of your nutrition.

Combining regular aerobic exercise with proper nutrition contributes to cardiovascular health as well as overall health.

The purpose of this lesson is to encourage you to develop a fitness portfolio, choreograph an aerobic exercise routine, participate in aerobic workouts, and plan for proper nutrition. **The Cardiovascular Endurance section of this manual includes the target heart rate zone formula and the Borg Rating of Perceived Exertion Scale to help you to determine if you are exercising for heart health.** You can also use available technology to monitor your pulse rate and intensity.

When beginning any exercise program, begin with workouts for your fitness level and then build accordingly. You want to feel refreshed after your exercise session, not exhausted. Use your pulse rate to monitor aerobic workouts.

 CAUTION: Wear proper equipment and follow activity-specific safety rules.

AEROBIC EXERCISE AND PROPER NUTRITION

Develop a fitness portfolio and make a commitment to aerobic exercise. Your fitness portfolio should include the following.

- endurance walk/run fitness score
- goals for improvement
- 4-week exercise plan (See below.)

TYPES OF AEROBIC EXERCISE

Sports: Examples include soccer, basketball, volleyball, swimming, hockey, lacrosse, tennis, badminton, pickleball, handball, gymnastics, dance, martial arts, wrestling, track and field, and so on.

Outdoor pursuits: Examples include walking, jogging, biking, canoeing, kayaking, golfing, fly fishing, hiking, rock climbing, horseback riding, skiing, and so on.

Fitness gyms: Find a gym that is convenient for you to attend where you can complete circuit exercises, use aerobic machines, take classes, and more.

Stationary exercise equipment: Examples include using a jump rope, treadmill, elliptical trainer, bike, mini trampoline, and so on.

Exercise apps or videos: Use a workout tutorial on an app, website, video, or other digital source.

Your own sequence workouts: You can also design your own workout sequences by following the steps below.

- Create your personal aerobic workout routines by blending activities that involve basic locomotor skills such as jogging in place, jumping jacks, high knees, and so on.
- Design the intensity and duration of the exercise according to your level of fitness.
- Perform your personal routine for some or all your aerobic workouts.

Choreograph a personal aerobic workout routine by blending basic locomotor skills. This is a workout that can be done at home for convenience. The suggested time for each skill is from 20 to 60 seconds with a 30-second rest every 4 to 5 minutes. Repeat for a 20- to 60-minute workout. Most important, exercise at your level of fitness and rest accordingly. Use the following skills to choreograph your routine, or use skills of your choice.

- Jogging in place: Run slowly in place.
- Jumping jacks: Stand with your feet apart with arms up, then feet together with arms at your sides.
- High knees: Alternate lifting your knees to waist height.
- Burpees: Jump vertically, then bend your knees and transition to a push-up position.
- Side slides: Step to the right. Bring the other foot over in a step-together motion. Repeat left.
- Squat jumps: Jump and land softly into a squat (hips even with knees).
- March in place: Alternate lifting knees to waist height.
- Carioca: Step to the side with 1 foot and cross with your other foot in a step-cross-step-cross movement. Alternate the step-cross movement with a cross behind the lead foot and a cross in front of the lead foot.
- Front kicks: Alternate lifting your legs forward.

EXTENSION: Work with a friend to create aerobic routines. Evaluate each other's level of fitness and schedule (school/work) to create and plan personalized workouts.

Plan your exercise. The following is an example of how to schedule and track aerobic exercise for 1 week. Plan for 4 weeks.

WARM UP BEFORE EACH WORKOUT.

Week 1	Exercise	Time of Day	Exercise Time (min.)	Heart Rate (bpm)
Mon.	jump rope	morning	20	160
Tues.				
Wed.	my routine	morning	30	155
Thurs.	volleyball	evening	60	145
Fri.				
Sat.	tennis	evening	45	140
Sun.				

COOL DOWN AFTER EACH WORKOUT.

EXTENSION: Use your exercise plan as training for a community event such as a 5K (walk or jog).

Plan your nutrition. Keep track of the food you eat each day for 1 week. Include food from the grain group, the fruit group, the vegetable group, the dairy group, and the protein group each day. Drink water daily. Limit high-fat and sugary foods. Exercise burns calories, so it is important to get food from all of the food groups. Plan for and eat healthful snacks. Review what you eat each day, discuss your diet with a trusted adult, and adjust so that you are getting a well-rounded, healthful diet. Be aware of false diet claims and rely on your doctor for advice.

 CAUTION: Do not consume foods to which you are allergic.

EXAMPLE

Day 1	Time	Servings	Total Servings
Grain	breakfast	2	6
	lunch	2	
	dinner	2	
Fruit	breakfast	1	4
	lunch	2	
	dinner	1	
Vegetable	breakfast	0	5
	lunch	2	
	dinner	3	
Dairy	breakfast	2	4
	lunch	1	
	dinner	1	
Protein	breakfast	0	3
	lunch	1	
	dinner	2	
Snacks	granola bar	1	2
	apple	1	

RESEARCH INTEGRATION

Research the connection of exercise, nutrition, and body composition. Confirm your findings with a doctor.

HEALTH INTEGRATION

Use available technology to monitor your pulse rate and intensity. Apply the results to your overall fitness plan.

DANCE

Dance involves expressing yourself through repeated patterns of movement. It is usually set to music. Some forms of dance include creative, tap, ballet, hip-hop, modern, folk, square, jazz, line, Latin, ballroom, and social. Your lifetime exercise plan can include dance to aerobic exercise. You can take dance classes, follow along with videos, dance individually, dance with a partner, and dance in a group.

The purpose of this lesson is for you to perform basic locomotor movements using common dance concepts in rhythmic patterns to create your own dance for aerobic exercise.

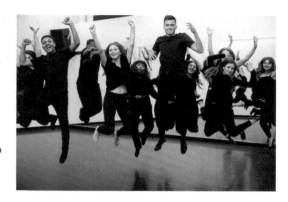

CREATIVE DANCE

PERSONAL DANCE ROUTINE

COMMON CONCEPTS OF DANCE TO USE FOR YOUR PERSONAL DANCE

- The concept of space includes the following.
  - ○ high, medium, or low **levels**
  - ○ forward, backward, right, or left **direction**
  - ○ curved, zigzag, straight, circle, or square **pathways**
- The concept of time includes the following.
  - ○ slow, medium, or fast **speeds**
  - ○ a pattern for **rhythm**
- The concept of force includes the following.
  - ○ applying light, moderate, or strong **weights**

CREATE A DANCE

Start with the 3 dance steps below. Then, complete the routine by adding your own dance steps. Set your dance to music.

1. Learn a sidestep.
   - Step to the right with your right foot.
   - Bring your left foot in to meet your right foot.
   - Touch your left toes to the floor with a light force, but do not put weight on them.
   - Repeat this to the left.

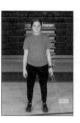 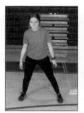 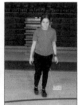

Sidestep

2. Learn a step-hop.
   - Step out to the right side with your right foot.
   - Bring your left foot in and simultaneously jump with a medium force.
   - Land with both feet together.
   - Clap your hands as you land.
   - Repeat to the left.

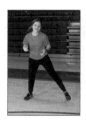 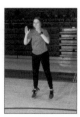

Step-hop

3. Combine the sidestep and step-hop for a double step (step together, step-hop, clap).
   - Step to the right with your right foot.
   - Bring your left foot in to meet your right foot.
   - Step out to the right side with your right foot.
   - Bring your left foot in and simultaneously jump, land, and clap.
   - Repeat this to the left.
4. Perform the double step 4 times.
5. Add your dance steps to complete the dance.
   - Choose locomotor skills to blend (slides, cariocas, turns, and so on).
   - Use your arms to accompany the footwork, for example: step, cross, step, clap.
   - Perform the skills at different levels.
   - Move in different directions.
   - Move in different pathways.
   - Move at slow, medium, and fast speeds.
   - Use light, moderate, and strong force to move your body.
   - Create a pattern.
   - Use an 8 count for each move.

Option: Dance with a partner or small group for a social experience.

RATE YOUR ENJOYMENT OF DANCE

On a scale from 1 to 4, where 1 is not enjoyable and 4 is very enjoyable, rate this activity.

1	It was not enjoyable, and I will not participate again.
2	It was not enjoyable, but I will participate again for exercise.
3	It was enjoyable, and I will dance again.
4	It was very enjoyable, and I will create more dances.

RESEARCH INTEGRATION

1. Research dance as a form of communication. Discuss your research with a friend or trusted adult.
2. Research and compare 2 dance types: ballet and tap.
3. Join a dance from the USB if provided in your PE program.

HEALTH INTEGRATION

Count your pulse to determine if you are exercising in your personal target heart rate zone. Apply the results to your overall fitness plan. Many people choose to get their aerobic workouts through dance.

JUMP ROPE

A jump rope is an inexpensive piece of exercise equipment. It can be used indoors, outdoors, and in a small space. A jump rope promotes adherence to participation in physical activity by eliminating cost and space barriers. It is also an effective sport-training tool that improves balance, agility, and coordination.

The purpose of this lesson is for you to use jumping rope to improve in areas of fitness that are important to you: cardiovascular, skill-related, or both.

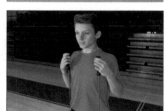

JUMP ROPE BASICS

FIT THE JUMP ROPE FOR YOUR HEIGHT

- Place a jump rope handle in each hand.
- Stand on the middle of the rope with 1 foot.
- Move the handles straight up, making sure that the rope is straight and pulled tight.
- The tops of the handles should reach close to your shoulders.

Fitting the jump rope to your height

ELEMENTS OF JUMP ROPE

- Keep your eyes forward.
- When turning the rope, keep your elbows near your sides, maintaining a 45-degree angle and making 2-inch circles with your wrists.
- Leave just enough space for the rope to pass under your feet when you jump.
- Stay on the balls of your feet.
- Land softly, keeping your knees slightly bent.

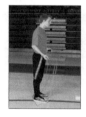 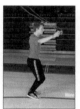 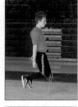

BASIC SKILLS

BASIC JUMP

- Pick up the rope. Holding a handle in each hand, rest the rope behind your feet. Stand on the balls of your feet. This is the ready position.
- Your hands should be just above the height of your waist.
- Swing the rope up and over your head.
- Jump over the rope when it approaches your toes.
- Continue as long as you can without stopping.

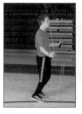 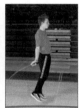

Basic jump

BACKWARD JUMP

- Begin with the rope in front of your feet.
- Swing the rope up and over your head.
- Jump over the rope when it approaches your feet.
- Jump a little higher than 1 inch off the ground. Stay on the balls of your feet.
- Continue as long as you can without stopping.

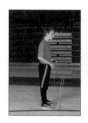 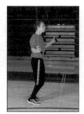 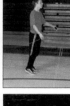

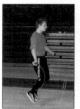 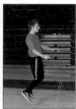

Backward jump

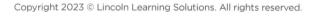

ALTERNATE-FOOT JUMP

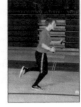
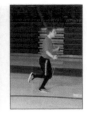

- Pick up the rope. Holding a handle in each hand, rest the rope behind your feet. Stand on the balls of your feet. This is the ready position. Note that 1 foot will be lifted off the ground during each turn of the rope before the other foot jumps.

- Turn the rope from behind you up over your head. When the rope reaches your toes, jump over it with your right foot.

Alternate-foot jump

- Turn the rope again from behind you up over your head. When the rope reaches your toes this time, jump over it with your left foot.

- Continue turning the rope and alternating feet as if you were running in place. Try it jumping backward.

Practice the basic jump rope skills until competent. Next, design a jump rope routine using basic jump rope skills that will improve footwork speed.

SAMPLE OF A WORKOUT TO IMPROVE FOOTWORK SPEED	
• basic jump 1 minute at a medium pace	• rest 30 seconds
• basic jump 30 seconds at a fast pace	• alternate-foot jump 1 minute at a medium pace
• rest 30 seconds	• alternate-foot jump 30 seconds at a fast pace
• backward jump 1 minute at a medium pace	• rest 30 seconds
• backward jump 30 seconds at a fast pace	• repeat as needed

DESIGN YOUR PERSONAL FOOTWORK SPEED ROUTINE

CHALLENGE SKILLS

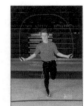
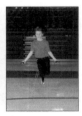

The following challenges are for students who have mastered the basic jump rope skills. The challenge level is recommended to learn advanced skills and add a variety of skills to your workout.

HOP ON 1 FOOT

Hop on 1 foot

- Perform the basic jump on your right foot.

- Perform the basic jump on your left foot.

SKIER

- With both feet together, hop side to side while turning the rope.

Skier

CROSSOVERS

- After the rope moves over your head, cross the rope in front of you, jump, and uncross the rope.

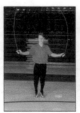
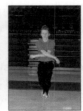
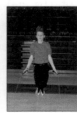

Crossovers

FRONT KICKS

- Kick 1 foot forward as the rope passes under your feet with a skip-step in between.
- Alternate kicks.

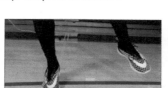

SIDE KICKS

- Kick 1 foot and then the other out to the side with a skip-step in between.

Front kicks

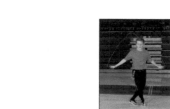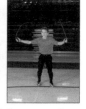

CRISSCROSS FEET

- Cross and uncross your feet while jumping.

Side kicks

FIGURE-8 JUMPS

- Hold a handle in each hand. Swing the rope from side to side in a figure-8 pattern. Then, open it to regular form and step over it. When you master that, practice jumping over the rope.

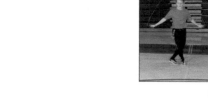

Crisscross feet

Practice the challenge jump rope skills until competent. Next, design your personal aerobic jump rope routine by blending the basic jump rope skills and the challenge skills. Set your routine to music. Monitor your pulse rate.

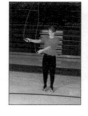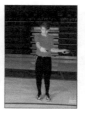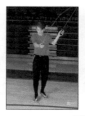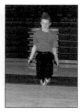

BLENDING: Perform 1 jump rope skill and transition smoothly to another jump rope skill without stopping between moves. Blend after a 4 count, an 8 count, or a 16 count. Mix it up so that it works for you.

Figure-8 jumps

SAMPLE OF A CARDIOVASCULAR CONDITIONING WORKOUT

- blend basic jump/crossovers/basic jump **2 minutes**
- march or jog in place **30 seconds**
- blend backward jump/hop on 1 foot/backward jump **2 minutes**
- march or jog in place **30 seconds**
- blend alternate-foot jump/basic jump/crisscross feet **2 minutes**
- walk or jog in place **30 seconds**
- blend skier/front kicks/side kicks **2 minutes**
- march or jog in place **30 seconds**
- repeat for a 20-minute workout

DESIGN YOUR PERSONAL CARDIOVASCULAR JUMP ROPE ROUTINE. SET IT TO MUSIC.

 ## HEALTH INTEGRATION

Count your pulse during and after jumping rope to determine if you are exercising in your personal target heart rate zone for health benefits.

FITNESS BALL

Including a fitness ball (or exercise ball) in your exercise routine is a fun, efficient way to improve muscular strength, muscular endurance, flexibility, and balance. Your core muscles work to balance on an unstable ball while exercising a variety of muscle groups.

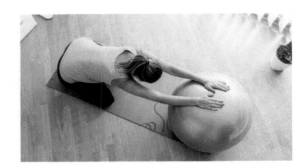

The purpose of this lesson is to exercise leg, back, and core muscles using a stability ball.

 CAUTION: Do not overinflate the ball.

FITNESS BALL STRENGTH-BUILDING EXERCISES

TIPS FOR USING A FITNESS BALL

- Exercises done on a firmer ball are more challenging.
- A beginner should start with a slightly-deflated ball.
- When you are seated on the ball, your feet should be flat on the floor.

Practice each of the following exercises, concentrating on proper form, prior to engaging in a workout.

SQUATS

muscle focus: quadriceps, hamstrings, and glutes

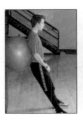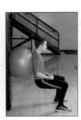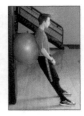

Squats

- Place the fitness ball against your lower back, between you and the wall.
- Holding the ball against the wall, place your feet shoulder-width apart and slightly out in front of you. Your body should be at an angle.
- Slide your body down into a seated position (the fitness ball should now be against your upper back), making sure your knees do not go past your toes.
- Stand back up to the starting position. The fitness ball should still be between you and the wall against your lower back.

BACK EXTENSIONS

muscle focus: erector spinae (iliocostales, longissimi, and spinales)

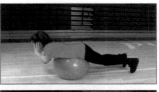

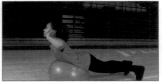

Back extensions

- Place the fitness ball on the floor.
- Place your abdomen on the ball. Your legs should be extended behind you and about shoulder-width apart for balance.
- Place your hands behind your head on your neck (like when doing a crunch).
- Lift your upper body so that you are hyperextending your back.
- Come back down to the starting position.

CRUNCHES

muscle focus: recti abdominis and oblique abdominal muscles

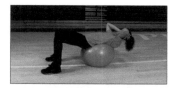

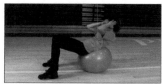

- Place the fitness ball on the floor.
- Place yourself on the fitness ball so that your lower back is on the ball. You do not want your shoulders on the ball.
- Your feet should be shoulder-width apart for balance.
- Place your hands behind your head on your neck.
- Bend your torso upward, performing a crunch.
- Come back down to the starting position, making sure your abdomen is still tight. Do not extend back the whole way as that would release the tension in your abdomen.

Crunches

SIDE CRUNCHES

muscle focus: abdominal muscles and erector spinae

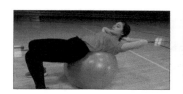

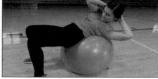

- Place the fitness ball on the ground behind you.
- Place your lower back on the ball. Do not let your shoulders touch the ball.
- Place your feet shoulder-width apart on the floor and in front of you for balance.
- Place your hands behind your head on your neck.
- Bend your torso upward and twist to the right. Your left elbow should almost touch your right thigh.
- Come back to the starting position, making sure your abdomen is still tight. Do not extend back the whole way; this would release the tension in your abdomen.
- Repeat this to the left.

Side crunches

HAMSTRING CURLS

muscle focus: abdominal muscles, erector spinae, hamstrings, and glutes

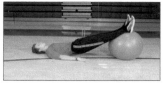

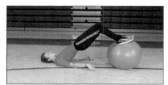

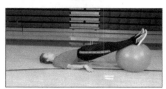

- Place the fitness ball on the floor.
- Lie down with your hands slightly out to your sides.
- Put your lower calves and ankles on the ball. Your feet should be together, and your glutes should be lifted off the ground.
- Bring your knees in toward your chest, moving the ball toward your glutes. The bottoms of your feet should be resting on the ball.
- Straighten your legs to return to the starting position.

Hamstring curls

LEG EXTENSIONS

muscle focus: quadriceps, hamstrings, and glutes

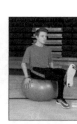
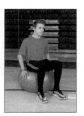
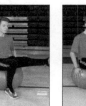

- Sit on the ball with both feet firmly on the ground.
- Lift your right leg so your calf is parallel to the ground.
- Lower your right leg slowly back to the starting position.
- Lift your left leg so your calf is parallel to the ground.
- Lower your left leg slowly back to the starting position.
- Alternate legs.

Leg extensions

Have a trusted adult or friend evaluate you for correct form for the previous exercises. Did you respond positively to the feedback?

Reciprocate and evaluate your friend. Were you able to provide feedback in a positive manner?

The following is a suggested use of the fitness ball in a strength-building workout. Exercise to your level of fitness.

- Warm up and cool down.

- Perform each exercise 2 to 3 days per week.

- Begin with 1 set of 10 repetitions. Increase sets and the number of repetitions when the current number is too easy.

- Your goal should be to reach 3 sets of 10 to 15 repetitions.

RESEARCH INTEGRATION

Research benefits of using a fitness ball.

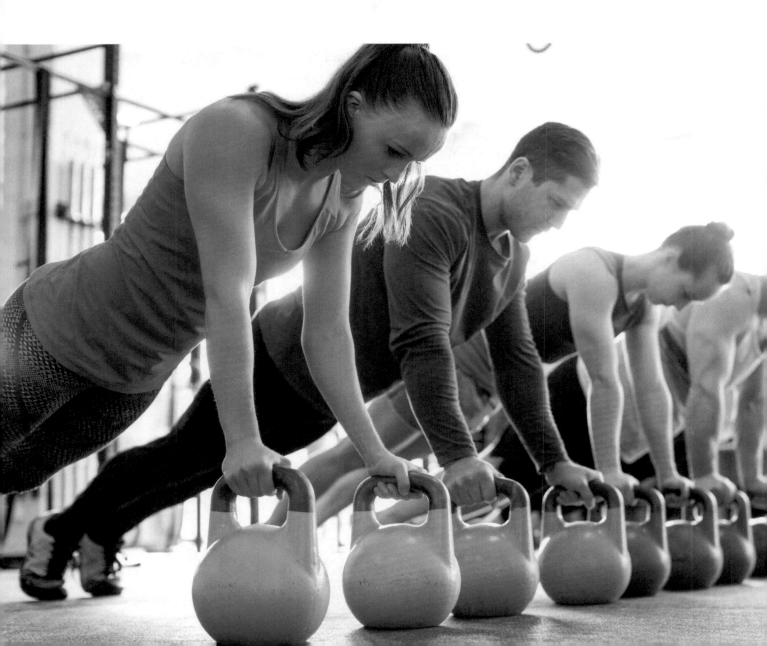

RESISTANCE BANDS

Resistance bands keep resistance maintained throughout every part of the motions that are being performed. Regular use of resistance bands helps to improve muscular strength, muscular endurance, and flexibility. When using resistance bands, start with the lightest resistance and gradually increase to a higher resistance as you get stronger.

The purpose of this lesson is to increase muscular strength and endurance using resistance bands.

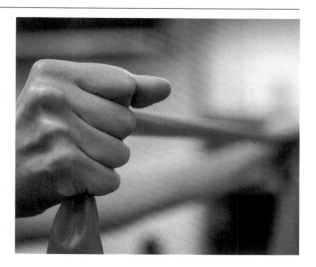

FITNESS TIP: When using resistance bands, you should make sure that the band is secured in a way that the length is appropriate to give resistance for the entire exercise. Wrap the band around your hands if you need an increased resistance level.

CAUTION: Check the resistance bands for damage or wear before exercising. When exercising, secure the band before adding any resistance.

RESISTANCE BANDS STRENGTH-BUILDING EXERCISES

BENEFITS OF STRENGTH TRAINING WITH RESISTANCE BANDS

- is an effective overall strength workout that does not require weights
- offers a variety of resistance adjustments for beginner through advanced levels
- requires inexpensive pieces of equipment
- requires equipment that is easy to carry with you when you are traveling

CHEST PRESSES

muscle focus: pectoralis majors, pectoralis minors, biceps, triceps, and front fibers of deltoid muscles

- Sit up straight in a chair or stand with your feet shoulder-width apart.
- Wrap the band around your upper body so that the band is resting across the middle of your shoulder blades and under your arms. You should have an end in each hand.
- Rotate your forearms and wrists so that your thumbs are facing each other but are not touching.

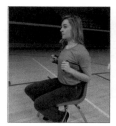 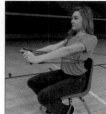

Chest presses

- Bend your elbows, making them level with your chest. Then lift them so your elbows and shoulders are in a straight line and your wrists and elbows are in alignment. (This is where you will adjust your resistance. If the resistance is not enough, wrap the band around your hands until the resistance is comfortable.)
- Straighten your elbows out in front of you so that your hands are almost touching.
- Bend your elbows slowly back to the starting position. Make sure your elbows and shoulders are in a straight line; your wrists and elbows should also be in alignment.

TRICEPS EXTENSIONS

muscle focus: triceps and biceps

- Sit on the exercise ball with the middle of the band under you. You should be sitting on the band.
- Hold the right handle in your right hand and the left handle in your left hand.
- Place both hands over your head with your elbows bent.
- Extend both hands above your head, straightening your elbows.

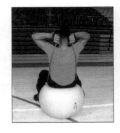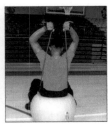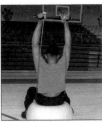

Tricep extensions

BICEPS HAMMER CURLS

muscle focus: biceps and triceps

- Stand on the middle of the exercise band with your feet shoulder-width apart.
- Hold both ends of the resistance band with your palms facing in toward your body.
- Bend at your elbows, and slowly bring each hand toward the respective shoulder while keeping your elbows by your sides and your palms toward your body.
- Return your arms slowly back to the starting position without fully straightening your elbows.

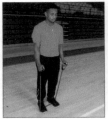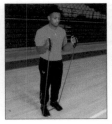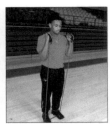

Biceps hammer curls

LATERAL RAISES

muscle focus: deltoids

- Place an end of the resistance band under your right foot and hold the other end in your right hand.
- Keep your arm straight at your side and make sure that the tension of the resistance band is at a good level. If the resistance is not enough, wrap the band around your hand until the resistance is comfortable.
- Keep your arm straight and raise it out to your side so that it is parallel with the floor.
- Bring your arm slowly back down to your side. Make sure you are keeping your arm straight during the entire exercise.

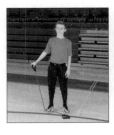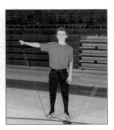

Lateral raises

SEATED ROWS

muscle focus: erector spinae, trapezii, rhomboids, and latissimi dorsi

- Sit on the ground. Your feet and legs should be straight out in front of you.
- Place the middle of the band around the bottom of both feet. The resistance band should be across the instep of both feet. Hold an end in each hand.
- Start with your arms straight out in front of you. Make sure there is good tension with the resistance band.
- Make sure your forearms and wrists are rotated so that your thumbs are on top of the grip. Your palms should be facing each other.
- Keep your back upright. In a single motion, bend your elbows back and pinch your shoulder blades together. Do not bring your elbows so far back that they are almost touching; bring them back so that they are slightly behind you.
- Bring your arms slowly straight in front of you, back to the starting position.

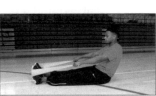
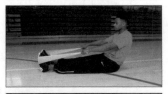
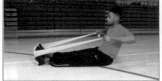

Seated rows

CALF RAISES

muscle focus: gastrocnemii and solei

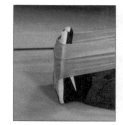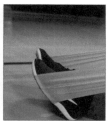

Calf raises

- Sit on the ground. Your feet and legs should be straight out in front of you.

- Place the middle of the resistance band around the bottom of both feet. The band should be across the balls of your feet (closer to the toes, but not on the toes). Hold an end in each hand.

- Flex your feet and point your toes away from your leg.

- Bring your toes slowly up toward your leg.

Have a trusted adult or friend evaluate you for correct form for the previous exercises. Did you respond positively to the feedback?

Reciprocate and evaluate your friend. Were you able to provide feedback in a positive manner?

The following is a suggested use of resistance bands in a strength-building workout. Exercise to your level of fitness.

- Warm up before your workout. Cool down after your workout.

- Perform each resistance band exercise 2 to 3 days per week. Do not exercise the same muscle group on consecutive days.

- Begin with 1 set of 10 repetitions for each exercise. Increase sets and the number of repetitions when the current number is too easy.

- Your goal should be to reach 3 sets of 10 to 15 repetitions.

- Wrap the band to increase resistance as necessary.

🖥 RESEARCH INTEGRATION

Research resistance band full body workouts.

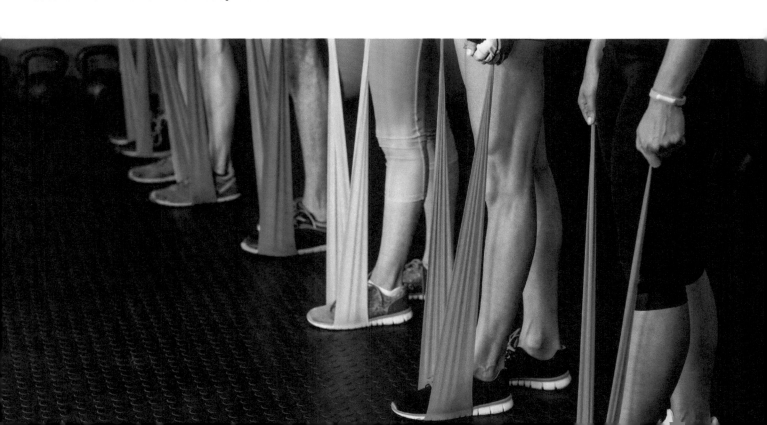

WEIGHTED BALL

Exercising with a weighted ball will help you with muscular strength and core stabilization. The weighted ball helps strengthen your legs, arms, back, and abs. Having good core strength helps reduce back problems.

The purpose of this lesson is to increase muscular strength and endurance using a weighted ball.

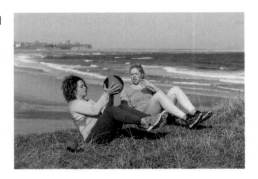

🏃 **FITNESS TIP: Have a certified trainer plan for you and supervise you when you are working with any type of weights.**

⚠️ **CAUTION: Make sure nobody is close to you before using the weighted ball. Do not walk into the path of another person using a weighted ball. Make sure to hold the ball and maneuver it without dropping it. Have a good grip on the ball before exercising. Keep the weighted ball movements controlled to avoid injury.**

BENEFITS OF STRENGTH TRAINING WITH A WEIGHTED BALL

- requires only 1 piece of equipment
- can be done almost anywhere
- is time effective and provides an overall workout in a short time
- combines cardio and strength training
- works your core and many muscles
- boosts metabolism and burns fat even after the exercise is over
- improves focus and coordination

Practice each of the following exercises, concentrating on proper form, prior to engaging in a workout.

WEIGHTED BALL STRENGTH-BUILDING EXERCISES

FIGURE-8s

muscle focus: erector spinae, trapezii, deltoids, hamstrings, quadriceps, and abdominal muscles

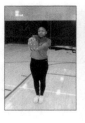
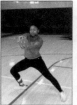
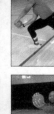
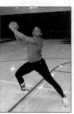
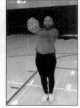

- Stand with your feet shoulder-width apart.
- Hold the weighted ball out in front of you with your right hand on top of it and your left hand under it. Extend your arms at chest level.
- Step out into a side lunge with your left leg.
- Bring the ball down to the outside of your left thigh in a smooth motion.
- Come back to the standing position and quickly move into a side lunge to the right.
- Make a figure-8 with the ball, moving the ball to the outside of your right thigh. This is 1 repetition.
- Continue to make a figure-8 with the ball as you lunge from side to side.

Figure-8s

SQUATTING SHOULDER PRESSES

muscle focus: quadriceps, hamstrings, deltoids, and triceps

- Hold the weighted ball with both hands—1 on either side of the ball—in the middle of your chest.

- Stand with your feet shoulder-width apart.

- Bend your knees and lower your buttocks toward the ground so you are in a squatting position. Do not let your knees go past your toes.

- Straighten your knees and hips while lifting the ball straight up in the air in a single motion.

- Return to the squatting position while bringing the ball back to your chest.

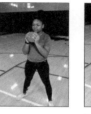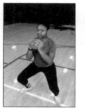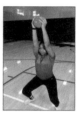
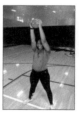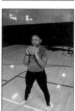

Squatting shoulder presses

LUNGES WITH PASSES

muscle focus: quadriceps, hamstrings, gastrocnemii, soleus, glutes, biceps, and triceps

- Stand with your feet together.

- Hold the weighted ball close to your chest with both hands.

- Step forward with your right foot. Bend your right knee so it is over your toes, not past them. Bend your left knee so it is almost touching the ground; lift your heel.

- Pass the ball from your left hand to your right hand under your right leg.

- Grab the ball with both hands and come back to the starting position.

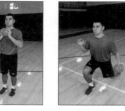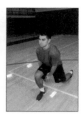
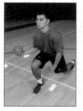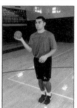

Lunges with passes

BACK EXTENSION WITH ROLLS

muscle focus: erector spinae, deltoids, and triceps

- Lie face down on the ground with the weighted ball in front of you.

- Extend your arms and legs. Your arms should be shoulder-width apart, and your legs should be hip-width apart.

- Place your right hand on the ball.

- Extend your spine and lift your chest and thighs off the ground. As you do this, roll the ball from your right hand to your left hand.

- Continue rolling the ball back and forth while keeping your chest and thighs off the ground.

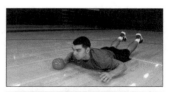
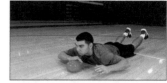
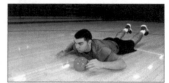
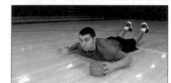

Back extensions with rolls

Have a trusted adult or friend evaluate you for correct form for the previous exercises. Did you respond positively to the feedback?

Reciprocate and evaluate your friend. Were you able to provide feedback in a positive manner?

The following is a suggested use of the weighted ball in strength-building and aerobic workouts. Exercise to your level of fitness.

Warm up and cool down.

Perform each weighted ball exercise 2 to 3 days per week. Do not exercise the same muscle group on consecutive days.

Begin with 15 seconds per exercise (per side). Increase to 30 seconds per exercise when ready.

Your goal should be to reach 3 sets of 30 seconds per exercise.

 ## RESEARCH INTEGRATION

Research weighted ball workouts.

♥ HEALTH INTEGRATION

Count your pulse to determine if you are exercising in your personal target heart rate zone. Apply the results to your overall fitness plan.

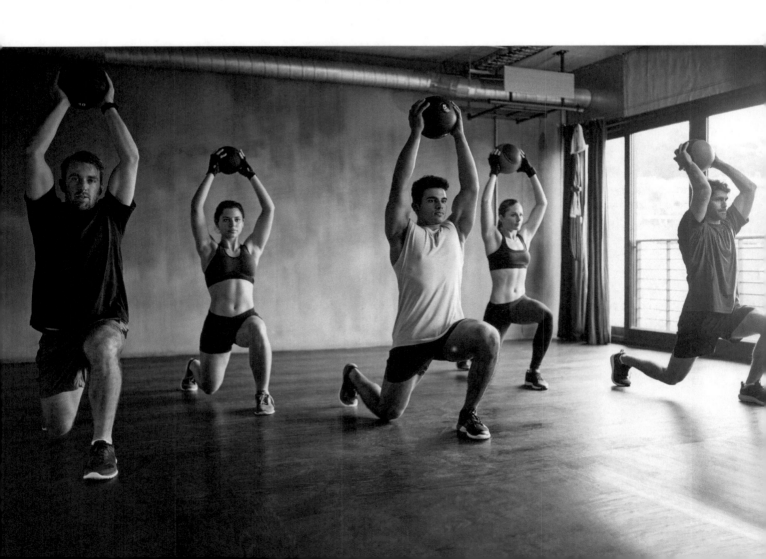

STRENGTH-TRAINING PROGRAM: USING WHAT YOU HAVE LEARNED

There are 3 types of muscle tissue: skeletal, cardiac, and smooth. Skeletal muscles are attached to bones and contract and relax to move the skeleton. The heart is made of cardiac muscles. Smooth muscles are found in the walls of the body's organs and blood vessels.

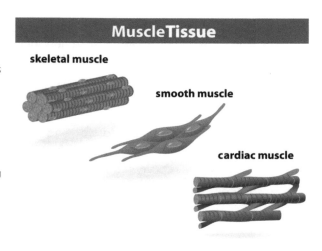

MuscleTissue

skeletal muscle

smooth muscle

cardiac muscle

Exercise directly affects skeletal and cardiac muscles. Aerobic exercise strengthens the heart muscles. Strength training, also known as resistance training, builds strength and endurance in the skeletal muscles.

Fibers that make up your skeletal muscles break down during the exercise phase. After your strength workout, when your muscles are resting, the fibers repair and strengthen. It is recommended that you allow 24 hours between training the same muscle group to allow the muscle fibers to repair and strengthen.

The purpose of this lesson is to encourage you to design your personal strength-training program and perform exercises 2 to 3 days per week to obtain health benefits. A certified trainer should help you set up a balanced, effective strength program.

 CAUTION: Have a certified trainer plan for you and supervise you when you are working with weights.

STRENGTH-TRAINING PROGRAM

There are a variety of exercises from which to choose. Do strength exercises for the muscles of your upper body, lower body, and core. Opposing muscles (antagonistic muscles), such as biceps and triceps, should be equally trained because they work together. Choose the intensity of the exercise to fit your fitness level. For example, if you are struggling doing a right-angle push-up, switch to a knee push-up. Limit excuses and make a commitment to exercise!

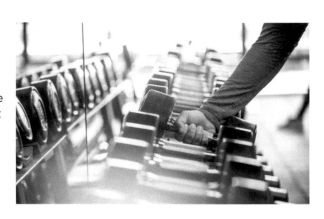

STRENGTH-TRAINING EXERCISE IDEAS

Weightlifting machines: You can use large stationary machines like those typically found in gyms.

Free weights: You can use free-weight equipment such as dumbbells, barbells, medicine balls, kettlebells, resistance bands, and weighted ropes to perform strength-training exercises.

Pilates or yoga: Pilates and yoga sessions are excellent workouts for muscle lengthening and muscle strengthening.

Personal workouts: You can use your own body weight as a source of resistance and create your own strength-training workouts. Create a personal workout by blending basic strength-building exercises such as sit-ups, push-ups, pull-ups, planks, and so on, and design the intensity and duration of each exercise according to your level of fitness. Include upper-body, lower-body, and core exercises in your workout. Perform your personal routine for some or all your strength-training workouts.

MUSCULAR STRENGTH AND MUSCULAR ENDURANCE SAMPLE WORKOUT

The following workout regimen is strictly an example of how to use the FITT principle to increase muscular strength and muscular endurance. The exercises are described in the Flexibility section, Muscular Endurance section, and PE Equipment Kit section of your PE Manual.

In the following chart, you will find a block plan for a weekly schedule based on increasing your muscular strength and muscular endurance. The chart includes the days of the week, muscle groups, exercises, sets and repetitions (for example, 3 · 10 = 3 sets of 10 repetitions), and the type of equipment used.

There is a column on the chart for you to design your personal workout. You can use fitness equipment or your own body weight. The plan you design should be for your fitness level. Personalized exercise plans work for all fitness levels and body types.

- Have a certified trainer plan for you and supervise you when you are working with any type of weights.
- Before working out, warm up properly to prepare your body. The warm-up should increase your heart rate, breathing rate, and body temperature.
- Never begin vigorous exercise with cold muscles.
- Cool down after working out to allow your body to return to its baseline.

Warm-up: Complete 3 sets of this warm-up before exercising.

Exercise	Duration
• basic jump rope	• 1 minute
• high knees	• 30 seconds
• forward arm circles	• 30 seconds
• backward arm circles	• 30 seconds
• rear kicks	• 30 seconds

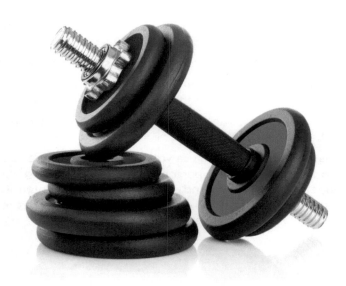

Day	Muscle Group	Exercise Sample	Sets/ Reps	Equipment	Personal Workout for Each Muscle Group
Mon. Wed.	chest shoulders	chest presses	3 · 15	resistance band	
		lateral raises	3 · 15	resistance band	
		squatting shoulder presses	3 · 10	weighted ball	
		wide-arm push-ups	3 · 15	body weight	
		wide-arm push-ups	3 · 15	body weight	
Mon. Wed.	biceps triceps	triceps extensions	3 · 15	resistance band	
		biceps hammer curls	3 · 15	resistance band	
		lunges with passes	3 · 10	weighted ball	
		triceps push-ups (narrow push-ups)	3 · 10	body weight	
Tue. Thur.	legs	squats	3 · 15	fitness ball	
		calf raises	3 · 15	resistance band	
		lunges with passes	3 · 10	weighted ball	
		lunges	3 · 15	body weight	
Tue. Thur.	back	back extensions	3 · 15	fitness ball	
		seated rows	3 · 15	resistance band	
		back extension rolls	3 · 10	weighted ball	
		pull-ups	3 · 10	body weight	
Mon. Wed. Fri.	core	crunches	3 · 15	fitness ball	
		side crunches	3 · 15	fitness ball	
		figure-8s	3 · 10	weighted ball	
		planks	3 · 30 seconds	body weight	

Cool-down: Complete this cool-down after exercising.

Exercise	Duration
• hamstring stretch	• 30 seconds
• quadriceps stretch	• 30 seconds
• shoulder/triceps stretch	• 30 seconds
• side stretch	• 30 seconds
• lower back/hip stretch	• 30 seconds
• groin stretch	• 30 seconds

List at least 1 response to each of the following questions about strength training.

Question	Response
What positive emotional response did you experience by participating in strength training?	
What type of strength training do you enjoy the most?	
How would the previously mentioned activity lead to good physical and mental health?	

RESEARCH INTEGRATION

Research and describe isometric, concentric, and eccentric contractions in a push-up.

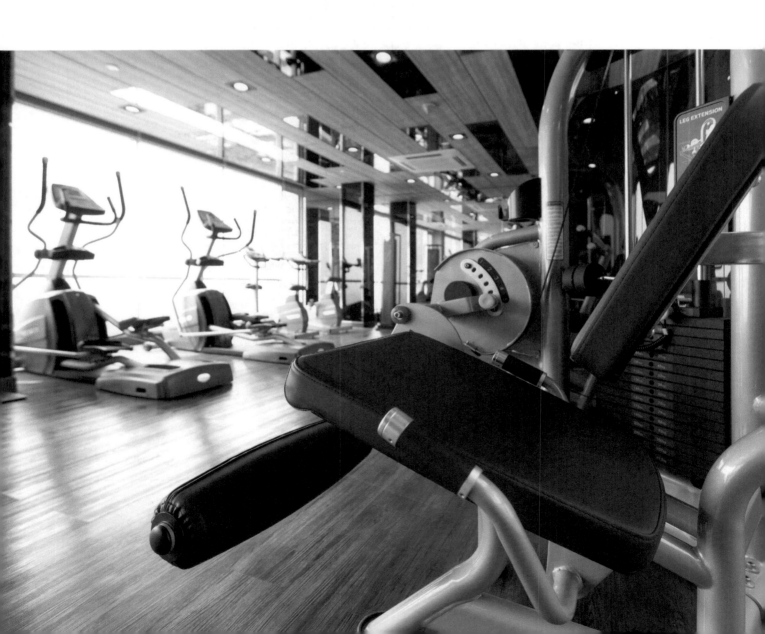

CROSS-TRAINING CARDIOVASCULAR AND STRENGTH CIRCUIT: USING WHAT YOU HAVE LEARNED

For efficient use of time, you can do a cross-training circuit. This cross-training circuit alternates strength exercises with aerobic movements. Cross-training saves time by giving you a single workout that has both strength and aerobic benefits. It is important for you to set your own goals based on your ability level and determine your intensity and duration based on your individual target heart rate zone.

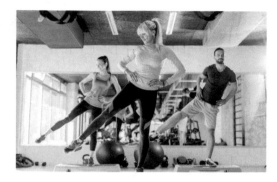

The purpose of this lesson is to encourage you to create and implement a cross-training circuit workout. The workout would be included in the recommended 60 minutes of daily physical activity and would count as both an aerobic and a strength workout. **The Cardiovascular Endurance section of this manual includes the target heart rate zone formula and the Borg Rating of Perceived Exertion Scale to help you to determine if you are exercising for heart health.** You can also use available technology to monitor your pulse rate and intensity.

CROSS-TRAINING CIRCUIT WORKOUT: CARDIOVASCULAR AND STRENGTH

Review the following example and use the information to establish a workout regimen that fits into your schedule. Adhere to the FITT principle (frequency, intensity, time, and type of exercise). This workout requires a jump rope, fitness ball, resistance bands, and kettlebell. You should have a mat or cushioned surface for sit-ups and push-ups.

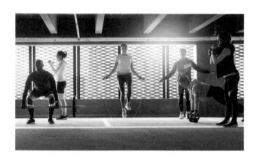

SAMPLE CROSS-TRAINING CIRCUIT WORKOUT

Build cardiovascular endurance, strength, and flexibility in a cross-training circuit workout using exercises from the appropriate sections of your manual: Cardiovascular Endurance, Muscle Strength, Muscle Endurance, and Flexibility. Review the Aerobic Exercise and Proper Nutrition, Jump Rope, Fitness Ball, Resistance Bands, and Weighted Ball sections to practice correct forms for the skills.

Warm-up: Perform 5 to 10 minutes of light cardio to increase your heart rate, breathing rate, and body temperature. Do some dynamic stretches to increase flexibility.

Perform each exercise for 30 seconds. Rest and hydrate when necessary. Set the workout to music.

1. **jumping jacks**
2. **sit-ups**
3. **high knees**
4. **weighted ball figure-8s**
5. **jump rope**
6. **resistance band biceps hammer curls**
7. **rear kicks**
8. **fitness ball back extensions**
9. **jog in place**
10. **right-angle push-ups**
11. **jump rope**
12. **weighted ball squatting shoulder presses**
13. **¼-squat jumps**
14. **weighted ball lunges with passes**
15. **march in place**
16. **resistance band seated rows**
17. **jump rope**
18. **fitness ball crunches**
19. **burpees**
20. **weighted ball extensions with rolls**

Repeat for a 20-minute workout.

Cool-down: Walk slowly until your heart rate, breathing rate, and body temperature have returned to baseline. Do some static stretches to increase flexibility.

CREATE A PERSONAL WORKOUT

Use the cross-training information to create a personal circuit workout you would enjoy.

CREATE A PERSONAL WORKOUT FOR A PERSON WITH A JOB

Objective: to overcome exercise barriers you may face when you are finished with school and ready for a career

Create a cross-training workout for a family member who works full time. A job is often a barrier to exercise, and many people have trouble fitting exercise into their schedules. Try to help your family member find the time to exercise.

- Make sure the family member has a doctor's approval to exercise.
- Interview the family member to evaluate the level of fitness and plan accordingly.
- Use exercises and equipment that the family member prefers. A beginner may need to march in place and use the resistance bands only.
- Review the family member's daily and weekly schedules to find at least 3 available times for regular exercise.
- Establish an exercise plan that may work for your family member.

EXTENSION: Exercise with your family member.

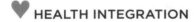 **RESEARCH INTEGRATION**

Research exercise and its connection to emotional health.

HEALTH INTEGRATION

Use available technology to monitor your pulse rate and intensity. Apply the results to your overall fitness plan.

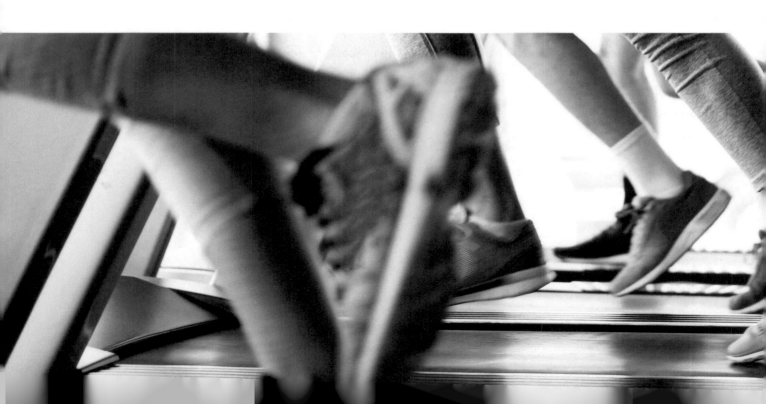

SPORTS-RELATED AND SKILL-RELATED ACTIVITIES

🏃 **FITNESS TIP:** Prior to beginning your physical education activities, read the following safety information that applies to every lesson, review the timeline, and review the assessment rubric.

⚠️ **SAFETY ALERT:** Before you exercise, make sure that you are properly warmed up and have enough room to perform each activity. Wear proper equipment and follow activity-specific safety rules. Stay hydrated and take breaks as needed. Exercise only if you are healthy, and always exercise at your own pace. If an exercise starts to hurt, if you feel dizzy, or if you feel light-headed, stop the exercise completely and get help. Upon completion of any workout, cool down and stretch.

TIMELINE

Review all of the activity information before beginning. Use the scoring rubrics as assessment tools. You may ask a trusted adult or friend to observe your performance and provide feedback. Progress according to your skill level. The time that it takes you to complete a module will depend on your personal progress.

Practice and assess the first skill until competent.

Apply skills in a game situation.

Continue to progress until you have practiced and assessed each skill until competent.

ASSESSMENT RUBRIC

You will find a rubric assessment tool following some of the basic skills. Use this tool to evaluate and score your progress in learning the elements of a new skill.

SKILL	PROGRESSING	COMPETENT	PROFICIENT
skill 1	1 or 2 of the elements	3 or 4 out of 5 elements	all elements met

CAM JAM

Can jam is played by 2 opposing teams, each made up of 2 players. Points are scored by throwing a flying disc to a can (goal). The rules are easy to follow, but the game is challenging and competitive. Can jam is a fun, social game that provides exercise, improves coordination, and is easy to set up.

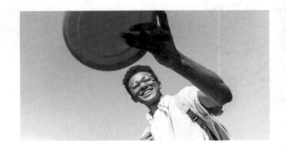

The purpose of this lesson is for you to practice disc-throwing skills and to encourage participation in games for physical activity.

CAM JAM SKILLS

BACKHAND GRIP

- Hold the disc in your dominant hand.
- Hold the disc parallel to the ground with your thumb on top.
- Rest your index finger on the edge of the disc, and curl your remaining fingers under the disc.

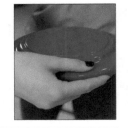

SKILL	PROGRESSING	COMPETENT	PROFICIENT
grip	1 of the elements	2 out of 3 elements	all elements met

BACKHAND THROW

- Hold the disc in your dominant hand.
- Bend your elbow and keep the disc close to your body so it is touching your forearm. The back of your hand should be facing the target.
- Step toward the target with your dominant foot.
- Snap your wrist and release the disc while extending your arm.

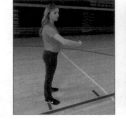 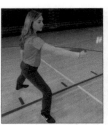 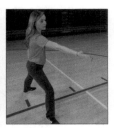

SKILL	PROGRESSING	COMPETENT	PROFICIENT
throw	1 or 2 of the elements	3 out of 4 elements	all elements met

DEFLECTING

- Use your hands to move the disc to the target without catching, carrying, or double hitting the disc.
- Make quick contact and release the disc with your hands.
- Tap or push it to the target.

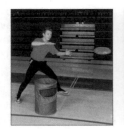 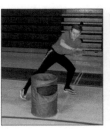 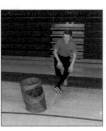

SKILL	PROGRESSING	COMPETENT	PROFICIENT
deflecting	1 of the elements	2 out of 3 elements	all elements met

PRACTICE THE SKILLS

- Using the backhand grip, practice throwing toward the target.
- Increase your distance as you improve.
- Pass and deflect with a partner.

PLAYING THE GAME

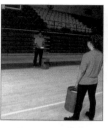
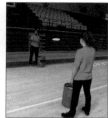

- The game requires 4 players (2 per team).
- Set the goals 50 feet apart.
- Mark a throw line with cones set 25 feet from each goal.
- For each team, 1 player (the deflector) stands near the goal and the other player (the thrower) stands at the throw line.
- Each team gets 1 disc.
- The thrower throws the disc toward the goal.
- The deflector redirects the disc toward the goal or into the goal.
- Switch roles with your teammate.
- After both players from the starting team throw and deflect, it is the other team's turn.
- Continue to alternate throws until a team reaches 21 points.

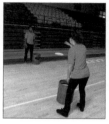
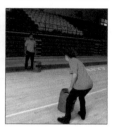

SCORING

dinger	1 point	redirected hit	Deflector redirects the thrown disk to hit any side of the goal.
deuce	2 points	direct hit	Thrower hits the side of the goal, unassisted by partner.
bucket	3 points	slam dunk	Deflector redirects the thrown disk and it lands inside the goal.
instant win	game over	direct entry	Thrower lands the disk inside the goal, unassisted by partner. The disk can enter through the slot opening on the side or through the top of the goal. When an instant win occurs, the throwing team is declared the winner and the opposing team does not receive a "last toss" option.

RULES

1. Players must remain behind the line when throwing. No points are awarded if the player crosses the line.

2. No points are awarded when a throw hits the ground before hitting the goal.

3. Deflectors can move anywhere within the playing area to redirect the disc.

4. No points are awarded if a deflector double-hits, catches, or carries the disc.

5. If an opponent interferes with a play or defends the goal, 3 points will be awarded. If the score is 19 or 20, 1 or 2 points are awarded.

6. A team must reach an exact score of 21 points to win. If a play places a team's score above 21 points, the points from that play are deducted from the team's current score, and play continues. For example, if a team has 20 points and scores a bucket (3 points), that team's score is reduced to 17.

7. Teams must complete an equal number of turns before the game is over. Unless an instant win is thrown, the team with the hammer (last toss) will always get to throw last.

8. If the game is tied, the winner is decided in a tiebreaker method of overtime. Each team completes 1 round of throws, and the team to score first wins. Overtime rounds continue until the tie is broken.

DEMONSTRATE POSITIVE GAME BEHAVIOR

- Follow the rules.
- Make no physical contact with an opposing player.
- Be supportive and encouraging to your teammate.
- Treat your opponents with respect.

SKILL	PROGRESSING	COMPETENT	PROFICIENT
game behavior	1 or 2 of the elements	3 out of 4 elements	all elements met

RATE YOUR ENJOYMENT OF CAN JAM

On a scale from 1 to 4, where 1 is not enjoyable and 4 is very enjoyable, rate this activity.

1	It was not enjoyable, and I will not participate again.
2	It was not enjoyable, but I will participate again for exercise.
3	It was enjoyable, and I will play again.
4	It was very enjoyable, and I will initiate future games.

💻 RESEARCH INTEGRATION

Research the cultural role of casual sports games in society.

❤️ HEALTH INTEGRATION

Count and analyze your pulse during and after playing can jam to determine if you are exercising in your personal target heart rate zone. Apply the results to your overall fitness plan. Many people choose to get their aerobic workouts by playing in casual games with friends.

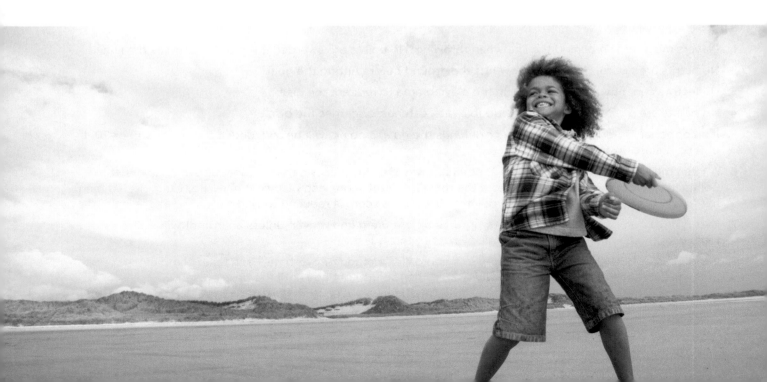

TENNIS

Tennis is a sport played by striking a ball with a racket over a net. It is played against a single opponent or as a doubles game. You may play tennis as a competitive sport or as an opportunity for social play. Find tennis courts in your community where you can play for fun and fitness.

The purpose of this lesson is for you to practice tennis skills and encourage participation in games for a lifetime of physical activity.

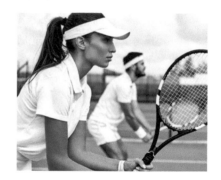

⚠ **CAUTION: Make sure nobody is close to you before you swing the racket. Do not walk into the path of another person swinging a racket.**

RACKET SKILLS

READY POSITION

The ready position allows a player to move quickly in any direction.

- Bend your knees and stand with your feet shoulder-width apart.
- Keep your head up.
- Keep your weight on the balls of your feet.
- Hold the racket in your dominant hand.

SKILL	PROGRESSING	COMPETENT	PROFICIENT
ready position	1 or 2 of the elements	3 out of 4 elements	all elements met

HANDSHAKE GRIP

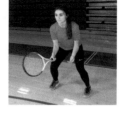

- Hold the racket in your dominant hand like you are about to shake someone's hand.
- Place your 4 fingers around the racket, and then wrap your thumb around the racket.
- Hold the racket so that the head is vertical to the ground. Make sure that the strings on the racket head are facing front and back.
- Point the handle toward your belly button.

SKILL	PROGRESSING	COMPETENT	PROFICIENT
handshake grip	1 or 2 of the elements	3 out of 4 elements	all elements met

FOREHAND STROKE

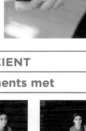
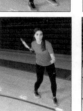
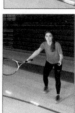

- Begin in the ready position.
- Pivot to bring the racket back on the same side of your body as your dominant hand.
- Face the palm of your hand forward.
- Shift your weight from your back foot to your front foot while stepping forward and swinging the racket with your dominant hand.
- Extend your arm and flick your wrist to hit the ball, pointing the face of the racket up to get the ball over the net.
- Follow through to your target.

SKILL	PROGRESSING	COMPETENT	PROFICIENT
forehand stroke	1, 2, or 3 of the elements	4 or 5 out of 6 elements	all elements met

BACKHAND STROKE

- Begin in the ready position.
- Rotate the racket and extend it across your body.
- Rotate your feet and shoulders in the same direction as the racket.
- Face the back of your hand (the side that your knuckles are on) forward.
- Step forward with your non-dominant foot while swinging the racket.
- Flick your wrist when hitting the ball with the center of the racket.
- Follow through to your target.

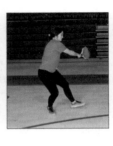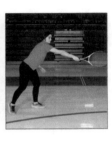

SKILL	PROGRESSING	COMPETENT	PROFICIENT
backhand stroke	1, 2, 3, or 4 of the elements	5 or 6 out of 7 elements	all elements met

2-HANDED BACKHAND STROKE

- Place your non-dominant hand below your dominant hand on the racket handle.
- Rotate the racket and extend it across your body.
- Rotate your feet and shoulders in the same direction as the racket.
- Flick your wrists when you are hitting the ball with the center of the racket.
- Follow through to your target.

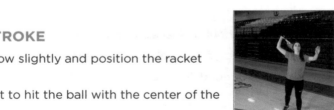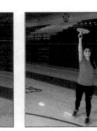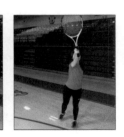

OVERHAND STROKE

- Bend your elbow slightly and position the racket under the ball.
- Flick your wrist to hit the ball with the center of the racket.
- Extend your arm as you make contact.
- Follow through to your target.

SKILL	PROGRESSING	COMPETENT	PROFICIENT
overhand stroke	1 or 2 of the elements	3 out of 4 elements	all elements met

SERVES

Every game starts with a serve

PUNCH SERVE

Stand behind the service line at a 45-degree angle to the net.

A punch serve is an excellent stroke to use as a beginner.

- If you are right-handed, place your left foot forward; if you are left-handed, place your right foot forward. Put your weight on your back foot.
- Hold the racket with a forehand grip in your dominant hand. Raise the racket over your head and slightly back.

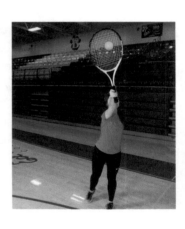

- Hold the ball with your fingertips in your non-dominant hand.
- Toss the ball slightly in front of you and high above the racket. Look up at the ball.
- As the ball comes back down, hit it up and forward with the racket. Extend your arm and the racket while you are hitting the ball.
- Follow through to your target. Swing out, across, and down.

SKILL	PROGRESSING	COMPETENT	PROFICIENT
punch serve	1 or 2 of the elements	4 out of 6 elements	all elements met

OVERHAND SERVE

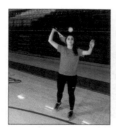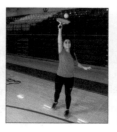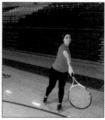

- Hold the racket with your dominant hand.
- Place your non-dominant foot toward the opposite post of the net and your dominant foot parallel to the court.
- Toss the ball into the air just above your head.
- Bring your dominant arm back with the head of the racket pointing toward the sky.
- Watch for the ball to begin to fall.
- Extend your arm up over your head and contact the ball with the head of the racket.

SKILL	PROGRESSING	COMPETENT	PROFICIENT
overhand serve	1, 2, or 3 of the elements	4 or 5 out of 6 elements	all elements met

SKILL PRACTICE

AGAINST A WALL

- Practice the various strokes and serves by hitting the ball against a wall with the racket. Catch the ball each time and repeat.
- Allow the ball to bounce before hitting it against the wall.
- Volley against the wall, aiming at and hitting certain spots.

WITH A PARTNER

- You can use a jump rope to separate each side if a net is unavailable.
- Have a partner stand on 1 side of the net and toss the ball toward your forehand. Return with a proper forehand stroke.
- Have a partner stand on 1 side of the net and toss the ball toward your backhand. Return with a proper backhand stroke.
- Have a partner stand on 1 side of the net and toss the ball, mixing up forehand and backhand shots. Return with a proper forehand stroke or backhand stroke.
- Use the various strokes to hit the ball back and forth with a partner. Stand 15 feet away from your partner when you are volleying back and forth.

ANALYZE AND IMPROVE STROKES AND SERVE

- Practice several times a week to improve skills and game play.
- Concentrate on proper body rotation and pivot to execute the forehand and backhand strokes.
- Use various amounts of force and speed to improve the placing of shots and serves.
- Practice the overhand serve without the ball. Keep your arm loose as you drop it back, and rotate your wrist before contact; follow through to the target.
- Practice the overhand serve with the ball.

GAME

OFFICIAL SINGLES GAME

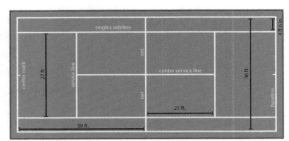

- You will need traditional tennis balls for this game.
- Start with an overhand serve from the right side of the court. Serve from behind the baseline to your opponent on the left.
- Get the ball into your opponent's service box. You have 2 tries to get the ball into the service box. If you hit the ball into your opponent's service box and your opponent cannot return it, you win that volley and get a point.
- Serve from the left side of the court next. When your score is an even number, serve from the right side of the court. When your score is an odd number, serve from the left side of the court.
- Continue serving the ball until the game is over. The receiver becomes the server during the next game.
- You may only hit the ball 1 time on each side.
- You score if your opponent does not have a successful serve, fails to return a serve, or hits the ball out of bounds.
- You lose a volley if you or the racket touch the net.

SCORING

- The server's score is always announced first.
- The point system is as follows.
    o no points or love = 0 points
    o 1 point = 15 points
    o 2 points = 30 points
    o 3 points = 40 points
    o 4 points = win
- To win a game, you must lead by at least 2 points.
- If the score is tied at 40 points (a deuce), you must earn 2 consecutive points (an advantage point) to win the game.
- You must win at least 6 games in a set. You must lead by 2 sets to win a match.

DEMONSTRATE POSITIVE GAME BEHAVIOR

- Follow the rules.
- There is to be no intentional hitting of an opposing player with the ball. You forfeit a point if you hit the opposing player with a ball.
- Be supportive and encouraging to your teammate.
- Treat your opponents with respect.

SKILL	PROGRESSING	COMPETENT	PROFICIENT
game behavior	1 or 2 of the elements	3 out of 4 elements	all elements met

RATE YOUR ENJOYMENT OF TENNIS

On a scale from 1 to 4, where 1 is not enjoyable and 4 is very enjoyable, rate this activity.

1	It was not enjoyable, and I will not participate again.
2	It was not enjoyable, but I will participate again for exercise.
3	It was enjoyable, and I will play again.
4	It was very enjoyable, and I will initiate future games.

 RESEARCH INTEGRATION

1. Research tennis serves such as the flat serve, slice serve, kick serve, and underhand serve.
2. Attend a tennis game or watch a tennis game on television.

 HEALTH INTEGRATION

Count your pulse to determine if you are exercising in your personal target heart rate zone. Count your pulse after practicing skills and after playing in a game. Apply the results to your overall fitness plan. Many people choose to get their aerobic workouts by playing in games with friends.

VOLLEYBALL

The official game of volleyball is played by 2 teams of 6 players on an indoor volleyball court. Another popular version of volleyball is beach volleyball, which is played by 2 teams of 2 to 6 players on a sand surface. The object of the game is to strike a ball over a net onto the ground so that the opposing team cannot return it.

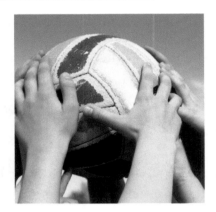

You may play volleyball as a competitive sport or as an opportunity for social play. Casual games of volleyball can be played by as few as 2 players and set up in a yard, park, beach, or gym.

The purpose of this lesson is for you to participate in aerobic exercise and in skill-building activities. When you play volleyball, be sure to follow the rules, communicate with teammates in a positive and effective manner, and exhibit appropriate behavior with your team and the opposing team.

 CAUTION: Do not overinflate the ball.

VOLLEYBALL SKILLS

The following striking skills will not only help to improve your volleyball game, but they may also enhance skills used in other sports and activities.

READY POSITION

The ready position will enable you to react quickly.

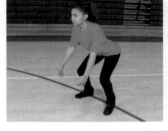

- Stand with your legs shoulder-width apart.
- Balance on the balls of your feet.
- Bend your knees slightly.
- Hold your shoulders rounded and slightly forward.
- Hold your arms in front of you and ready to react.

SKILL	PROGRESSING	COMPETENT	PROFICIENT
ready position	1 or 2 of the elements	3 or 4 out of 5 elements	all elements met

FOREARM GRIP

Try both of the following grips to decide which works better for you.

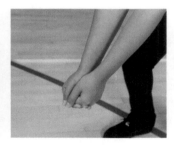

1. Right-handed players: Make a fist with your left hand, wrap the fingers of your right hand around your left hand, and line up your thumbs side by side on top.
   Left-handed players: Make a fist with your right hand, wrap the fingers of your left hand around your right hand, and line up your thumbs side by side on top.

2. Place 1 hand out flat with your palm up. Place the other hand underneath with the palm up. Curl your thumbs until they are next to each other, centered, and pointing down.

FOREARM PASS (BUMP)

- Stand in the ready position.
- Use the correct grip.
- Contact the ball with your forearm platform.
- Follow through toward your target.

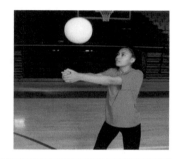

SKILL	PROGRESSING	COMPETENT	PROFICIENT
forearm pass	1 or 2 of the elements	3 out of 4 elements	all elements met

FOREARM PASS (BUMP) PRACTICE

- Forearm pass and catch: Toss the ball to yourself to begin. Pass it back up with your forearm platform, reaching toward your target and catching it. Do not allow your swing to be out of control.
- Forearm pass: Toss the ball to yourself to begin, then continue to pass it. How many times can you pass in a row?
- Wall forearm passes: Toss the ball to yourself to begin, then pass it against a wall. How many times can you pass in a row?
- Partner wall forearm passes: Take turns passing against a wall with a partner.
- Partner toss, forearm pass, and catch: Toss the ball to your partner. Your partner passes it back to you. You catch it. Switch roles.
- Partner forearm passes: How many times can you pass back and forth with a partner?

OVERHAND PASS (SET)

- Stand in the ready position.
- Hold your hands level with your forehead with your elbows bent. Form the size and shape of the ball with your fingers and thumbs.
- Contact the ball with your finger pads, not tips.
- Use a soft touch near your forehead and extend your elbows to push the ball up into the air.

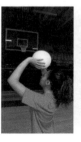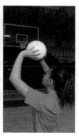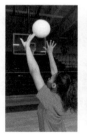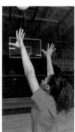

SKILL	PROGRESSING	COMPETENT	PROFICIENT
overhand pass	1 or 2 of the elements	3 out of 4 elements	all elements met

OVERHAND PASS (SET) PRACTICE

- Set and catch: Toss the ball to yourself to begin, set it back up with your finger pads, and catch it.
- Set: Toss the ball to yourself to begin, then continue to set it. How many times can you set in a row?
- Wall sets: Toss the ball to yourself to begin, then set it against a wall. How many times can you set in a row?
- Partner wall sets: Take turns setting against a wall with a partner.
- Partner toss, set, and catch: Toss the ball to your partner. Your partner sets it back to you. You catch it. Switch roles.
- Partner sets: How many times can you set back and forth with a partner?

UNDERHAND SERVE

- Put your non-dominant foot forward.
- Hold the ball on the palm of your non-dominant hand. Position that arm across your body at waist height.
- Make a fist with your striking hand.
- Bring your striking arm back and then forward, striking the ball with the heel of your hand.
- Shift your weight to your front foot.
- Serve successfully 70 percent of the time.

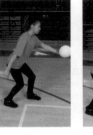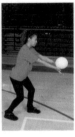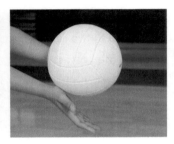

SKILL	PROGRESSING	COMPETENT	PROFICIENT
underhand serve	1 or 2 of the elements	4 or 5 out of 6 elements	all elements met

UNDERHAND SERVE PRACTICE

- Wall serves: Practice serving toward a wall.
- Partner serves: Serve to a partner and volley back and forth using the set and bump skills.

ANALYZE AND IMPROVE PASSES AND SERVES

- Practice several times a week to improve skills and game play.
- Concentrate on proper grip and arm position for the forearm pass.
- Concentrate on hand position for the set.
- Use various amounts of force and speed to improve the placing of shots and serves.
- Practice the underhand serve technique without the ball.
- Practice and refine the underhand serve with the ball.

CHALLENGING VOLLEYBALL SKILLS

The following advanced skills are for students who have mastered the basic skills. The challenge level is recommended if you want to further explore the volleyball activity.

OVERHAND SERVE

- Put your non-dominant foot forward.
- Turn the non-dominant side of your body slightly toward the net or target.
- Hold the ball in your non-dominant hand.
- Bend your striking arm with your hand cupped near your ear.

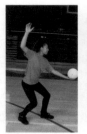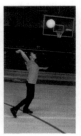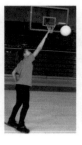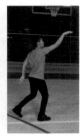

- Contact: Toss the ball 2 to 3 feet in the air, placing your weight on your back foot. Shift your weight to your front foot as you strike the ball approximately 12 inches above your head.
- Follow through in the direction of the ball.

SKILL	PROGRESSING	COMPETENT	PROFICIENT
overhand serve	1 or 2 of the elements	3, 4, or 5 out of 6 elements	all elements met

OVERHAND SERVE PRACTICE

Wall serves: Practice serving toward a wall.

Partner serves: Serve to a partner and volley back and forth using the set and bump skills.

OVERHAND HITTING (SPIKE)

1 player: Follow the overhand serve techniques.

2 players: A teammate hits the ball up high near the net.

- As a hitter, approach from behind using a 4-step approach.
- Place your dominant foot forward.
- Step forward with your non-dominant foot, then quick step with your dominant then non-dominant foot. For example, if you are right-handed, you would start with your right foot forward, step left, then right, then left.
- Begin with your arms at waist height in front of your body. Swing them backward then forward until both of your arms are reaching high with your dominant arm slightly forward.
- Strike the ball with the fleshy part of your dominant hand.
- Follow through, facing the direction in which you want the ball to go.

SKILL	PROGRESSING	COMPETENT	PROFICIENT
overhand hit (spike)	1 or 2 of the elements	3, 4, or 5 out of 6 elements	all elements met

EXTENSION

If you have an available outdoor wall or garage door and permission from your parent or guardian, you can place a horizontal line of tape or chalk mark 7 feet 4½ inches from the ground to represent the height of a net. Begin approximately 10 feet back and practice the underhand and overhand serves. When you are successful, move back farther. Continue this until you are able to serve from 30 feet back, which is the official serving distance.

VOLLEYBALL GAMES

REGULATION VOLLEYBALL GAME

- There are 6 people on a team: 3 front row players and 3 back row players.
- Players rotate in order to reach the serving position.
- The players from the same team all rotate 1 position clockwise when it is their team's turn to serve.
- The serving position is behind the end line. Most players will serve from the right end line; however, for left-handed servers, you may serve from anywhere behind the end line.
- The objective is to serve the ball across the net into the opponent's court within the boundaries. The ball can hit the net on the way over and still be playable.
- Each team is allowed 3 hits, but no player can hit the ball twice in a row.
- A player may not make contact with any part of the net.
- A ball contacting the net is considered playable.

SCORING

- A serve starts the game.
- When the serving team wins the rally, a point is scored.
- If the rally is won by the non-serving team, that team gets a point and a chance to serve.
- The first team to score 25 points and be ahead by at least 2 points wins the game.
- A match consists of either winning 2 out of 3 games or 3 out of 5 games.

ALTERNATIVE: A COOPERATIVE SCORING GAME

- You will need at least 2 players.
- Toss a coin to see which side serves first.
- There will be 1 person or team on each side of the net. You may use a jump rope or disc cones to separate each side if a net is unavailable.
- Rally back and forth.
- Count each time the ball goes over the net except for the serve.
- There are unlimited hits per side, but a point is scored only when it goes over the net.
- Continue until the ball is not in play.
- Indicate the score.
- Rotate sides and players for each serve.
- Count again and try to beat your previous score.

DEMONSTRATE POSITIVE GAME BEHAVIOR

- Follow the rules.
- Call out when you are attempting to strike the ball to avoid collisions.
- Be supportive and encouraging to your teammates.
- Treat your opponents with respect.

SKILL	PROGRESSING	COMPETENT	PROFICIENT
game behavior	1 or 2 of the elements	3 out of 4 elements	all elements met

RATE YOUR ENJOYMENT OF VOLLEYBALL

On a scale from 1 to 4, where 1 is not enjoyable and 4 is very enjoyable, rate this activity.

1	It was not enjoyable, and I will not participate again.
2	It was not enjoyable, but I will participate again for exercise.
3	It was enjoyable, and I will play again.
4	It was very enjoyable, and I will initiate future games.

🖥 RESEARCH INTEGRATION

Research beach volleyball.

Attend a volleyball game or watch a volleyball game on television and compare the skills you have practiced for the game of volleyball with the skills the players use.

♥ HEALTH INTEGRATION

Count your pulse to determine if you are exercising in your personal target heart rate zone. Count your pulse after practicing skills and after playing in a game. Apply the results to your overall fitness plan.

GRADE 11
PE EQUIPMENT KIT

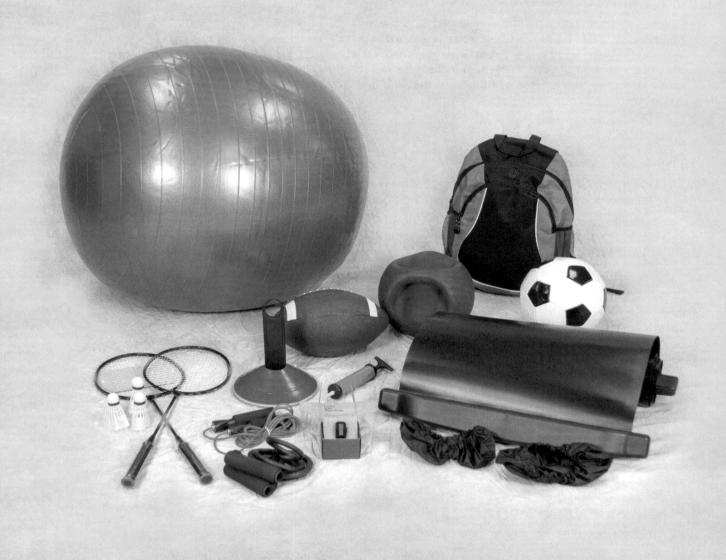

WARM-UP AND COOL-DOWN

⚠ **CAUTION: Stretching should not be painful; ease up if stretching hurts. See the Flexibility section of your PE Manual for more information.**

WARM-UP

The purpose of a warm-up is to gradually increase heart rate, breathing rate, body temperature, and muscle temperature. Warming up prior to exercising increases circulation and blood flow to your muscles. When your muscles are warmed up, their performance—such as in the areas of strength and speed—is enhanced and risk of injury is decreased.

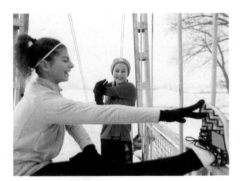

Stretching your muscles helps to minimize risk of injury by making the muscle fibers pliable, which means easy to bend or move.

Before you begin any workout, you should always warm up. Getting your heart and muscles prepared for exercise is important. There are numerous ways to get your body ready to participate in physical activity. **The Flexibility section of your PE Manual includes a variety of dynamic and static stretches for each major body part that will help you increase your flexibility.**

Elements of a Warm-Up

1. **Low-intensity cardio**: Walk, slow jog, or slow swim for 5 to 10 minutes to increase your heart rate, breathing rate, and body temperature before your workout.

2. **Dynamic stretch**: Perform a repeated motion—such as kicks, high knees, lunges, or arm circles—that will loosen up your joints and prepare your muscles for the exercise that you are about to do. Perform each dynamic stretch for at least 30 seconds.

   • Choose dynamic stretches that will warm up the major muscles that you will be using in the activity. For example, you could perform arm circles as part of your warm-up prior to swimming.

3. **Static stretch**: Stretch your muscles slowly and hold each stretch for 20 to 30 seconds without bouncing in order to lengthen your muscles and increase your flexibility. Some important areas to stretch as a part of your warm-up are your neck, sides, shoulders, triceps, back, hamstrings, quadriceps, and groin.

Example 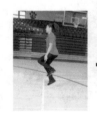 **+** 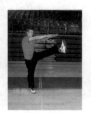 **+** 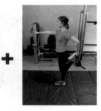 **= EFFECTIVE WARM-UP**

PERSONAL WARM-UP ACTIVITY

1. Select an exercise activity to participate in.

2. Design your personal warm-up plan for the activity that you selected. Any dynamic and static stretches that you choose to complete should be specific to the exercise activity that you chose.

3. Have a trusted adult or friend assess your stretches to make sure that you are using proper form.

4. Explain how the warm-up will decrease your risk of injury for this activity. _____

Procedure	Enter your personal warm-up regimen below.
1. **Low-intensity cardiovascular exercise:** Exercise for 5 to 10 minutes.	
2. **Dynamic stretches:** Perform dynamic stretches specifically for the selected activity.	
3. **Static stretches:** Perform static stretches specifically for the selected activity.	

COOL-DOWN

After you have finished your workout, exercise, or activity, it is imperative that your body returns to its normal state. You want to avoid stopping immediately and sitting down **unless you are in pain, dizzy, or injured**. Be sure to slow your heart rate and breathing rate back to or slightly above their resting rates. There are several ways to do this. You can simply walk or slow down your exercise for a few minutes, or you can find your own way to slow your body back down. You also may want to incorporate static stretches to increase flexibility and to avoid your muscles tightening. **The Flexibility section of your PE Manual includes a variety of static stretches for each major body part.** Always keep hydrated by drinking water before, during, and after exercise.

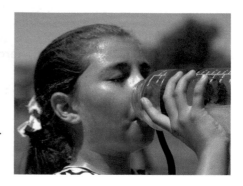

Elements of a Cool-Down

1. **Slow down**: Walk or gradually slow down your exercise—such as returning to a slow swim if you are swimming—until your heart rate, breathing rate, and body temperature are back to normal.

2. **Static stretch**: Stretch your muscles slowly and hold each stretch for 20 to 30 seconds without bouncing in order to lengthen your muscles and increase flexibility. Some important areas to stretch as part of your cool-down are your neck, sides, shoulders, triceps, back, hamstrings, quadriceps, and groin.

WALK + STATIC STRETCHES = EFFECTIVE COOL-DOWN

Design your personal cool-down plan. You can perform the same cool-down each time you finish a physical activity or you can change each time in order to reflect the exercise activity, such as by slowing your pedaling if you are biking.

Procedure	Enter your personal cool-down regimen below.
1. **Slow down:** Perform this slowed activity for 5 to 10 minutes.	
2. **Static stretches:** Perform several lower-body and upper-body stretches.	

AEROBIC EXERCISE AND PROPER NUTRITION

It is important that your commitment to aerobic exercise and proper nutrition continues throughout your lifetime. College and work environments can increase your workload and increase your stress. Exercising regularly and eating healthfully can help reduce stress and its adverse effects. Because any exercise done in your target heart rate zone and performed for 20 to 60 minutes 3 to 5 days per week is aerobic exercise, you can find something that fits into your current and future schedules.

You are more likely to commit to healthful eating if you plan and keep track of your nutrition. Eating proper portions from the grain group, the fruit group, the vegetable group, the dairy group, and the protein group is essential to proper nutrition. Limit high-fat and sugary foods.

Combining regular aerobic exercise with proper nutrition contributes to cardiovascular health as well as overall health. It should be a lifelong commitment.

The purpose of this lesson is to encourage you to develop a fitness portfolio, choreograph an aerobic exercise routine, participate in aerobic workouts, and plan for proper nutrition. **The Cardiovascular Endurance section of this manual includes the target heart rate zone formula and the Borg Rating of Perceived Exertion Scale to help you to determine if you are exercising for heart health.** You can also use available technology to monitor your pulse rate and intensity.

When beginning any exercise program, begin with workouts for your fitness level and then build accordingly. You want to feel refreshed after your exercise session, not exhausted. Use your pulse rate to monitor aerobic workouts.

 CAUTION: Wear proper equipment and follow activity-specific safety rules.

AEROBIC EXERCISE AND PROPER NUTRITION

Develop a fitness portfolio and make a commitment to aerobic exercise. Your fitness portfolio should include the following.

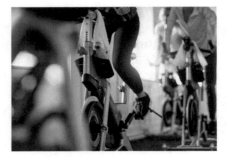

- endurance walk/run fitness score
- goals for improvement
- 4-week exercise plan (See below.)

TYPES OF AEROBIC EXERCISE

Sports: Examples include soccer, basketball, volleyball, swimming, hockey, lacrosse, tennis, badminton, pickleball, handball, gymnastics, dance, martial arts, wrestling, track and field, and so on.

Outdoor pursuits: Examples include walking, jogging, biking, canoeing, kayaking, golfing, fly fishing, hiking, rock climbing, horseback riding, skiing, and so on.

Fitness gyms: Find a gym that is convenient for you to attend where you can complete circuit exercises, use aerobic machines, take classes, and more.

Stationary exercise equipment: Examples include using a jump rope, treadmill, elliptical trainer, bike, mini trampoline, and so on.

Exercise apps or videos: Use a workout tutorial on an app, website, video, or other digital source.

Your own sequence workouts: You can also design your own workout sequences by following the steps below.

- Create your personal aerobic workout routines by blending activities that involve basic locomotor skills such as jogging in place, jumping jacks, high knees, and so on.
- Design the intensity and duration of the exercise according to your level of fitness.
- Perform your personal routine for some or all your aerobic workouts.

Choreograph a personal aerobic workout routine by blending basic locomotor skills. This is a workout that can be done at home for convenience. The suggested time for each skill is from 20 to 60 seconds with a 30-second rest every 4 to 5 minutes. Repeat for a 20- to 60-minute workout. Most important, exercise at your level of fitness and rest accordingly. Use the following skills to choreograph your routine, or use skills of your choice.

- Jogging in place: Run slowly in place.
- Jumping jacks: Stand with your feet apart with arms up, then feet together with arms at your sides.
- High knees: Alternate lifting your knees to waist height.
- Burpees: Jump vertically, then bend your knees and transition to a push-up position.
- Side slides: Step to the right. Bring the other foot over in a step-together motion. Repeat left.
- Squat jumps: Jump and land softly into a squat (hips even with knees).
- March in place: Alternate lifting knees to waist height.
- Carioca: Step to the side with 1 foot and cross with your other foot in a step-cross-step-cross movement. Alternate the step-cross movement with a cross behind the lead foot and a cross in front of the lead foot.
- Front kicks: Alternate lifting your legs forward.

EXTENSION: Work with a friend to create aerobic routines. Evaluate each other's level of fitness and schedule (school/work) to create and plan personalized workouts.

Plan your exercise. The following is an example of how to schedule and track aerobic exercise for 1 week. Plan for 4 weeks.

WARM UP BEFORE EACH WORKOUT.

Week 1	Exercise	Time of Day	Exercise Time (min.)	Heart Rate (bpm)
Mon.	jump rope	morning	20	160
Tues.				
Wed.	my routine	morning	30	155
Thurs.	soccer	evening	60	145
Fri.				
Sat.	badminton	evening	45	140
Sun.				

COOL-DOWN AFTER EACH WORKOUT

EXTENSION: Use your exercise plan as training for a community event such as a 5K (walk or jog). Predict what a week in your future college or career path would resemble. Create a weekly exercise plan for a possible college or career setting.

Plan your nutrition. Keep track of the food you eat each day for 1 week. Include food from the grain group, the fruit group, the vegetable group, the dairy group, and the protein group each day. Drink water daily. Limit high-fat and sugary foods. Exercise burns calories, so it is important to get food from all of the food groups. Plan for and eat healthful snacks. Review what you eat each day, discuss your diet with a trusted adult, and adjust so that you are getting a well-rounded, healthful diet. Be aware of false diet claims and rely on your doctor for advice.

 CAUTION: Do not consume food to which you are allergic or sensitive.

EXAMPLE

Day 1	Time	Servings	Total Servings
Grain	breakfast lunch dinner	2 2 2	6
Fruit	breakfast lunch dinner	1 2 1	4
Vegetable	breakfast lunch dinner	0 2 3	5
Dairy	breakfast lunch dinner	2 1 1	4
Protein	breakfast lunch dinner	0 1 2	3
Snacks	granola bar apple	1 1	2

🖥 RESEARCH INTEGRATION

Research the connection of regular exercise and healthful eating to performing well in college or a career.

♥ HEALTH INTEGRATION

Use available technology to monitor your pulse rate and intensity. Apply the results to your overall fitness plan.

HIP-HOP DANCE

Dancing is an exercise option for aerobic workout, for competition, or just for fun. You can dance independently, with a partner, or in groups. Dancing on your own at home for exercise is fun, inexpensive, and does not require a lot of space.

Dancing is expressing yourself through repeated patterns of movement which are usually set to music. Some forms of dance include creative, tap, ballet, hip-hop, modern, folk, square, jazz, line, Latin, ballroom, and social.

Hip-hop is an energetic dance type that originated when the hip-hop style of music surfaced. Hip-hop dancing was first performed within a subculture and is now also practiced in dance studios.

The purpose of this lesson is for you to perform basic hip-hop steps and locomotor movements using common dance concepts in rhythmic patterns to create your own dance for aerobic exercise.

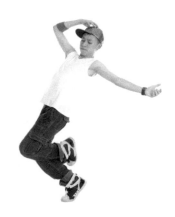

HIP-HOP DANCE
HIP-HOP DANCE: CREATE YOUR PERSONAL DANCE ROUTINE
COMMON CONCEPTS OF DANCE TO USE FOR YOUR PERSONAL DANCE

- The concept of space includes the following.
  - high, medium, or low **levels**
  - forward, backward, right, or left **directions**
  - curved, zigzag, straight, circle, or square **pathways**
- The concept of time includes the following.
  - slow, medium, or fast **speeds**
  - a pattern for **rhythm**
  - The concept of force includes the following.
  - applying light, moderate, or strong **weights**

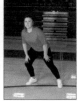
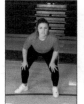
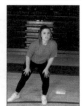

CREATE A HIP-HOP DANCE

Start with the dance steps below. Then, complete the routine by adding your own dance steps. Set your dance to music.

1. Learn a scoop.
   - Face forward, with your feet a little more than shoulder-width apart.
   - Place your hands lightly on your thighs.
   - Simultaneously bend your knees and lean to the right.
   - Repeat this to the left.
   - Do these 4 times.

2. Learn a circle.
   - Face forward, with your feet a little more than shoulder-width apart.
   - Place your hands lightly on your thighs.
   - Simultaneously bend your knees, lean to the right, and do a complete circle to the right with your upper body.
   - Repeat this to the left.
   - Do these 4 times.

Scoop

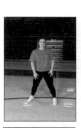
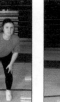
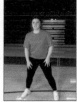

Circle

3. Learn a walk step with an arm pump.
   - Walk to the right with your right foot leading; step right, left, right, left.
   - At the last left step, simultaneously pump your right arm; reach above your head and pull your hand down to shoulder level with your elbow bent.
   - Repeat this to the left.
   - Do these 4 times.
4. Combine the scoop, circle, and walk step, doing them 4 times each.
5. Next, choreograph your dance steps to complete the dance. Create the steps, write a description of each step, and practice the steps.
   - Choose locomotor skills to blend (steps, jumps, slides, turns, and so on).
   - Use your arms to accompany the footwork, for example: step, cross, step, clap.
   - Perform each skill at different levels.
   - Move in different directions.
   - Move in different pathways.
   - Move at slow, medium, and fast speeds.
   - Use light, moderate, and strong force to move your body.
   - Create a pattern.
   - Use an 8 count for each move.

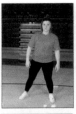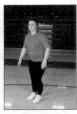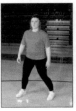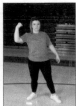

Walk step with arm pump

Option: Dance with a partner or small group for a social experience. You can also perform your dance for friends or family.

PREDICT IF DANCE IS AN EXERCISE THAT YOU WILL PURSUE IN COLLEGE OR A CAREER SETTING

1	I will not consider dance as an exercise option in college or a career setting.
2	I will consider dance as an exercise option in college or a career setting.

RESEARCH INTEGRATION

1. Research hip-hop dance and some hip-hop moves you can safely use in your dance.
2. Research and compare 2 dance types: jazz and Latin.
3. Research dance classes in your local area.

HEALTH INTEGRATION

Count your pulse to determine if you are exercising in your personal target heart rate zone. Apply the results to your overall fitness plan. Many people choose to get their aerobic workouts through dance.

JUMP ROPE

A jump rope is an inexpensive piece of exercise equipment. It can be used indoors, outdoors, and in a small space. A jump rope promotes adherence to participation in physical activity by eliminating cost and space barriers. It is also an effective sport-training tool that improves balance, agility, and coordination.

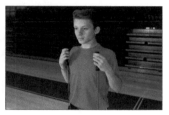

The purpose of this lesson is for you to use jumping rope to improve in areas of fitness that are important to you: cardiovascular, skill-related, or both.

JUMP ROPE BASICS

FITTING THE JUMP ROPE TO YOUR HEIGHT

- Place a jump rope handle in each hand.
- Stand on the middle of the rope with 1 foot.
- Move the handles straight up, making sure that the rope is straight and pulled tight.
- The tops of the handles should reach close to your shoulders.

Fitting the jump rope to your height

ELEMENTS OF JUMP ROPE

- Keep your eyes forward.
- When turning the rope, keep your elbows near your sides, maintaining a 45-degree angle and making 2-inch circles with your wrists.
- Leave just enough space for the rope to pass under your feet when you jump.
- Stay on the balls of your feet.
- Land softly, keeping your knees slightly bent.

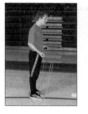 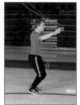 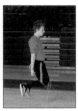

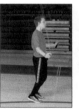 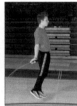

BASIC SKILLS

BASIC JUMP

- Pick up the rope. Holding a handle in each hand, rest the rope behind your feet. Stand on the balls of your feet. This is the ready position.
- Your hands should be just above the height of your waist.
- Swing the rope up and over your head.
- Jump over the rope when it approaches your toes.
- Continue as long as you can without stopping.

Basic jump

BACKWARD JUMP

- Begin with the rope in front of your feet.
- Swing the rope up and over your head.
- Jump over the rope when it approaches your feet.
- Jump a little higher than 1 inch off the ground. Stay on the balls of your feet.
- Continue as long as you can without stopping.

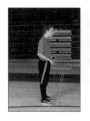 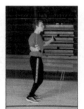

 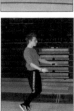

Backward jump

ALTERNATE-FOOT JUMP

- Pick up the rope. Holding a handle in each hand, rest the rope behind your feet. Stand on the balls of your feet. This is the ready position. Note that 1 foot will be lifted off the ground during each turn of the rope before the other foot jumps.

- Turn the rope from behind you up over your head. When the rope reaches your toes, jump over it with your right foot.

- Turn the rope again from behind you up over your head. When the rope reaches your toes this time, jump over it with your left foot.

- Continue turning the rope and alternating feet as if you were running in place. Try it jumping backward.

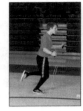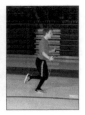

Alternate-foot jump

Practice the basic jump rope skills until competent. Next, design a jump rope routine using basic jump rope skills that will improve footwork speed.

SAMPLE OF A WORKOUT TO IMPROVE FOOTWORK SPEED	
• basic jump 1 minute at a medium pace	• rest 30 seconds
• basic jump 30 seconds at a fast pace	• alternate-foot jump 1 minute at a medium pace
• rest 30 seconds	• alternate-foot jump 30 seconds at a fast pace
• backward jump 1 minute at a medium pace	• rest 30 seconds
• backward jump 30 seconds at a fast pace	• repeat as needed

DESIGN YOUR PERSONAL FOOTWORK SPEED ROUTINE

CHALLENGE SKILLS

The following challenges are for students who have mastered the basic jump rope skills. The challenge level is recommended to learn advanced skills and add a variety of skills to your workout.

HOP ON 1 FOOT

- Perform the basic jump on your right foot.
- Perform the basic jump on your left foot.

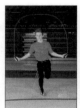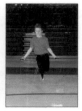

Hop on 1 foot

SKIER

- With both feet together, hop side to side while turning the rope.

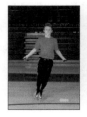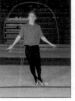

Skier

CROSSOVERS

- After the rope moves over your head, cross the rope in front of you, jump, and uncross the rope.

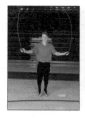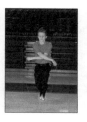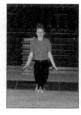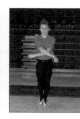

Crossovers

FRONT KICKS

- Kick 1 foot forward as the rope passes under your feet with a skip-step in between.

- Alternate kicks.

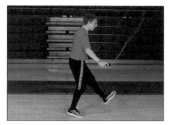

Front kicks

SIDE KICKS

- Kick 1 foot and then the other out to the side with a skip-step in between.

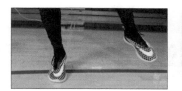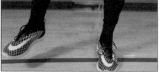

Side kicks

CRISSCROSS FEET

- Cross and uncross your feet while jumping.

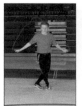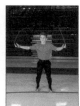

Crisscross feet

FIGURE-8 JUMPS

- Hold a handle in each hand. Swing the rope from side to side in a figure-8 pattern. Then, open it to regular form and step over it. When you master that, practice jumping over the rope.

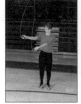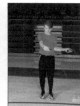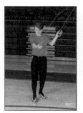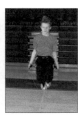

Figure-8 jumps

STRADDLE JUMPS

- Turn the rope from behind you up over your head. When the rope reaches your toes, jump over it with both feet. Split your legs apart as you jump. On the next turn, land with your feet together.

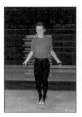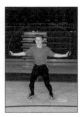

Straddle jumps

Practice the challenge jump rope skills until competent. Next, design your personal aerobic jump rope routine by blending the basic jump rope skills and the challenge skills. Set your routine to music. Monitor your pulse rate.

BLENDING: Perform 1 jump rope skill and transition smoothly to another jump rope skill without stopping between moves. Blend after a 4 count, an 8 count, or a 16 count. Mix it up so that it works for you.

SAMPLE OF A CARDIOVASCULAR CONDITIONING WORKOUT

- blend basic jump/crossovers/basic jump **2 minutes**
- march or jog in place **30 seconds**
- blend figure-8s/backward jump/figure-8s **2 minutes**
- march or jog in place **30 seconds**
- blend alternate-foot jumps/figure-8s/crisscross feet **2 minutes**
- march or jog in place **30 seconds**
- blend skier/front kicks/side kicks **2 minutes**
- march or jog in place **30 seconds**
- repeat for a 20-minute workout

DESIGN YOUR PERSONAL CARDIOVASCULAR JUMP ROPE ROUTINE. SET IT TO MUSIC.

PREDICT IF JUMPING ROPE IS AN EXERCISE THAT YOU WILL PURSUE IN COLLEGE OR A CAREER SETTING

1	I will not consider jumping rope as an exercise option in college or a career setting.
2	I will consider jumping rope as an exercise option in college or a career setting.

♥ **HEALTH INTEGRATION**

Count your pulse during and after jumping rope to determine if you are exercising in your personal target heart rate zone for health benefits. Apply the results to your overall fitness plan.

FITNESS BALL

Including a fitness ball (or exercise ball) in your exercise routine is a fun, efficient way to improve muscular strength, muscular endurance, flexibility, and balance. Your core muscles work to balance on an unstable ball while exercising a variety of muscle groups.

The purpose of this lesson is to exercise leg, back, and core muscles using a stability ball.

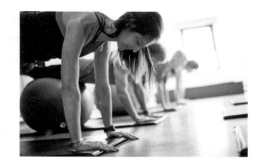

 CAUTION: Do not overinflate the ball.

FITNESS BALL STRENGTH-BUILDING EXERCISES

TIPS FOR USING A FITNESS BALL

- Exercises done on a firmer ball are more challenging.
- A beginner should start with a slightly-deflated ball.
- When you are seated on the ball, your feet should be flat on the floor.

Practice each of the following exercises, concentrating on proper form, prior to engaging in a workout.

SINGLE-LEG SQUATS

muscle focus: hamstrings and quadriceps

- Stand up straight and place the fitness ball against your lower back between yourself and the wall.
- Place your feet shoulder-width apart and slightly out in front of you. Your body should be at an angle.
- Lift your right leg straight out in front of you.
- Slide your body down into a sitting position; the ball should now be against your upper back. Make sure that your knees do not go past your toes.
- Stand back up to the starting position. The ball should return against your lower back.
- Switch sides after completing your repetitions.

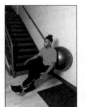 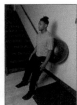

Single-leg squats

CHEST PRESSES WITH MEDICINE BALL

muscle focus: pectoralis majors, pectoralis minors, deltoids, and triceps

- Place the fitness ball on the ground behind you.
- Place your upper back on the ball. Make sure that your head and neck do not touch the ball.
- Place your feet shoulder-width apart.
- Bend your knees to form 90-degree angles. Place your feet under your knees.
- Hold the weighted ball close to your chest with both hands. If the weighted ball is too heavy, you can use a resistance band. Wrap the band around your upper back and hold an end of the band in each hand.
- Stabilize yourself on the fitness ball and raise the weighted ball or resistance band toward the ceiling. Then, bring the weighted ball or resistance band back to your chest.

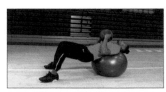
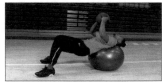
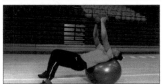

Chest presses with medicine ball

PLANK ROLLOUTS

muscle focus: abdominal muscles

- Place the fitness ball on the ground in front of you.
- Place your knees on the ground and your forearms on the ball.
- Hold your body at a slight angle. There should be about 2 feet between your knees and the ball.
- Roll the ball forward with your forearms until half of your forearms are off the ball. Tighten your abdominal muscles while doing this.
- Roll the ball back to the starting position with your forearms.

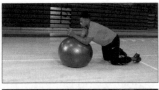
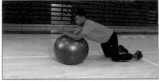
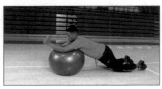

Plank rollouts

SQUATS WITH TWISTS

muscle focus: abdominal muscles, quadriceps, hamstrings, and triceps

- Hold the fitness ball straight out in front of you at chest level.
- Stand with your feet shoulder-width apart.
- Get into a squat position. Bend your knees and lower your buttocks toward the ground. Make sure that your knees do not go past your toes.
- Twist your torso to the right while in the squat position and while still holding the ball out in front of you.
- Stand up to the starting position.
- Repeat this to the left side.

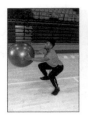
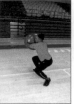
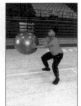
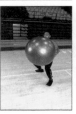
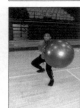

Squats with twists

BACK EXTENSIONS

muscle focus: erector spinae (iliocostales, longissimi, and spinales)

- Place the fitness ball on the floor.
- Place your abdomen on the ball. Your legs should be extended behind you and about shoulder-width apart for balance.
- Place your hands behind your head on your neck (like when doing a crunch).
- Lift your upper body so that you are hyperextending your back.
- Come back down to the starting position.

Have a trusted adult or friend evaluate you for correct form for the previous exercises. Did you respond positively to the feedback?

Reciprocate and evaluate your friend. Were you able to provide feedback in a positive manner?

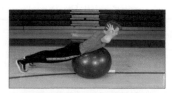
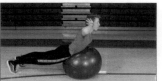

Back extensions

The following is a suggested use of the fitness ball in a strength-building workout. Exercise to your level of fitness.

- Warm up and cool down.
- Perform each exercise 2 to 3 days per week.
- Begin with 1 set of 10 repetitions. Increase sets and the number of repetitions when the current number is too easy.
- Your goal should be to reach 3 sets of 10 to 15 repetitions.

PREDICT IF USING A FITNESS BALL IS AN EXERCISE THAT YOU WILL PURSUE IN COLLEGE OR A CAREER SETTING

1	I will not consider the fitness ball as an exercise option in college or a career setting.
2	I will consider the fitness ball as an exercise option in college or a career setting.

🖥 RESEARCH INTEGRATION

Research and discuss with a friend or trusted adult the connection between strong abdominal muscles and a healthy back.

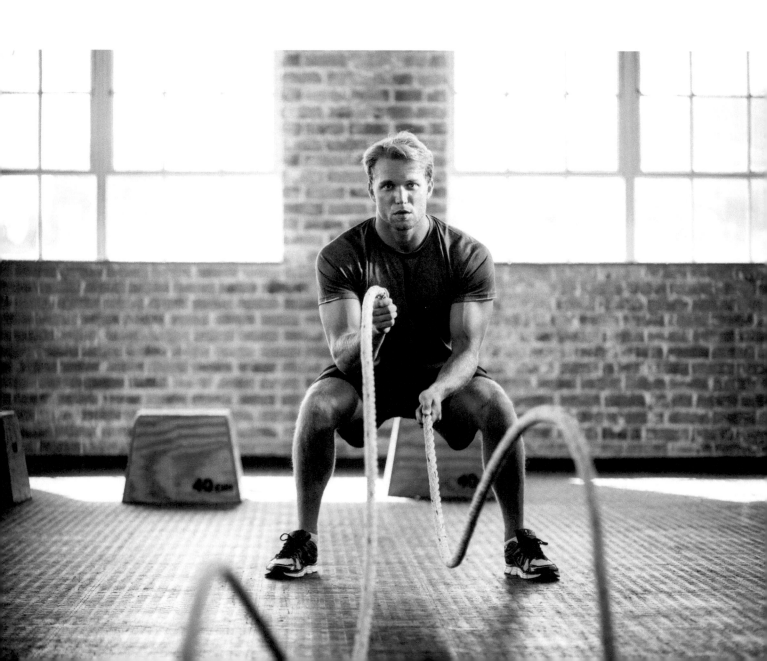

RESISTANCE BANDS

Regular use of resistance bands helps to improve muscular strength, muscular endurance, and flexibility while being easy on your joints. They can be used for isometric strengthening by keeping the joint in 1 position or for isotonic strengthening by moving the band through the joint's range of motion. When using resistance bands, start with the lightest resistance and gradually increase to a higher resistance as you get stronger.

The purpose of this lesson is to increase muscular strength and endurance using resistance bands.

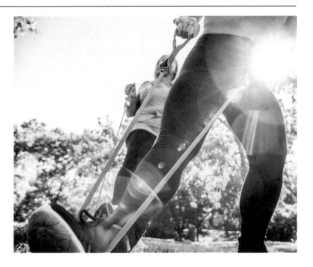

FITNESS TIP: When using resistance bands, you should make sure that the band is secured in a way that the length is appropriate to give resistance for the entire exercise. Wrap the band around your hands if you need an increased resistance level.

⚠ CAUTION: Check the resistance bands for damage or wear before exercising. When exercising, secure the band before adding any resistance.

RESISTANCE BANDS STRENGTH-BUILDING EXERCISES

BENEFITS OF STRENGTH TRAINING WITH RESISTANCE BANDS

- is an effective overall strength workout that does not require weights
- offers a variety of resistance adjustments for beginner through advanced levels
- requires inexpensive pieces of equipment
- requires equipment that is easy to carry with you when you are traveling

Practice each of the following exercises. Concentrate on proper form prior to engaging in a workout.

BENT-OVER FLIES

muscle focus: trapezii, rhomboids, deltoids, and biceps

- Stand in the middle of the resistance band with your feet shoulder-width apart.
- Grab the left handle of the band with your right hand and the right handle of the band with your left hand. The band should now be crisscrossed.
- Bend your knees slightly and bend at the waist.
- Begin with your arms slightly bent.
- Lift both arms up and out to your sides.
- Bend your arms slowly down to the starting position.

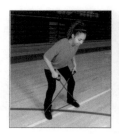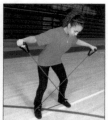

Bent-over files

RESISTANCE PUSH-UPS

muscle focus: pectoralis majors, pectoralis minors, deltoids, triceps, and abdominal muscles

- Tie the resistance band around your chest, making sure that you have 2 even ends.

- Place a handle in each hand. You may need to wrap the band around your hands to get the proper tension.

- Get into a push-up position. Lie face down on the floor or yoga mat with your palms flat on the floor and shoulder-width apart. Bend your elbows and straighten your legs out behind you with your toes on the floor.

- Straighten your elbows as you push your body up off the floor. Keep your back straight and look straight ahead.

- Lower yourself slowly back to the starting position.

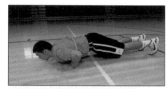
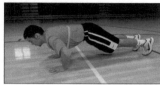
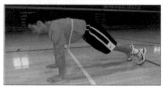

Resistance Push-ups

MONSTER WALK

muscle focus: hip abductors and glutes

- Stand with your feet shoulder-width apart.

- Tie the resistance band around both ankles.

- Bend your knees and waist into a squatting position.

- Hold your arms at your sides with your elbows bent.

- Take a step to the right with your right foot. Bring your left foot to meet your right foot. Make sure that your knees are aligned over top of your feet.

- Repeat to the left after completing the repetitions to the right.

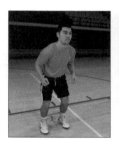
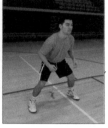

Monster walk

BAND EXPLOSIONS

muscle focus: glutes, hamstrings, quadriceps, gastrocnemii, solei, triceps, and deltoids

- Stand with your feet shoulder-width apart.

- Place a handle of the resistance band under your right foot and hold the other handle with your right hand.

- Bend your elbow so that your fist is at shoulder level. Your palm should be facing forward.

- Bend your knees, making sure that they do not go past your toes. Bend at the waist into a squatting position.

- Straighten your elbow and lift the band as you stand back up, bringing your upper arm to touch your ear.

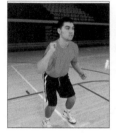
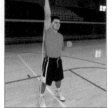

Band explosions

Have a trusted adult or friend evaluate you for correct form for the previous exercises. Did you respond positively to the feedback?

Reciprocate and evaluate your friend. Were you able to provide feedback in a positive manner?

The following is a suggested use of resistance bands in a strength-building workout. Exercise to your level of fitness.

- Warm up before your workout. Cool down after your workout.
- Perform each resistance band exercise 2 to 3 days per week. Do not exercise the same muscle group on consecutive days.
- Begin with 1 set of 10 repetitions for each exercise. Increase sets and the number of repetitions when the current number is too easy.
- Your goal should be to reach 3 sets of 10 to 15 repetitions.
- Wrap the band to increase resistance as necessary.

PREDICT IF USING RESISTANCE BANDS IS AN EXERCISE THAT YOU WILL PURSUE IN COLLEGE OR A CAREER SETTING

1	I will not consider using resistance bands as an exercise option in college or a career setting.
2	I will consider using resistance bands as an exercise option in college or a career setting.

RESEARCH INTEGRATION

Research resistance band exercises and how they are used to improve athletic performance.

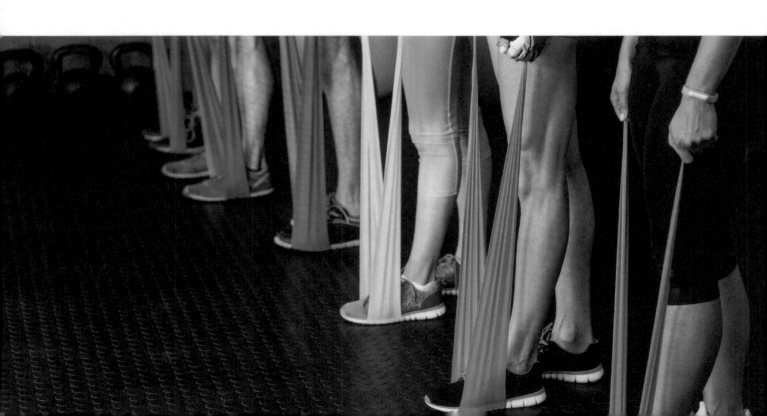

SLIDER AND BOOTIES

The slider and booties work together as a unique exercise tool that improves muscular endurance and strength. Sliding on the smooth board while wearing the special booties is an exercise option that uses your body weight to strength train.

Sliding is a low-impact, full-body workout. The slippery surface forces you to use many muscles to maintain control. Regular use of the slider helps to improve muscular strength, muscular endurance, power, balance, and flexibility while being easy on your joints. When using the slider, start each movement slowly and maintain control throughout each movement. Increase your range of motion as your balance improves.

The purpose of this lesson is to increase muscular strength and endurance using the slider and booties.

⚠ **CAUTION: When using the slider and booties, be careful stepping onto the slider as it will be slippery. Step off of the slider before putting on and taking off your booties.**

SLIDER AND BOOTIES STRENGTH-BUILDING EXERCISES
BENEFITS OF STRENGTH TRAINING WITH A SLIDER

- is an effective overall strength workout that does not require weights
- is a unique approach to strength training
- can be done almost anywhere
- does not require a lot of space

Practice each of the following exercises. Concentrate on proper form prior to engaging in a workout.

SLIDE LUNGES

muscle focus: hip abductors and adductors, glutes, and quadriceps

- Place the slider on a hard, flat surface.
- Position yourself horizontally on the slider with your right foot on the left end of the slider and your left foot on the floor.
- Slide your right foot into a side lunge toward the opposite end of the slider.
- Remember that your right knee should not go past your toes.
- Slide your right foot back to the starting position.
- Switch to the other side after completing the repetitions.

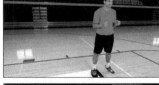
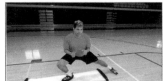

Side lunges

DYNAMIC SUMO SQUATS

muscle focus: hip abductors and adductors, quadriceps, hamstrings, glutes, gastrocnemii, and solei

- Place the slider on a hard, flat surface.
- Position yourself horizontally on the slider, standing in the middle.
- Slide your feet outward as you lower your buttocks into a sitting position.
- Slide your feet inward back to the starting position.
- Make sure that your knees do not go past your toes.

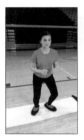
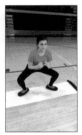

Dynamic sumo squats

HAMSTRING CURLS

muscle focus: hamstrings and glutes

- Place the slider on a hard, flat surface.
- Position yourself vertically on the slider and lie flat on your back with your feet at 1 end and your head near the opposite end.
- Keep your shoulders on the ground and bring your heels to your buttocks as you lift your buttocks off the ground.
- Slide your heels back to the starting position, lowering your buttocks back to the ground.

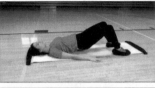
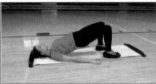

Hamstring curls

PIKES

muscle focus: abdominal muscles

- Place the slider on a hard, flat surface.
- Position yourself vertically on the slider with your feet on the far end of the slider.
- Get into a push-up position with your hands shoulder-width apart.
- Slide your feet upward on the slider toward your chest. Do not bend your knees.
- Go back down to a push-up position.

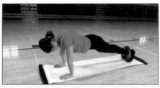
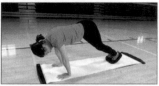
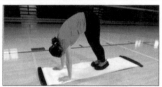

Pikes

KNEE-TUCK PUSH-UPS

muscle focus: abdominal muscles, pectoralis majors, pectoralis minors, triceps, biceps, and deltoids

- Place the slider on a hard, flat surface.
- Position yourself vertically on the slider with your feet on the far end of the slider.
- Get into a push-up position with your hands shoulder-width apart.
- Do a push up.
- Slide your feet up the slider so that your knees are bent into your chest after you come up.

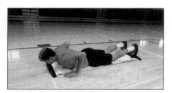
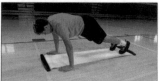
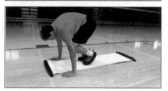

Knee-tuck push-ups

AEROBIC EXTENSION

- Place the slider on a hard, flat surface.
- Position yourself horizontally on the slider, standing with both feet in the middle.
- Slide your right foot into a side lunge toward the right end of the slider.
- Slide your right foot back to the starting position.
- Slide your left foot into a side lunge toward the left end of the slider.
- Slide your left foot back to the starting position.
- Continue going back and forth from your right foot to your left foot. Increase your speed and time as is appropriate to your fitness level.
- Make sure that your knees do not go past your toes.

Have a trusted adult or friend evaluate you for correct form for the previous exercises. Did you respond positively to the feedback?

Reciprocate and evaluate your friend. Were you able to provide feedback in a positive manner?

The following is a suggested use of the slider in a strength-building workout. Exercise to your level of fitness.

- Warm up before exercising and cool down after exercising.
- Perform each slider exercise 2 to 3 days per week. Do not exercise the same muscle group on consecutive days.
- Begin with 1 set of 10 repetitions. Increase sets and the number of repetitions when the current number is too easy.
- Your goal should be to reach 3 sets of 10 to 15 repetitions.

PREDICT IF USING A SLIDER WITH BOOTIES IS AN EXERCISE THAT YOU WILL PURSUE IN COLLEGE OR A CAREER SETTING

1	I will not consider using the slider as an exercise option in college or a career setting.
2	I will consider using the slider as an exercise option in college or a career setting.

RESEARCH INTEGRATION

Research and discuss with a friend or trusted adult the benefits of strength training.

HEALTH INTEGRATION

Count your pulse to determine if you are exercising in your personal target heart rate zone. Apply the results to your overall fitness plan.

DOUBLE-GRIP MEDICINE BALL

Exercising with a double-grip medicine ball will help you to improve overall muscular strength and endurance. Gripping the ball makes it easier to control.

The purpose of this lesson is to increase muscular strength and endurance using the double-grip medicine ball.

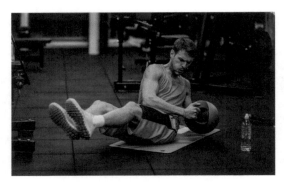

FITNESS TIP: have a certified trainer plan for you and supervise you when you are working with any type of weights.

⚠ **CAUTION: Make sure that nobody is close to you before you use the double-grip medicine ball. Do not walk into the path of another person who is using a medicine ball. Make sure to hold the ball and maneuver it without dropping it. Have a good grip on the ball before exercising. Keep the medicine ball movements controlled to avoid injury.**

DOUBLE-GRIP MEDICINE BALL STRENGTH-BUILDING EXERCISES
BENEFITS OF STRENGTH TRAINING WITH A DOUBLE-GRIP MEDICINE BALL

- requires only 1 piece of equipment
- provides a convenient grip
- can be done almost anywhere
- boosts metabolism and burns fat even after the workout is over

Practice each of the following exercises. Concentrate on proper form prior to engaging in a workout.

LUNGES WITH TWISTS

muscle focus: oblique abdominal muscles, quadriceps, hamstrings, and glutes

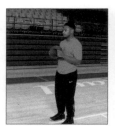
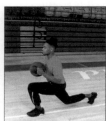
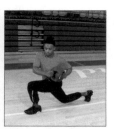
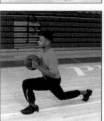
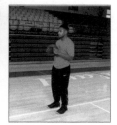

- Place your feet shoulder-width apart and relax your shoulders.
- Hold the medicine ball a few inches in front of your chest with both hands.
- Step forward into a lunge with your right leg. Make sure that your knee does not go past your toes.
- Make sure that your right thigh is parallel to the floor once you are in the lunge position. Then, extend your arms in front of you with the ball in both hands.
- Rotate your torso to the right, moving the ball in the same direction at the same time.
- Hold this for 2 seconds and come back to the starting position.
- Do the same with the left leg.

Lunges with twists

CHEST PRESSES WITH SIT-UPS

muscle focus: pectoralis majors, pectoralis minors, deltoids, triceps, and abdominal muscles

- Lie flat on a bench or the floor.
- Hold the medicine ball in front of your chest with both hands.
- Hold the ball and extend your hands straight up from your chest.
- Bring the ball back down to the starting position.
- Do a sit-up and come back down.
- Repeat from the beginning.

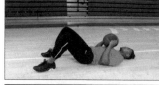
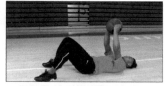
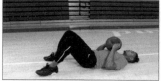
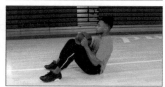
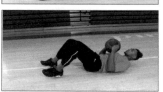

Chest presses with sit-ups

SHOULDER PRESSES

muscle focus: deltoids, triceps, and biceps

- Sit in a chair with your back straight or stand with your feet shoulder-width apart.
- Hold the medicine ball in front of your chest with both hands.
- Extend your arms to the ceiling with the ball in your hands.
- Lower the ball slowly back to the starting position.

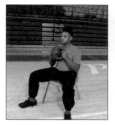
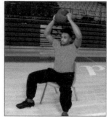
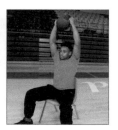

Shoulder presses

TRICEPS EXTENSIONS

muscle focus: triceps

- Stand with your feet shoulder-width apart.
- Extend your arms over your head with the medicine ball in both hands. Your inner arms should be almost touching your ears.
- Bend your elbows and lower the ball behind your head. Your arms should make 45-degree angles.
- Straighten your arms and bring the ball back up to the starting position.

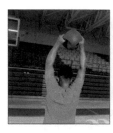
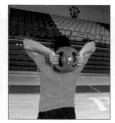
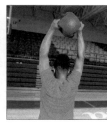

Triceps presses

BICEPS CURLS

muscle focus: biceps

- Stand with your feet shoulder-width apart.
- Hold the medicine ball with both hands and extend your arms down toward the ground.
- Bring the ball slowly up to your chest.
- Lower the ball down to the starting position. Do not lock your elbows when doing this.

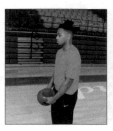
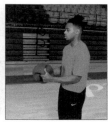
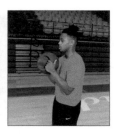

Biceps curls

SINGLE-HANDED BICEPS CURLS

muscle focus: biceps

- Stand with your feet shoulder-width apart.
- Hold the medicine ball with your right hand and extend your arm down toward the ground.
- Bring the ball slowly up to your chest.
- Lower the ball back to the starting position. Make sure that you do not lock your elbows when doing this.
- Repeat with your left hand after completing the repetitions.

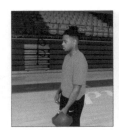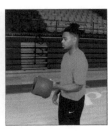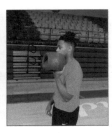

Single-handed biceps curls

Have a trusted adult or friend evaluate you for correct form for the previous exercises. Did you respond positively to the feedback?

Reciprocate and evaluate your friend. Were you able to provide feedback in a positive manner?

The following is a suggested use of the double-grip medicine ball in a strength-building workout. Exercise to your level of fitness.

- Warm up before exercising and cool down after exercising.
- Perform each medicine ball exercise 2 to 3 days per week. Do not exercise the same muscle group on consecutive days.
- Begin with 1 set of 10 repetitions. Increase sets and the number of repetitions when the current number is too easy.
- Your goal should be to reach 3 sets of 10 to 15 repetitions.

🖥 RESEARCH INTEGRATION

Research medicine ball workouts.

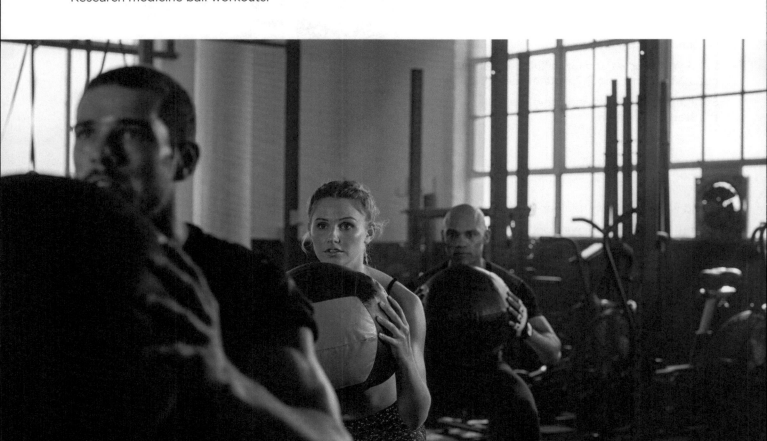

STRENGTH-TRAINING PROGRAM: USING WHAT YOU HAVE LEARNED

Strength training, also known as resistance training, builds strength and endurance in the skeletal muscles. Building muscle increases your body's metabolism. A purpose of metabolism is to convert food to energy. Regular strength training at light, moderate, or intense levels will help you achieve or maintain a healthy body weight.

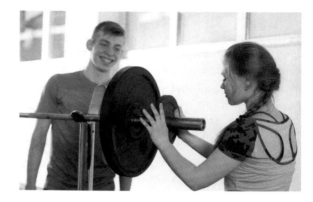

Using body-weight exercises, a fitness ball, resistance bands, a medicine ball, a slider, or other portable strength-training equipment provides you with exercise opportunities in dorm rooms, at home, or in limited spaces. Access to equipment in a convenient location will help you commit to your strength-training routine.

Fibers that make up your skeletal muscles break down during the exercise phase. After your strength workout, when your muscles are resting, the fibers repair and strengthen. It is recommended that you allow 24 hours between training the same muscle group to allow the muscle fibers to repair and strengthen.

The purpose of this lesson is to encourage you to design your personal strength-training program and perform exercises 2 to 3 days per week to obtain health benefits. A certified trainer should help you set up a balanced, effective strength program.

 CAUTION: Have a certified trainer plan for you and supervise you when you are working with weights.

STRENGTH-TRAINING PROGRAM

There are a variety of exercises from which to choose. Do strength exercises for the muscles of your upper body, lower body, and core. Opposing muscles (antagonistic muscles), such as biceps and triceps, should be equally trained because they work together. Choose the intensity of the exercise to fit your fitness level. For example, if you are struggling doing a right-angle push-up, switch to a knee push-up. Limit excuses and make a commitment to exercise!

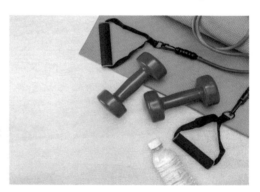

STRENGTH-TRAINING EXERCISE IDEAS

Weightlifting machines: You can use large stationary machines like those typically found in gyms.

Free weights: You can use free-weight equipment such as dumbbells, barbells, medicine balls, kettlebells, resistance bands, and weighted ropes to perform strength-training exercises.

Pilates or yoga: Pilates and yoga sessions are excellent workouts for muscle lengthening and muscle strengthening.

Personal workouts: You can use your own body weight as a source of resistance and create your own strength-training workouts. Create a personal workout by blending basic strength-building exercises such as sit-ups, push-ups, pull-ups, planks, and so on, and design the intensity and duration of each exercise according to your level of fitness. Include upper-body, lower-body, and core exercises in your workout. Perform your personal routine for some or all your strength-training workouts.

MUSCULAR STRENGTH AND MUSCULAR ENDURANCE SAMPLE WORKOUT

The following workout regimen is strictly an example of how to use the FITT principle to increase muscular strength and muscular endurance. The exercises are described in the Flexibility section, Muscular Endurance section, and PE Equipment Kit section of your PE Manual.

In the following chart, you will find a block plan for a weekly schedule based on increasing your muscular strength and muscular endurance. The chart includes the days of the week, muscle groups, exercises, sets and repetitions (for example, 3 · 10 = 3 sets of 10 repetitions), and the type of equipment used.

There is a column on the chart for you to design your personal workout. You can use fitness equipment or your own body weight. The plan you design should be for your fitness level. Personalized exercise plans work for all fitness levels and body types.

- Have a certified trainer plan and supervise you when you are working with weights.
- Before working out, warm up properly to prepare your body. The warm-up should increase your heart rate, breathing rate, and body temperature.
- Never begin vigorous exercise with cold muscles.
- Cool down after working out to allow your body to return to its baseline.

Warm-up: Complete 3 sets of this warm-up before exercising.

Exercise	Duration
• basic jump rope	• 1 minute
• high knees	• 30 seconds
• forward arm circles	• 30 seconds
• backward arm circles	• 30 seconds
• rear kicks	• 30 seconds

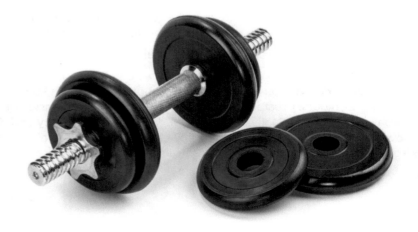

Day	Muscle Group	Exercise Sample	Sets/Reps	Equipment	Personal Workout for Each Muscle Group
Mon. Wed.	chest shoulders	resistance push-ups	3 · 15	resistance band	
		knee-tuck push-ups	3 · 15	slider	
		chest presses with sit-ups	3 · 15	weighted ball	
		wide-arm push-ups	3 · 15	body weight	
Mon. Wed.	biceps triceps	chest presses	3 · 15	fitness ball	
		bent-over flies	3 · 15	resistance band	
		triceps extensions	3 · 15	weighted ball	
		biceps curls	3 · 15	weighted ball	
		narrow-arm push-ups	3 · 10	body weight	
Tue. Thur.	legs	single-leg squats	3 · 15	fitness ball	
		band explosions	3 · 15	resistance band	
		lunges with twists	3 · 15	weighted ball	
		side lunges	3 · 15	slider	
		dynamic sumo squats	3 · 15	slider	
		lunges	3 · 15	body weight	
Tue. Thur.	back	back extensions	3 · 15	fitness ball	
		pull-ups	3 · 10	body weight	
Mon. Wed. Fri.	core	plank rollouts	3 · 15	fitness ball	
		squats with twists	3 · 15	fitness ball	
		pikes	3 · 15	slider	
		planks	3 · 30 seconds	body weight	

Cool-down: Complete this cool-down after exercising.

Exercise	Duration
• hamstring stretch	• 30 seconds
• quadriceps stretch	• 30 seconds
• shoulder/triceps stretch	• 30 seconds
• side stretch	• 30 seconds
• lower back/hip stretch	• 30 seconds
• groin stretch	• 30 seconds

RESEARCH INTEGRATION

Research how strength training is beneficial to your health and daily living.

CROSS-TRAINING CARDIOVASCULAR AND STRENGTH CIRCUIT: USING WHAT YOU HAVE LEARNED

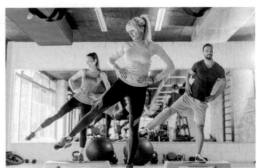

A convenient workout is a cross-training circuit. The following cross-training circuit alternates strength exercises with aerobic movements. Cross-training saves you time by providing a single workout that has both strength and aerobic benefits. This type of workout can be done in a small place at home or in a college dorm room. It is important for you to set your own goals based on your ability level and determine your intensity and duration based on your individual target heart rate zone.

The purpose of this lesson is to encourage you to create and implement a cross-training circuit workout. The workout would be included in the recommended 60 minutes of daily physical activity and would count as both an aerobic and a strength workout. **The Cardiovascular Endurance section of this manual includes the target heart rate zone formula and the Borg Rating of Perceived Exertion Scale to help you to determine if you are exercising for heart health.** You can also use available technology to monitor your pulse rate and intensity.

CROSS-TRAINING CIRCUIT WORKOUT: CARDIOVASCULAR AND STRENGTH

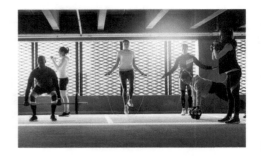

Review the following example and use the information to establish a workout regimen that fits into your schedule. Adhere to the FITT principle (frequency, intensity, time, and type of exercise). This workout requires a jump rope, fitness ball, resistance bands, and kettlebell. You should have a mat or cushioned surface for sit-ups and push-ups.

SAMPLE CROSS-TRAINING CIRCUIT WORKOUT

Build cardiovascular endurance, strength, and flexibility in a cross-training circuit workout using exercises from the appropriate sections of your manual: Cardiovascular Endurance, Muscle Strength, Muscle Endurance, and Flexibility. Review the Aerobic, Jump Rope, Fitness Ball, Resistance Band, Slider, and Weighted Ball sections to practice correct forms for the skills.

Warm-up: Perform 5 to 10 minutes of light cardio to increase your heart rate, breathing rate, and body temperature. Do some dynamic stretches to increase flexibility.

Perform each exercise for 30 seconds. Rest and hydrate when necessary. Set the workout to music.

1. **jumping jacks**
2. **sit-ups**
3. **high knees**
4. **weighted ball lunges**
5. **jump rope**
6. **resistance band monster walk**
7. **rear kicks**
8. **fitness ball chest presses**
9. **jog in place**
10. **right-angle push-ups**
11. **jump rope**
12. **slider hamstring curls**
13. **¼-squat jumps**
14. **weighted ball chest passes with sit-ups**
15. **march in place**
16. **resistance band push-ups**
17. **jump rope**
18. **fitness ball plank rollouts**
19. **burpees**
20. **slider pikes**

Repeat for a 20-minute workout.

Cool-down: Walk slowly until your heart rate, breathing rate, and body temperature have returned to baseline. Do some static stretches to increase flexibility.

CREATE A PERSONAL WORKOUT

Use the cross-training information to create a personal circuit workout you would enjoy.

CREATE A PERSONAL CIRCUIT WORKOUT WITHOUT EQUIPMENT

Objective: to overcome exercise barriers you may face now and in the future

Use the cross-training information to create a personal circuit workout without equipment. Design your own personal aerobic/strength workout that can be done almost anywhere to eliminate several barriers to exercise: insufficient time, lack of access to a gym, expense, and lack of enjoyment.

 RESEARCH INTEGRATION

Research the health triangle for balanced health.

HEALTH INTEGRATION

Use available technology to monitor your pulse rate and intensity. Apply the results to your overall fitness plan.

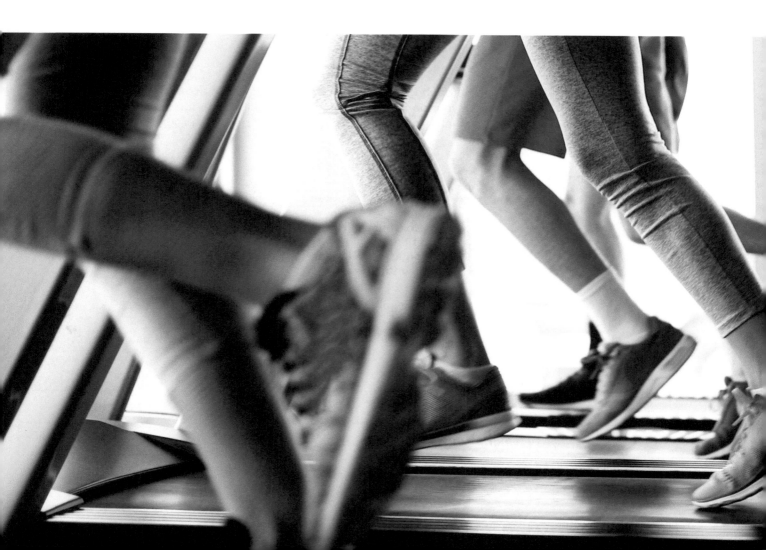

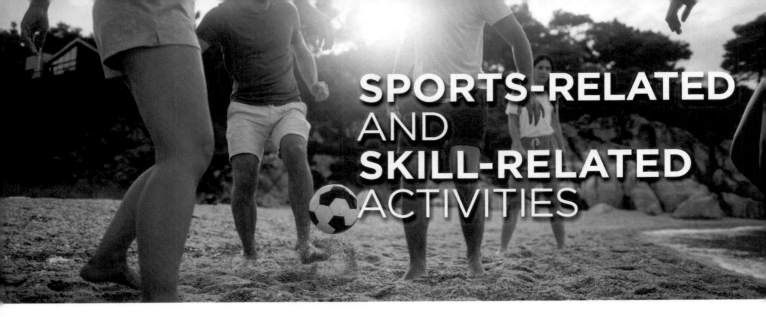

SPORTS-RELATED AND SKILL-RELATED ACTIVITIES

FITNESS TIP: Prior to beginning your physical education activities, read the following safety information that applies to every lesson, review the timeline, and review the assessment rubric.

SAFETY ALERT: Before you exercise, make sure that you are properly warmed up and have enough room to perform each activity. Wear proper equipment and follow activity-specific safety rules. Stay hydrated and take breaks as needed. Exercise only if you are healthy, and always exercise at your own pace. If an exercise starts to hurt, if you feel dizzy, or if you feel light-headed, stop the exercise completely and get help. Upon completion of any workout, cool down and stretch.

TIMELINE

Review all of the activity information before beginning. Use the scoring rubrics as assessment tools. You may ask a trusted adult or friend to observe your performance and provide feedback. Progress according to your skill level. The time that it takes you to complete a module will depend on your personal progress.

Practice and assess the first skill until competent.

Continue to progress until you have practiced and assessed each skill until competent.

Apply skills in a game situation.

ASSESSMENT RUBRIC

You will find a rubric assessment tool following some of the basic skills. Use this tool to evaluate and score your progress in learning the elements of a new skill.

SKILL	PROGRESSING	COMPETENT	PROFICIENT
skill 1	1 or 2 of the elements	3 or 4 out of 5 elements	all elements met

BADMINTON

If you are more likely to commit to exercise by playing in games with others, badminton may be a good choice for you. Badminton is a sport played by striking a shuttlecock (birdie) with a racket over a net. You may play badminton as a competitive sport or as an opportunity for social play.

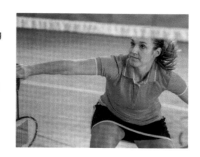

Badminton is considered a lifetime sport because it is not hard to learn and is not hard on your body. The equipment is easy to set up. You can look for badminton games in your local area or set up your own league.

The purpose of this lesson is for you to practice badminton skills and encourage participation in games for a lifetime of physical activity.

⚠ **CAUTION: Make sure that nobody is close to you before you swing the racket. Do not walk into the path of another person who is swinging a racket.**

BADMINTON STROKES

READY POSITION

- Bending your knees, stand with your feet shoulder-width apart.
- Keep your head up and your weight on the balls of your feet.
- Hold the racket in your dominant hand.
- React quickly.
- Anticipate direction.

SKILL	PROGRESSING	COMPETENT	PROFICIENT
ready position	1 or 2 of the elements	3 or 4 out of 5 elements	all elements met

HANDSHAKE GRIP (V GRIP)

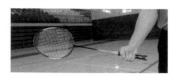
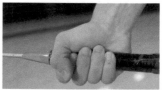

- Hold the handle of the racket in your dominant hand in a handshake grip.
- Form a V with your thumb and forefinger.
- Point the racket away from your body at waist height.
- Placing the head of the racket vertical to the ground, point the handle toward your belly button.
- Support the throat of racket lightly with your non-dominant hand.

SKILL	PROGRESSING	COMPETENT	PROFICIENT
grip	1 or 2 of the elements	3 or 4 out of 5 elements	all elements met

UNDERHAND STROKE

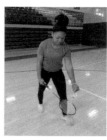

- Hold the racket so that the head is facing the ground and is under the birdie.
- Step forward with your non-dominant foot.
- Flick your wrist to hit the birdie with the center of the racket.
- Rotate your forearm so that it faces upward on contact.
- Follow through to your target.

SKILL	PROGRESSING	COMPETENT	PROFICIENT
underhand stroke	1 or 2 of the elements	3 or 4 out of 5 elements	all elements met

OVERHAND STROKE

- Bend your elbow so that your racket is in a back-scratching position.
- Reach up and position the racket under the birdie.
- Flick your wrist to hit the birdie with the center of the racket. Extend your arm when you make contact.
- Follow through to your target.

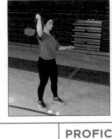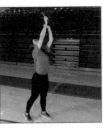

SKILL	PROGRESSING	COMPETENT	PROFICIENT
overhand stroke	1 or 2 of the elements	3 out of 4 elements	all elements met

FOREHAND STROKE

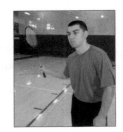

- The racket should be on the same side of your body as your dominant hand.
- Face the palm of your hand forward.
- Rotate your hips in the direction that you are hitting.
- Extend your arm and flick your wrist to hit the birdie.
- Point the face of the racket up to get the birdie over the net.
- Follow through to your target.

SKILL	PROGRESSING	COMPETENT	PROFICIENT
forehand stroke	1, 2, or 3 of the elements	4 or 5 out of 6 elements	all elements met

BACKHAND STROKE

- Rotate the racket and extend it across your body.
- Rotate your feet and shoulders in the same direction as the racket.
- Rotate your hips.
- Face the back of your hand (the side that your knuckles are on) forward.
- Flick your wrist when as you hit the shuttlecock with the center of the racket.
- Follow through to your target.

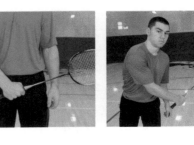

SKILL	PROGRESSING	COMPETENT	PROFICIENT
backhand stroke	1 or 2 of the elements	3, 4, or 5 out of 6 elements	all elements met

UNDERHAND SERVE

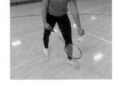

You may choose the low or high underhand serve. The low serve sends the shuttlecock to the front of your opponent's court. The high serve sends the shuttlecock to the back of your opponent's court. You must adjust the power of the shot and the arc. You would hit hard and high for the long serve or light and low for the low serve.

Create a 6-step rubric for the underhand serve using the following information. The concepts of force and direction are important to the underhand serve.

Hold the racket in your dominant hand. Hold the shuttlecock by the feathers in your non-dominant hand. Step forward with your non-dominant foot. Drop the shuttlecock slightly below your waist. Flick your wrist as you hit the shuttlecock with the center of the racket. End with a follow through.

PRACTICE THE STROKES

Practice independently by holding the birdie by the feathers in your non-dominant hand. Hold the racket appropriately for the stroke. Drop the birdie and make contact with the racket.

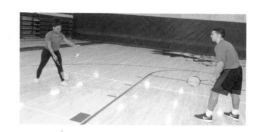

- Practice each stroke without using the shuttlecock.

- Then, practice each stroke using the birdie.

- Practice the underhand stroke by holding the head of the racket down toward the floor. Drop the birdie and make contact with the racket slightly below your waist. Flick your wrist and make contact with the birdie. How many times you can hit the birdie in a row?

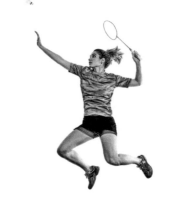

- Use the various strokes to strike the shuttlecock toward a target.

- Strike the shuttlecock toward a target using different levels of force.

- Aim and strike the shuttlecock to the left of the target.

- Aim and strike the shuttlecock to the right of the target.

- Practice with a partner. Hit the shuttlecock back and forth. How many times can you hit it?

BADMINTON SHOTS

CLEAR SHOT

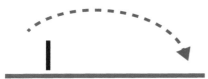

The overhead and underhand defensive clear shots arc or lob the birdie high and push your opponent to the rear of the court. This slows down the game to give you a chance to get ready for your opponent's shot.

DROP SHOT

The overhand drop shot keeps the pace of the game the same. It is sent at a steep angle, forcing your opponent to rush forward.

SMASH SHOT

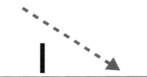

The overhand smash shot is a powerful hit at a severe angle. You need to contact the birdie high, which may even require you to jump to hit the birdie. This shot is often used to end a game.

PRACTICE THE SHOTS

Practice the shots independently by tossing the birdie at the appropriate height for each shot. Practice with a set-up net.

- Practice the clear shot with both the underhand and overhand strokes.

- Practice the drop shot.

- Practice the smash shot.

- Practice with a partner. Have a partner toss the shuttlecock for you. Practice each shot, and then switch roles. Be supportive and encouraging to your partner.

- Practice with a partner. Strike the shuttlecock to your partner using different levels of speed. Strike for accuracy, using the necessary speed for success. Discuss with your partner the speed you needed to use for each shot to achieve accuracy.

BADMINTON GAME

- Badminton is usually a singles game with 2 players or a doubles game with 4 players.
- Start with an underhand serve from the right side of the court. Serve from behind the end line to your opponent on the left.
- If you hit the birdie onto your opponent's side and your opponent cannot return it, you win the rally—which is the series of consecutive strokes back and forth until a point is earned—and get a point.
- Now, serve from the left side of the court.
- When your score is an even number, serve behind the right end line. When your score is an odd number, serve behind the left end line.
- In a doubles game, the same player serves, alternating serving sides, until losing the rally. The opponent then serves until the rally is lost. Partners alternate turns serving.
- You may only hit the shuttlecock 1 time on each side.
- You lose a rally if you or your racket touch the net.
- You lose a rally if you hit the birdie into the net, hit it out of bounds, or miss it when you swing.

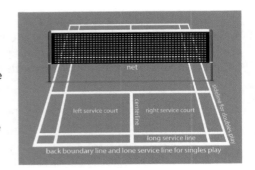

DEMONSTRATE POSITIVE GAME BEHAVIOR

- Follow the game rules.
- Call for the shot, when appropriate, to identify that you are going to hit the shot. This is for safety and game efficiency.
- Be supportive and encouraging to your teammate.
- Treat your opponents with respect.

SKILL	PROGRESSING	COMPETENT	PROFICIENT
game behavior	1 or 2 of the elements	3 out of 4 elements	all elements met

HOW TO SCORE

- You score a point when you hit the shuttlecock over the net and onto your opponent's side before your opponent can return it. You also score a point when your opponent hits the shuttlecock either into the net or out of bounds.
- A match consists of 3 games of 21 points.
- If you win a rally, you score a point.
- If the score is tied at 20 points, the first team to score 2 points wins the game.
- If the score is tied at 29 points, the first team to score 30 points wins the game.
- The winning team serves first in the next game.

PREDICT IF PLAYING BADMINTON IS AN EXERCISE THAT YOU WILL PURSUE IN COLLEGE OR A CAREER SETTING

1	I will not consider playing badminton as an exercise option in college or a career setting.
2	I will consider playing badminton as an exercise option in college or a career setting.

 RESEARCH INTEGRATION

Research terminology associated with the game of badminton.

HEALTH INTEGRATION

Count and analyze your pulse during and after playing badminton to determine if you are exercising in your personal target heart rate zone. Apply the results to your overall fitness plan. Many people choose to get their aerobic workouts by playing in casual games with friends.

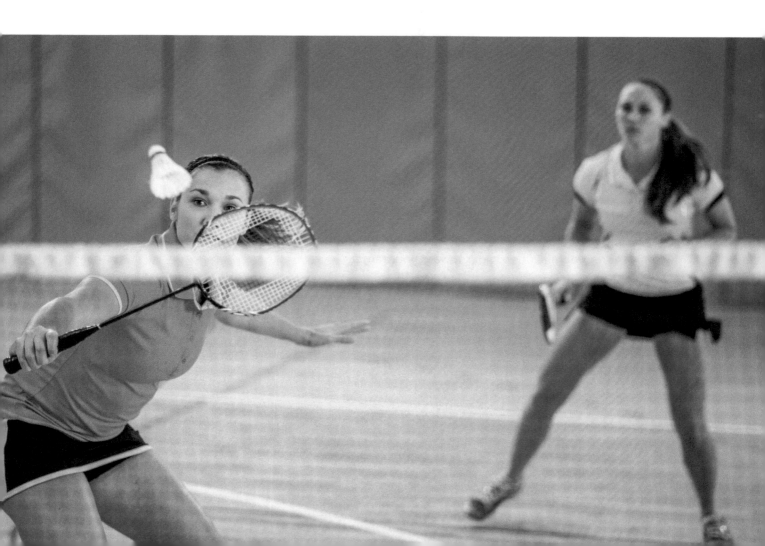

FOOTBALL FUN

Most people are familiar with the official American version of the game of football that is played from the youth level through the professional level. The official game of football requires players to have a high level of skill, wear protective equipment, and cooperate with coaches and referees. Casual, non-contact football activities can be fun, easy to learn, and good exercise.

The purpose of this lesson is for you to participate in casual, non-contact football activities for exercise.

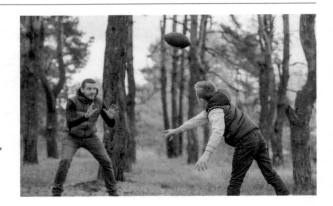

⚠️ **CAUTION: Wear appropriate safety equipment. Do not overinflate the ball.**

FOOTBALL SKILLS

THROWING A FOOTBALL

HAND PLACEMENT

- Hold the football in your dominant hand with your index finger closest to the tip of the ball.
- Place your middle finger between the first and second laces.
- Place your ring finger between the third and fourth laces.
- Place your pinky finger between the fifth and sixth laces.
- Wrap your thumb around the ball.

SKILL	PROGRESSING	COMPETENT	PROFICIENT
hand placement	1 or 2 of the elements	3 or 4 out of 5 elements	all elements

STANCE

- Stand with your feet shoulder-width apart.
- Point your non-dominant foot toward your target—where you are going to throw the football.
- Raise your dominant hand with the ball up to your ear. The laces should be facing away from you.
- Point your non-dominant shoulder toward your target.

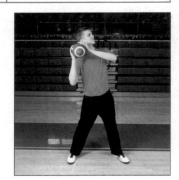

SKILL	PROGRESSING	COMPETENT	PROFICIENT
stance	1 or 2 of the elements	3 out of 4 elements	all elements

RELEASE

- Bend your non-dominant arm at chest level.
- Bring your dominant arm into a forward motion.
- Raise the football above your head and back.
- Bring your dominant arm into another forward motion and step forward toward your target with your non-dominant foot.
- Release the ball and allow it to roll off your fingers, starting with your pinky and ending with your index finger.
- Follow through by fully extending your dominant arm toward your target.

SKILL	PROGRESSING	COMPETENT	PROFICIENT
release	1, 2, or 3 of the elements	4 or 5 out of 6 elements	all elements

CATCHING A FOOTBALL

There are 2 basic hand positions for catching a football, depending on where the ball is located.

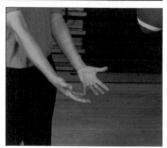

1. If the ball is above your shoulders, do the following.
   a. Make a diamond with your index fingers and thumbs.
   b. Extend your fingers and curve them slightly to receive the pass.
   c. Absorb the ball into your body until you have a good grasp on it.

2. If the ball is below your waist, do the following.
   a. Turn your fingers so that your pinkies are close together.
   c. Extend your fingers and curve them slightly to receive the pass.
   d. Absorb the ball into your body until you have a good grasp on it.

SKILL PRACTICE

Practice throwing routes.

- Find a partner.
- Create different running patterns.
- Practice throwing the football to your partner while your partner runs through the different patterns.
- Make your passes lead your partner.
- Try to time each pass so that the ball reaches the spot when your partner gets there.

DESIGN AND COACH/REFEREE YOUR OWN PRACTICE ACTIVITY GAME

Create a practice activity that will improve your throwing and catching skills.

- Determine the number of players.
- Determine the boundaries.
- Establish safety rules.
- Establish scoring for your game.

Prior to playing your practice game, establish and review the rules so that everyone understands them. If problems arise, work to solve them in a positive and effective manner. Appreciate each player's abilities. An example of a rule that you may want to decide upon is the boundaries.

Below are our game rules for safety and fairness.
1.
2.
3.
4.
5.

NON-CONTACT GAME

ULTIMATE FOOTBALL

- Gather with friends to play a game of ultimate football.
- Decide where you want your end zones to be. You can make the field as big as you want.
- Decide how many points you need to win the game.
- If you are an offensive player, stand behind your goal line. Then, take 5 steps—or hold the football for 5 seconds—before throwing the ball. Pass the ball to your teammates to advance the ball down the field. When you get the ball into your end zone, you have scored a point.
- If you are a defensive player, do not touch any of the offensive players.
- If a dropped pass or an interception occurs, the defensive team gets the ball and becomes the offensive team, and the offensive team becomes the defensive team.
- The first team to reach the points you have determined at the beginning of the game wins.

RESEARCH INTEGRATION

Count your pulse to determine if you are exercising in your personal target heart rate zone. Count your pulse after practicing skills and after playing in a game. Apply the results to your overall fitness plan.

SOCCER

Playing recreational soccer at your current age and into college or your career can help reduce stress, increase the opportunity to socialize, and provide exercise for good health. Playing official, competitive soccer requires high skill and fitness levels. People of all skill levels can enjoy playing casual games of soccer.

The purpose of this lesson is for you to participate in soccer activities. You will practice skills, learn game rules, be encouraged to communicate with teammates in a positive manner, and be reminded to exhibit appropriate behavior with your team and the opposing team.

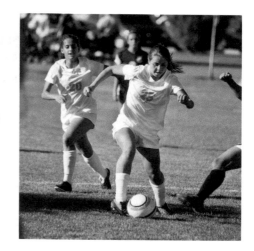

⚠ **CAUTION: Wear appropriate safety equipment. Do not overinflate the ball.**

SOCCER SKILLS

DRIBBLING

Use your peripheral vision, or your side vision, to watch the ball as you dribble it. Dribbling is a series of small, controlled touches that you complete in order to move with the ball in your possession. Dribble the ball with the insides and outsides of your feet as well as with the tops of your feet, where your shoelaces lay. Do not dribble the ball with your toes, otherwise, you risk losing control of the ball.

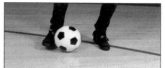
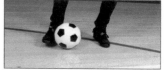

- Start with the ball positioned in front of you on the ground.
- Dribble forward, keeping the ball close—no more than 3 to 5 feet in front of you.
- Move the ball with the insides, outsides, and/or tops of both of your feet.
- Keep your head up.
- Match your speed to your skill.
- Change directions.

SKILL	PROGRESSING	COMPETENT	PROFICIENT
dribbling	1, 2, or 3 of the elements	4 or 5 out of 6 elements	all elements

PASSING

Passing the ball is an important part of soccer. Players pass the ball to each other in order to keep the other team from gaining control of the ball and to progress the ball up the field toward the other team's goal.

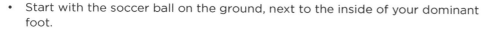
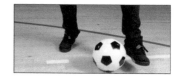

- Start with the soccer ball on the ground, next to the inside of your dominant foot.
- Position the inside of your kicking foot behind the middle of the soccer ball.
- Establish your non-kicking foot slightly behind you.
- Swing your kicking leg back, keeping it straight throughout your entire kick.
- Contact the middle of the ball with the inside of your foot. Follow through your kick with your foot and leg.
- Use appropriate force and direction to keep your pass on target.

SKILL	PROGRESSING	COMPETENT	PROFICIENT
passing	1, 2, or 3 of the elements	4 or 5 out of 6 elements	all elements

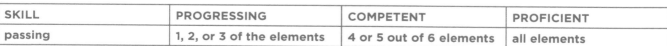

TRAPPING: OPTION 1

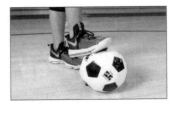

Trapping is a way of stopping the ball, receiving a pass, or gaining control of the ball.

- Start with the ball positioned in front of you on the ground.

- Place your dominant foot on top of the ball. To do this, lift your foot slightly off the ground, keeping your ankle locked and your toes up.

- Repeat this with your non-dominant foot.

SKILL	PROGRESSING	COMPETENT	PROFICIENT
trapping: option 1	1 of the elements	2 out of 3 elements	all elements

TRAPPING: OPTION 2

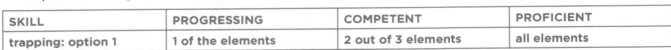

Trapping is also a way to stop the ball in order to quickly gain control and transition to your next move.

- When the soccer ball comes toward you, turn the ankle of whichever foot you are trapping with so that your instep, or the inside of your foot, is facing forward.

- Cushion the ball with your foot as you stop it lightly, as if you were catching an egg.

- Repeat this with your other foot.

SKILL	PROGRESSING	COMPETENT	PROFICIENT
trapping: option 2	1 of the elements	2 out of 3 elements	all elements

SHOOTING

The purpose of shooting is to get the soccer ball into your opponent's goal by striking it with your foot.

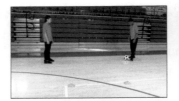
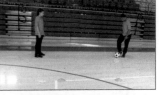
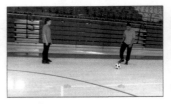
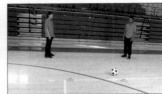

- Stand so that your dominant leg or kicking leg is pulled back behind you.

- Place your non-kicking foot alongside the soccer ball, pointing your toes at the target.

- Bend the knee of your kicking leg back; in a single motion, swing your leg forward, straightening it to kick the soccer ball.

- Kick the center of the soccer ball with the laces of your shoe, pointing your toes down. You do not want to kick the soccer ball with your toes; make contact with the ball with the top of your foot.

- Follow through, making sure that your toes are pointing toward the goal.

SKILL	PROGRESSING	COMPETENT	PROFICIENT
shooting	1 or 2 of the elements	3 or 4 out of 5 elements	all elements

SKILL PRACTICE

After mastering the skills above, put them all together in individual and group practice activities.

STRATEGIES TO REMEMBER

- When dribbling the soccer ball, keep it close to you.
- When passing the ball, kick with the instep of your foot.
- When trapping the ball, cushion it as if you were catching an egg.
- When shooting the soccer ball, point your toes down and kick the middle of the ball with the top of your foot. Your non-kicking foot should be next to the ball, pointing toward the target. When you follow through, make sure that your kicking toes are pointing toward the target as well.

INDEPENDENT PRACTICE ACTIVITY 1

- Place 2 discs about 4 feet apart to use as a goal. Place them about 10 to 20 feet away from you.
- Toss the soccer ball up in the air, trapping it with your foot, thigh, or chest, and guide it to the ground in front of you.
- Dribble the ball toward the goal.
- Shoot the ball through the discs when you get about 5 feet away from them.

INDEPENDENT PRACTICE ACTIVITY 2

- Place 2 discs about 4 feet apart to use as your goal.
- Add extra discs between you and the goal to dribble the ball around. This prompts you to change directions.
- Pass the ball to a wall. The ball will bounce off the wall so that you can trap it.
- Dribble the ball toward the goal.
- Shoot the ball between the discs.

DESIGN AND COACH/REFEREE YOUR OWN PRACTICE ACTIVITY GAME

Establish a skill that you want to improve upon and create a practice activity that will enhance your performance of that skill.

- Determine the number of players.
- Determine the boundaries.
- Establish safety rules.
- Establish scoring for your game.

Prior to playing your practice game, establish and review the rules so that everyone understands them. If problems arise, work to solve them in a positive and effective manner. Appreciate each player's abilities. An example of a rule you that may want to decide upon is the boundaries.

Below are our game rules for safety and fairness.
1.
2.
3.
4.
5.

SOCCER GAMES

SOCCER GOLF

- You need at least 2 players to play this game.
- Set up discs anywhere in an open space. Place them far apart from each another. These represent golf holes.
- Designate a starting spot.
- See who can kick the ball to the holes in the least amount of kicks.
- The team or player with the lowest score wins.

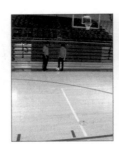 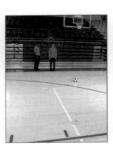 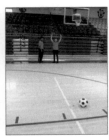

SOCCER GAME

ABOUT THE GAME

- To begin, 2 opposing teams of 11 players each including a goalie are established.
- All players must wear shin guards, socks that cover their shin guards, and appropriate cleats.
- The game is played on a rectangular grass or turf field.
- A goal is located at each end of the field.
- The object of the game is to move the ball down the field by passing or dribbling with your feet and to score by getting the ball into your opponent's goal.
- A game is divided into 45-minute halves.
- A goal is worth 1 point.
- The team with the most points at the end of the second half wins.

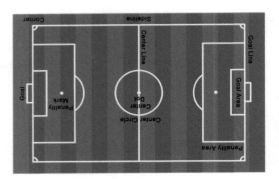

PLAYING THE GAME

- The game begins with a coin toss made by a referee at midfield.
- The team that possesses the ball is on offense and the other team is on defense.
- The first player to touch the ball at kickoff can only touch the ball once. They must kick the ball or pass it to another player who can dribble, pass, or kick the ball.
- No players except for the goalies or a player who is performing a throw-in can touch the ball with their hands. The entire arm counts as a hand in soccer, which means that a player cannot touch the ball anywhere from their fingertips to their upper arm.
- It is legal to use any body part other than a hand to contact the ball.
- If a player illegally uses their hands, which is referred to as a handball, the ball is turned over to the opposing team.
- The players on defense try to intercept, or take away, the ball from the offensive team to gain possession of the ball.

DEMONSTRATE POSITIVE GAME BEHAVIOR

- Follow all game rules.
- Do not conduct any fouls against another player (do not make illegal physical contact) and do not exhibit any unsportsmanlike behavior.
- Fouls and unsportsmanlike behavior can result in a free kick for the other team, a yellow card warning for the offending player, or a red card ejection from the game for the offending player.
- Be supportive and encouraging to your teammates.
- Treat your opponents with respect.

SKILL	PROGRESSING	COMPETENT	PROFICIENT
game behavior	1 of the elements	2 or 3 out of 4 elements	all elements met

PREDICT IF PLAYING SOCCER IS AN EXERCISE THAT YOU WILL PURSUE IN COLLEGE OR A CAREER SETTING

1	I will not consider playing soccer as an exercise option in college or a career setting.
2	I will consider playing soccer as an exercise option in college or a career setting.

RESEARCH INTEGRATION

Research local facilities to find where soccer is played in your community for your age group.

HEALTH INTEGRATION

Count your pulse to determine if you are exercising in your personal target heart rate zone. Count your pulse after practicing skills and after playing in a game. Compare the pulse rates of the goalie and a running player. Apply the results to your overall fitness plan. Many people choose to get their aerobic workouts by playing in fast-paced games like soccer.

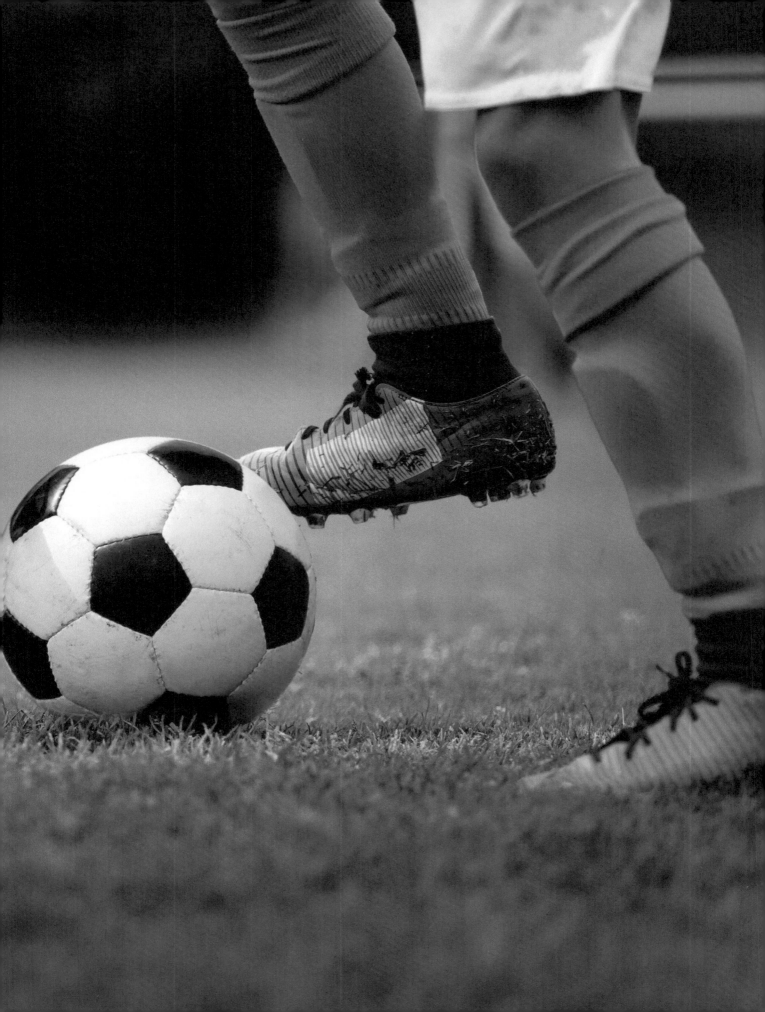

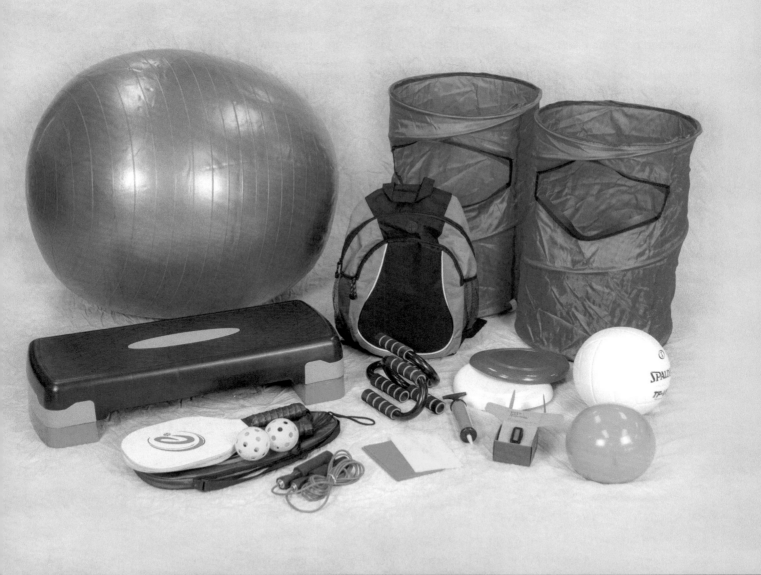

SAFETY ALERT!

Before you exercise, make sure that you are properly warmed up and have enough room to perform each activity. Wear proper equipment and follow activity-specific safety rules. Stay hydrated and take breaks as needed. Exercise only if you are healthy, and always exercise at your own pace. If an exercise starts to hurt, if you feel dizzy, or if you feel light-headed, stop the exercise completely and get help. Upon completion of any workout, cool down and stretch.

WARM-UP AND COOL-DOWN

⚠️ **CAUTION: Stretching should not be painful; ease up if stretching hurts. See the Flexibility section of your PE Manual for more information.**

WARM-UP

The purpose of a warm-up is to gradually increase heart rate, breathing rate, body temperature, and muscle temperature. Warming up prior to exercising increases circulation and blood flow to your muscles. When your muscles are warmed up, their performance—such as in the areas of strength and speed—is enhanced and risk of injury is decreased.

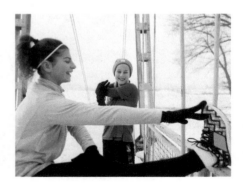

Stretching your muscles helps to minimize risk of injury by making the muscle fibers pliable, which means easy to bend or move.

Before you begin any workout, you should always warm up. Getting your heart and muscles prepared for exercise is important. There are numerous ways to get your body ready to participate in physical activity. **The Flexibility section of your PE Manual includes a variety of dynamic and static stretches for each major body part that will help you increase your flexibility.**

Elements of a Warm-Up

1. **Low-intensity cardio**: Walk, slow jog, or slow swim for 5 to 10 minutes to increase your heart rate, breathing rate, and body temperature before your workout.

2. **Dynamic stretch**: Perform a repeated motion—such as kicks, high knees, lunges, or arm circles—that will loosen up your joints and prepare your muscles for the exercise that you are about to do. Perform each dynamic stretch for at least 30 seconds.

   • Choose dynamic stretches that will warm up the major muscles that you will be using in the activity. For example, you could perform arm circles as part of your warm-up prior to swimming.

3. **Static stretch**: Stretch your muscles slowly and hold each stretch for 20 to 30 seconds without bouncing in order to lengthen your muscles and increase your flexibility. Some important areas to stretch as a part of your warm-up are your neck, sides, shoulders, triceps, back, hamstrings, quadriceps, and groin.

Example 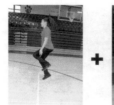 **+** 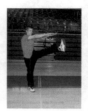 **+** 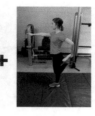 **= EFFECTIVE WARM-UP**

PERSONAL WARM-UP ACTIVITY

1. Select an exercise activity to participate in.

2. Design your personal warm-up plan for the activity that you selected. Any dynamic and static stretches that you choose to complete should be specific to the exercise activity that you chose.

3. Have a trusted adult or friend assess your stretches to make sure that you are using proper form.

4. Explain how the warm-up will decrease your risk of injury for this activity. _____

Procedure	Enter your personal warm-up regimen below.
1. **Low-intensity cardiovascular exercise:** Exercise for 5 to 10 minutes.	
2. **Dynamic stretches:** Perform dynamic stretches specifically for the selected activity.	
3. **Static stretches:** Perform static stretches specifically for the selected activity.	

COOL-DOWN

After you have finished your workout, exercise, or activity, it is imperative that your body returns to its normal state. You want to avoid stopping immediately and sitting down **unless you are in pain, dizzy, or injured**. Be sure to slow your heart rate and breathing rate back to or slightly above their resting rates. There are several ways to do this. You can simply walk or slow down your exercise for a few minutes, or you can find your own way to slow your body back down. You also may want to incorporate static stretches to increase flexibility and to avoid your muscles tightening. **The Flexibility section of your PE Manual includes a variety of static stretches for each major body part.** Always keep hydrated by drinking water before, during, and after exercise.

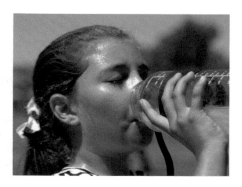

Elements of a Cool-Down

1. **Slow down**: Walk or gradually slow down your exercise—such as returning to a slow swim if you are swimming—until your heart rate, breathing rate, and body temperature are back to normal.

2. **Static stretch**: Stretch your muscles slowly and hold each stretch for 20 to 30 seconds without bouncing in order to lengthen your muscles and increase flexibility. Some important areas to stretch as part of your cool-down are your neck, sides, shoulders, triceps, back, hamstrings, quadriceps, and groin.

WALK + STATIC STRETCHES = EFFECTIVE COOL-DOWN

Design your personal cool-down plan. You can perform the same cool-down each time you finish a physical activity or you can change each time in order to reflect the exercise activity, such as by slowing your pedaling if you are biking.

Procedure	Enter your personal cool-down regimen below.
1. **Slow down:** Perform this slowed activity for 5 to 10 minutes.	
2. **Static stretches:** Perform several lower-body and upper-body stretches.	

AEROBIC EXERCISE AND PROPER NUTRITION

You want to make cardiovascular workouts a part of your daily life now and throughout your lifetime. Maintaining bone, muscle, and joint health is important. Varying your exercise routines helps to reduce the risk of injury. For example, if you enjoy high-impact workouts, intermingle them with low-impact workouts to reduce impact-related injuries. A runner can alternate running workouts with swimming or using an elliptical machine to minimize injury risks. Playing the same sport or performing the same workout year-round places continuous stress on the same bones, muscles, and joints. Switch up the types of exercises you do to avoid overuse injuries. Because any exercise done in your target heart rate zone and performed for 20 to 60 minutes 3 to 5 days per week is aerobic exercise, you can find several exercise activities that will fit into your current and future schedules.

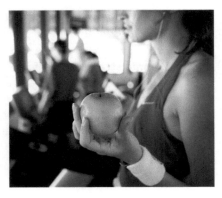

You are more likely to commit to healthful eating if you plan and keep track of your nutrition. Eating proper portions from the grain group, the fruit group, the vegetable group, the dairy group, and the protein group is essential to proper nutrition. Limit high-fat and sugary foods.

Combining regular aerobic exercise with proper nutrition contributes to cardiovascular health as well as overall health. It should be a lifelong commitment.

The purpose of this lesson is to encourage you to develop a fitness portfolio that includes a variety of exercise options and a plan for healthful nutrition. **The Cardiovascular Endurance section of this manual includes the target heart rate zone formula and the Borg Rating of Perceived Exertion Scale to help you to determine if you are exercising for heart health.** You can also use available technology to monitor your pulse rate and intensity.

When beginning any exercise program, begin with workouts for your fitness level and then build accordingly. You want to feel refreshed after your exercise session, not exhausted. Use your pulse rate to monitor aerobic workouts.

 CAUTION: Wear proper equipment and follow activity-specific safety rules.

AEROBIC EXERCISE AND PROPER NUTRITION

Develop a fitness portfolio and make a commitment to aerobic exercise. Your fitness portfolio should include the following.

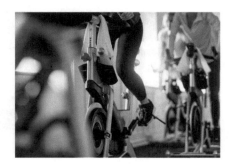

- endurance walk/run fitness score
- goals for improvement
- 4-week exercise plan (See below.)
- a plan for adjusting your exercise routine as your fitness level improves and when your schedule changes (for example, from high school to college or career)

Plan an exercise routine that includes more than 1 type of aerobic exercise.

TYPES OF AEROBIC EXERCISE

Sports: Examples include soccer, basketball, volleyball, swimming, hockey, lacrosse, tennis, badminton, pickleball, handball, gymnastics, dance, martial arts, wrestling, track and field, and so on.

Outdoor pursuits: Examples include walking, jogging, biking, canoeing, kayaking, golfing, fly fishing, hiking, rock climbing, horseback riding, skiing, and so on.

Fitness gyms: Find a gym that is convenient for you to attend where you can complete circuit exercises, use aerobic machines, take classes, and more.

Stationary exercise equipment: Examples include using a jump rope, treadmill, elliptical trainer, bike, mini trampoline, and so on.

Exercise apps or videos: Use a workout tutorial on an app, website, video, or other digital source.

Create your own movement sequence workout: Create your personal aerobic workout routines by blending basic locomotor skills such as jogging in place, jumping jacks, high knees, and so forth.

Choreograph a personal aerobic workout routine by blending basic locomotor skills. This is a workout that can be done at home for convenience. Suggested time for each skill is from 20 to 60 seconds with a 30-second rest every 4 to 5 minutes. Repeat for a 20- to 60-minute workout. Most important, exercise at your level of fitness and rest accordingly. Use the following skills to choreograph your routine, or use skills of your choice.

- Jogging in place: Run slowly in place.
- Jumping jacks: Stand with your feet apart with arms up, then feet together with arms at your sides.
- High knees: Alternate lifting your knees to waist height.
- Burpees: Jump vertically, then bend your knees and transition to a push-up position.
- Side slides: Step to the right. Bring the other foot over in a step-together motion. Repeat left.
- Squat jumps: Jump and land softly into a squat (hips even with knees).
- March in place: Alternate lifting knees to waist height.
- Carioca: Step to the side with 1 foot and cross with your other foot in a step-cross-step-cross movement. Alternate the step-cross movement with a cross behind the lead foot and a cross in front of the lead foot.
- Front kicks: Alternate lifting your legs forward.

The following is an example of how to schedule and track aerobic exercise for 1 week. Plan for 4 weeks.

WARM UP BEFORE EACH WORKOUT.

Week 1	Exercise	Time of Day	Exercise Time (min.)	Heart Rate (bpm)
Mon.	stepper	morning	20	160
Tues.				
Wed.	my routine	morning	30	155
Thurs.	pickleball	evening	60	145
Fri.				
Sat.	volleyball	evening	45	140
Sun.				

COOL-DOWN AFTER EACH WORKOUT.

EXTENSION: Use your exercise plan as training for a community event such as a 5K (walk or jog). Predict what a week in your future college or career path would resemble. Create a weekly exercise plan for college or career settings.

Plan your nutrition. Keep track of the food you eat each day for 1 week. Include food from the grain group, the fruit group, the vegetable group, the dairy group, and the protein group each day. Drink water daily. Limit high-fat and sugary foods. Exercise burns calories, so it is important to get food from all of the food groups. Plan for and eat healthful snacks. Review what you eat each day, discuss your diet with a trusted adult, and adjust so that you are getting a well-rounded, healthful diet. Be aware of false diet claims and rely on your doctor for advice.

 CAUTION: Do not consume food to which you are allergic or sensitive.

EXAMPLE

Day 1	Time	Servings	Total Servings
Grain	breakfast	2	6
	lunch	2	
	dinner	2	
Fruit	breakfast	1	4
	lunch	2	
	dinner	1	
Vegetable	breakfast	0	5
	lunch	2	
	dinner	3	
Dairy	breakfast	2	4
	lunch	1	
	dinner	1	
Protein	breakfast	0	3
	lunch	1	
	dinner	2	
Snacks	granola bar	1	2
	apple	1	

💻 RESEARCH INTEGRATION

1. Research proper portion sizes for you according to your weight and your level of exercise.

2. Research healthful snacking for before and after workouts.

💜 HEALTH INTEGRATION

Use available technology to monitor your pulse rate and intensity. Apply the results to your overall fitness plan.

DANCE

Dance involves expressing yourself through repeated patterns of movement. It is usually set to music. Some forms of dance include creative, tap, ballet, hip-hop, modern, folk, square, jazz, line, Latin, ballroom, and social.

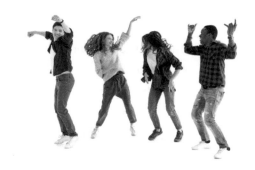

Social dance involves dancing with a partner or a group in a social situation for enjoyment. Social dancing is common at events such as weddings and parties. Freestyle dancing with a partner and following a choreographed line dance are some examples of social dancing.

The purpose of this lesson is for you to perform basic locomotor movements using common dance concepts in rhythmic patterns to create your own line dance that you can do now and in your future. Put your favorite music on and get moving for a convenient, fun workout!

SOCIAL DANCE

PERSONAL DANCE ROUTINE

COMMON CONCEPTS OF DANCE TO USE FOR YOUR PERSONAL DANCE

- The concept of space includes the following.
  - o high, medium, or low **levels**
  - o forward, backward, right, or left **directions**
  - o curved, zigzag, straight, circle, or square **pathways**
- The concept of time includes the following.
  - o slow, medium, or fast **speeds**
  - o a pattern for **rhythm**
- The concept of force includes the following.
  - o applying light, moderate, or strong **weights**

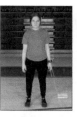
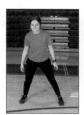
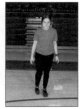
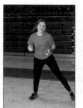
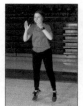
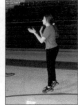

CREATE A LINE DANCE

Start with the dance steps described below. Start moving to the right. When you jump, turn, and clap, turn to the right as you step and land. Continue this pattern until you complete the square. Next, complete the routine by adding your own dance steps. Set the dance to music.

1. Combine the sidestep and step-hop for a double step (step together then step-hop and clap).

   - Step to the right with your right foot.
   - Bring your left foot in to meet your right foot.
   - Step out to the right side with your right foot.
   - Bring your left foot in, simultaneously jumping and clapping.
   - Step to the right with your right foot.
   - Bring your left foot in to meet your right foot.
   - Step out to the right side with your right foot.
   - Bring your left foot in and simultaneously **jump, turn, and clap**.
   - Repeat these steps until you complete a square pattern.

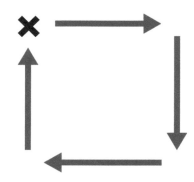

2. Next, add your own dance steps to complete the dance. Create the steps, write a description of each step, and practice the steps.

- Choose locomotor skills to blend (slides, cariocas, turns, and so on).
- Use your arms to accompany the footwork, for example: step, cross, step, clap.
- Perform the skills at different levels.
- Move at medium and fast speeds.
- Use light, moderate, and strong force to move your body.
- Create a pattern.
- Use an 8 count for each move.

Option: Line dance with friends outside of PE class, or dance with a partner at a social function.

PREDICT IF DANCE IS AN EXERCISE THAT YOU WILL PURSUE IN COLLEGE OR A CAREER SETTING

1	I will not consider dance as an exercise option in college or a career setting.
2	I will consider dance as an exercise option in college or a career setting.

💻 RESEARCH INTEGRATION

1. Research current dance trends.
2. Research and compare 2 dance types: square and modern.
3. Research dance classes in your local area.

♥ HEALTH INTEGRATION

Count your pulse to determine if you are exercising in your personal target heart rate zone. Apply the results to your overall fitness plan. Many people choose to get their aerobic workouts through dance.

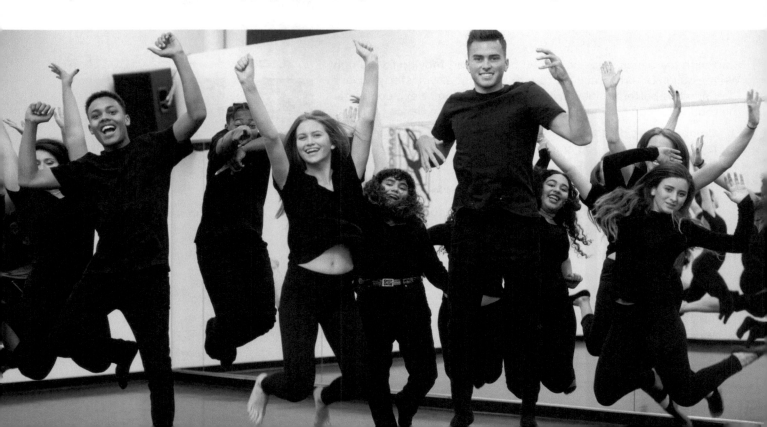

JUMP ROPE

A jump rope is an inexpensive piece of exercise equipment. It can be used indoors, outdoors, and in a small space. A jump rope promotes adherence to participation in physical activity by eliminating cost and space barriers. It is also an effective sport-training tool that improves balance, agility, and coordination.

The purpose of this lesson is for you to use jumping rope to improve in areas of fitness that are important to you: cardiovascular, skill-related, or both.

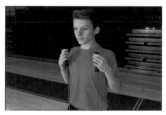

JUMP ROPE BASICS

FITTING THE JUMP ROPE TO YOUR HEIGHT

- Place a jump rope handle in each hand.
- Stand on the middle of the rope with 1 foot.
- Move the handles straight up, making sure that the rope is straight and pulled tight.
- The tops of the handles should reach close to your shoulders.

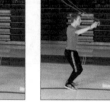

Fitting the jump rope to your height

ELEMENTS OF JUMP ROPE

- Keep your eyes forward.
- When you are turning the rope, keep your elbows near your sides, maintaining a 45-degree angle and making 2-inch circles with your wrists.
- Leave just enough space for the rope to pass under your feet when you jump.
- Stay on the balls of your feet.
- Land softly, keeping your knees slightly bent.

BASIC SKILLS

BASIC JUMP

- Pick up the rope. Holding a handle in each hand, rest the rope behind your feet. Stand on the balls of your feet. This is the ready position.
- Your hands should be just above the height of your waist.
- Swing the rope up and over your head.
- Jump over the rope when it approaches your toes.
- Continue as long as you can without stopping.

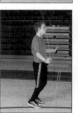
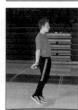

Basic jump

BACKWARD JUMP

- Begin with the rope in front of your feet.
- Swing the rope up and over your head.
- Jump over the rope when it approaches your feet.

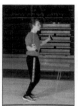
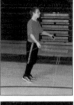
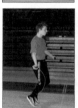
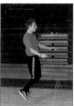

Backward jump

ALTERNATE-FOOT JUMP

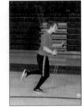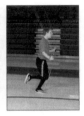

- Pick up the rope. Holding a handle in each hand, rest the rope behind your feet. Stand on the balls of your feet. This is the ready position. Note that 1 foot will be lifted off the ground during each turn of the rope before the other foot jumps.

- Turn the rope from behind you up over your head. When the rope reaches your toes, jump over it with your right foot.

Alternate-foot jump

- Turn the rope again from behind you up over your head. When the rope reaches your toes this time, jump over it with your left foot.

- Continue turning the rope and alternating feet as if you were running in place. Try it jumping backward.

Practice the basic jump rope skills until competent. Next, design a jump rope routine using basic jump rope skills that will improve footwork speed.

SAMPLE OF A WORKOUT TO IMPROVE FOOTWORK SPEED

- basic jump 1 minute at a medium pace
- basic jump 30 seconds at a fast pace
- rest 30 seconds
- backward jump 1 minute at a medium pace
- backward jump 30 seconds at a fast pace

- rest 30 seconds
- alternate-foot jump 1 minute at a medium pace
- alternate-foot jump 30 seconds at a fast pace
- rest 30 seconds
- repeat as needed

DESIGN YOUR PERSONAL FOOTWORK SPEED ROUTINE

CHALLENGE SKILLS

The following challenges are for students who have mastered the basic jump rope skills. The challenge level is recommended to learn advanced skills and add a variety of skills to your workout.

TOES UP/HEELS UP

This is a basic skill that helps a beginner learn how to jump rope. It is also a skill that is used to give you a rest during an aerobic workout so that you can continue the flow of the routine without stopping.

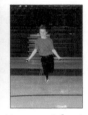

- Hold the rope with a handle in each hand.
- Place the rope behind your feet.
- Keep your feet on the ground.
- Turn the rope forward and over your head. Lift your toes and capture the rope under your feet.
- Standing on your toes, lift your heels and bring the rope over your head.

Toes up/heels up

HOP ON 1 FOOT

- Perform the basic jump on your right foot.
- Perform the basic jump on your left foot.

Hop on 1 foot

SKIER

- With both feet together, hop side to side while turning the rope.

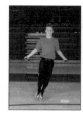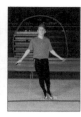

Skier

CROSSOVERS

- After the rope moves over your head, cross the rope in front of you, jump, and uncross the rope.

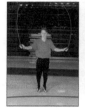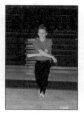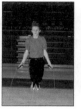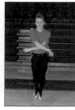

Crossovers

FRONT KICKS

- Kick 1 foot forward as the rope passes under your feet with a skip-step in between.
- Alternate kicks.

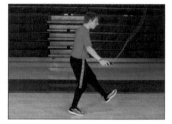

Front kicks

SIDE KICKS

- Kick 1 foot and then the other out to the side with a skip-step in between.

CRISSCROSS FEET

- Cross and uncross your feet while jumping.

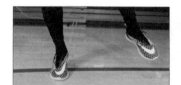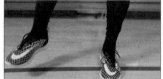

Side kicks

FIGURE-8 JUMPS

- Hold a handle in each hand. Swing the rope from side to side in a figure-8 pattern. Then, open it to regular form and step over it. When you master that, practice jumping over the rope.

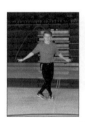

Crisscross feet

STRADDLE JUMPS

- Turn the rope from behind you up over your head. When the rope reaches your toes, jump over it with both feet. Split your legs apart as you jump. On the next turn, land with your feet together.

DOUBLE UNDER

- Allow the rope to pass under your feet 2 times before your feet touch the ground.

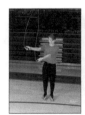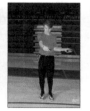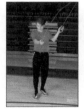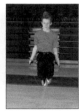

Figure-8 jumps

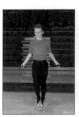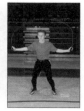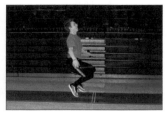

Straddle jumps *Double under*

Practice the challenge jump rope skills until competent. Next, design your personal aerobic jump rope routine by blending the basic jump rope skills and the challenge skills. Set your routine to music. Monitor your pulse rate.

BLENDING: Perform 1 jump rope skill and transition smoothly to another jump rope skill without stopping between moves. Blend after a 4 count, an 8 count, or a 16 count. Mix it up so that it works for you.

SAMPLE OF A CARDIOVASCULAR CONDITIONING WORKOUT

- blend basic jump/crossovers/basic jump **2 minutes**
- toes up/heels up **30 seconds**
- blend figure-8s/backward jump/figure-8s **2 minutes**
- toes up/heels up **30 seconds**
- blend alternate-foot jumps/figure-8s/crisscross feet **2 minutes**
- toes up/heels up **30 seconds**
- blend skier/front kicks/side kicks **2 minutes**
- toes up/heels up **30 seconds**
- repeat for a 20-minute workout

DESIGN YOUR PERSONAL CARDIOVASCULAR JUMP ROPE ROUTINE. SET IT TO MUSIC.

PREDICT IF JUMPING ROPE IS AN EXERCISE THAT YOU WILL PURSUE IN COLLEGE OR A CAREER SETTING

| 1 | I will not consider jumping rope as an exercise option in college or a career setting. |
| 2 | I will consider jumping rope as an exercise option in college or a career setting. |

♥ HEALTH INTEGRATION

Count your pulse during and after jumping rope to determine if you are exercising in your personal target heart rate zone for health benefits. Apply the results to your overall fitness plan.

STEPPER

Exercising on a stepper is good for improving your cardiovascular endurance. You can also incorporate a stepper into your strength-training program; between each weight-lifting exercise, you can use the stepper to enhance your program. A stepper is also a great calorie burner, and it helps with muscular endurance. Focusing on your footwork while exercising on a stepper may help to reduce stress.

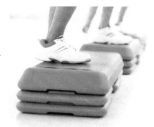

A stepper is a portable piece of equipment that can be used for an aerobic workout in a small space such as a dorm room or an office. The convenience of a stepper may help you commit to regular exercise.

The purpose of this lesson is for you to use a stepper for an aerobic workout now and in the future.

⚠️ **CAUTION: Set up the stepper on a solid surface and lock it in place. Make sure that you step fully on the step and not on the side. When stepping up, step higher than the step to avoid injury. Stop immediately if you feel dizzy or light-headed at any time.**

STEPPER EXERCISES

Practice each of the following exercises. Concentrate on proper form prior to engaging in a workout.

QUICK STEP-UPS

- Place the stepper horizontally in front of you.
- Step up on the stepper with your left foot and then your right foot.
- Step off the stepper with your left foot and then your right foot.
- Increase your pace when you feel comfortable.
- Repeat this exercise, starting with your right foot, after the desired amount of time.

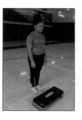
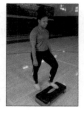
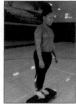
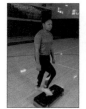
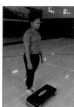

Quick step-ups

STEP-UP PUSH-UPS

- Place the stepper horizontally in front of you. For more stability, place the opposite side of the stepper against a wall.
- Get into a push-up position in front of the stepper with your hands shoulder-width apart.
- Keeping your hands shoulder-width apart, place your left hand and then your right hand on the stepper.
- Do a push-up.
- Come up from your push-up. Bring your left hand off the stepper and then your right hand.

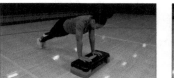
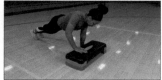
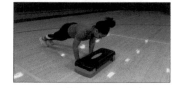

Step-up push-ups

SIDE STEP-UP

- Place the stepper vertically on the ground to your left. Stand on the ground to the right side of the stepper.
- Step up onto the stepper with your left foot, placing your foot in the middle of the stepper.
- Switch feet quickly so that your right foot is now on the stepper. Bring your left foot down off the opposite side of the stepper.
- Stand on the left side of the stepper and step on it with your right foot placed in the middle of the stepper.
- Switch feet quickly so that your left foot is now on the stepper. Bring your right foot down off the opposite side of the stepper.
- Continue the side-to-side pattern. Start to increase the speed with which you switch legs.

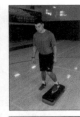
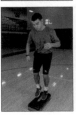
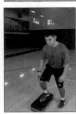
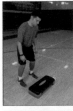
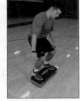

Side step-up

STEPPER SQUAT JUMP

- Place the stepper horizontally in front of you.
- Stand with your feet shoulder-width apart.
- Jump with both feet onto the stepper, do a squat, and jump back down.

EXTENSION: Place the stepper horizontally in front of you and perform the following steps while alternating your feet.

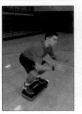
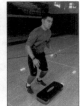

Stepper squat jump

ALTERNATING QUICK STEPS

- Step up onto the stepper with your left foot and then your right foot.
- Step off the stepper with your left foot and then your right foot.
- Step up onto the stepper with your right foot and then your left foot.
- Step off the stepper with your right foot and then your left foot.

KNEE-UPS

- Step up onto the stepper with your left foot and lift your right knee.
- Step off the stepper with your right foot and then your left foot.
- Step up onto the stepper with your right foot and lift your left knee.
- Step off the stepper with your left foot and then your right foot.

SIDE KICKS

- Step up onto the stepper with your left foot and lift your right leg straight to the side.
- Step off the stepper with your right foot and then your left foot.
- Step up onto the stepper with your right foot and lift your left leg straight to the side.
- Step off the stepper with your left foot and then your right foot.

BACK LEG LIFTS

- Step up onto the stepper with your left foot and lift your right leg straight behind you.
- Step off the stepper with your right foot and then your left foot.
- Step up onto the stepper with your right foot and lift your left leg straight behind you.
- Step off the stepper with your left foot and then your right foot.

The following is a suggested use of the stepper in an aerobic workout. Exercise to your level of fitness.

Warm up before your workout. Cool down after your workout.

Begin each movement slowly until you feel comfortable increasing your speed.

Repeat each move for 30 seconds or to your level of fitness.

Your goal should be to reach 1 minute per exercise and continue to alternate moves for an aerobic workout.

PREDICT IF USING A STEPPER IS AN EXERCISE THAT YOU WILL PURSUE IN COLLEGE OR A CAREER SETTING

| 1 | I will not consider the stepper as an exercise option in college or a career setting. |
| 2 | I will consider the stepper as an exercise option in college or a career setting. |

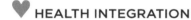 **RESEARCH INTEGRATION**

Research additional stepper exercises to incorporate into your stepper workout.

 HEALTH INTEGRATION

Count your pulse to determine if you are exercising in your personal target heart rate zone. Apply the results to your overall fitness plan.

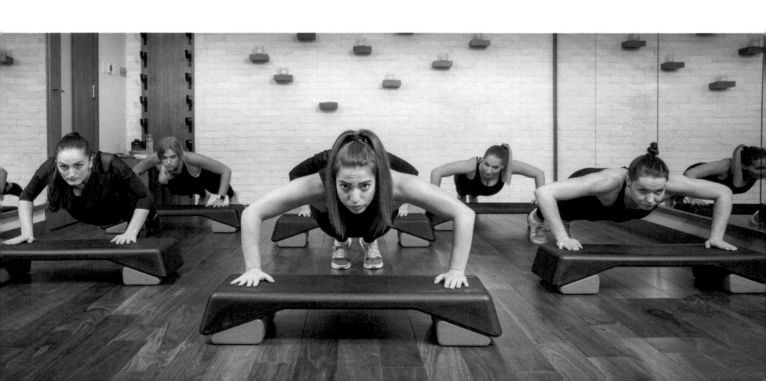

FITNESS BALL

Exercising with a fitness ball forces your core muscles to engage to balance your body throughout the exercise. Working out with a fitness ball improves muscular strength and endurance. Approximately at age 35, if you do not exercise, you will begin to naturally lose muscle strength. Strength training with a fitness ball or other resistance methods can reverse this physiological process and help maintain and improve muscle strength. Make strength training a lifelong habit to prevent the loss of muscle strength as you get older.

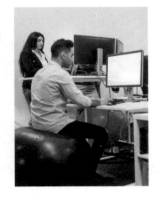

You can strength train with a fitness ball almost anywhere. A fitness ball is portable and does not require a lot of space to use.

The purpose of this lesson is to exercise leg, back, and core muscles using a fitness ball.

 CAUTION: Do not overinflate the ball.

FITNESS BALL STRENGTH-BUILDING EXERCISES
TIPS FOR USING A FITNESS BALL

- Exercises done on a firmer ball are more challenging.
- A beginner should start with a slightly deflated ball.
- When you are seated on the ball, your feet should be flat on the floor.

Practice each of the following exercises. Concentrate on proper form prior to engaging in a workout.

SINGLE-LEG SQUATS

muscle focus: hamstrings and quadriceps

- Stand up straight and place the fitness ball against your lower back between yourself and the wall.
- Place your feet shoulder-width apart and slightly out in front of you. Your body should be at an angle.
- Lift your right leg straight out in front of you.
- Slide your body down into a sitting position; the ball should now be against your upper back. Make sure that your knees do not go past your toes.
- Stand back up to the starting position. The ball should return against your lower back.
- Switch sides after completing your repetitions.

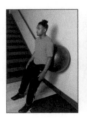 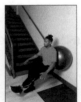 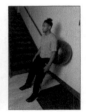

Single-leg squats

HAMSTRING CURLS

muscle focus: abdominal muscles, erector spinae, hamstrings, glutes

- Place the fitness ball on the floor.
- Lie down with your hands slightly out to your sides.
- Put your lower calves and ankles on the ball. Your feet should be together, and your glutes should be lifted off the ground.
- Bring your knees in toward your chest, moving the ball toward your glutes. The bottoms of your feet should be resting on the ball.
- Straighten your legs to return to the starting position.

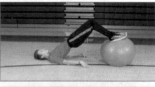 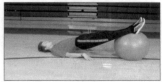

Hamstring curls

LEG EXTENSIONS

muscle focus: quadriceps, hamstrings, and glutes

- Sit on the ball with both feet firmly on the ground.
- Lift your right leg so your calf is parallel to the ground.
- Lower your right leg slowly back to the starting position.
- Lift your left leg so your calf is parallel to the ground.
- Lower your left leg slowly back to the starting position.
- Alternate legs.

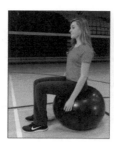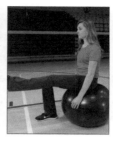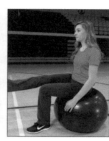

Leg extensions

SQUATS WITH TWISTS

muscle focus: abdominal muscles, quadriceps, hamstrings, triceps

- Hold the fitness ball straight out in front of you at chest level.
- Stand with your feet shoulder-width apart.
- Get into a squat position. Bend your knees and lower your buttocks toward the ground. Make sure that your knees do not go past your toes.
- Twist your torso to the right while in the squat position and while still holding the ball out in front of you.
- Stand up to the starting position.
- Repeat this to the left side.

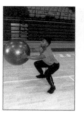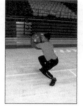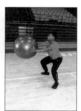

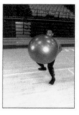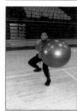

Squats with twists

CHEST PRESSES WITH MEDICINE BALL

muscle focus: pectoralis majors, pectoralis minors, deltoids, and triceps

- Place the fitness ball on the ground behind you.
- Place your upper back on the ball. Make sure that your head and neck do not touch the ball.
- Place your feet shoulder-width apart.
- Bend your knees to form 90-degree angles. Place your feet under your knees.
- Hold the weighted ball close to your chest with both hands. If the weighted ball is too heavy, you can use a resistance band. Wrap the band around your upper back and hold an end of the band in each hand.
- Stabilize yourself on the fitness ball and raise the weighted ball or resistance band toward the ceiling. Then, bring the weighted ball or resistance band back to your chest.

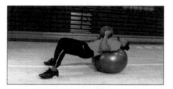

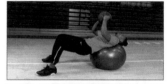

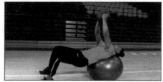

Chest presses with medicine ball

PLANK ROLLOUTS

muscle focus: abdominal muscles

- Place the fitness ball on the ground in front of you.
- Place your knees on the ground and your forearms on the ball.
- Hold your body at a slight angle. There should be about 2 feet between your knees and the ball.
- Roll the ball forward with your forearms until half of your forearms are off the ball. Tighten your abdominal muscles while doing this.
- Roll the ball back to the starting position with your forearms.

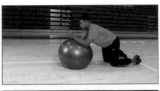
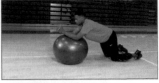
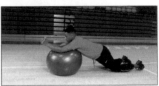

Plank rollouts

CRUNCHES

muscle focus: recti abdominis and oblique abdominal muscles

- Place the fitness ball on the floor.
- Place yourself on the fitness ball so that your lower back is on the ball. Do not let your shoulders touch the ball.
- Place your feet shoulder-width apart for balance.
- Place your hands behind your head on your neck.
- Bend your torso upward, performing a crunch.
- Come back down to the starting position, making sure that your abdomen is still tight. Do not extend back the whole way as that would release the tension in your abdomen.

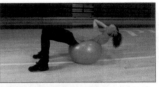
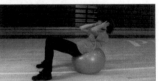

Crunches

SIDE CRUNCHES

muscle focus: abdominal muscles and erector spinae

- Place the fitness ball on the ground behind you.
- Place your lower back on the ball. Do not let your shoulders touch the ball.
- Place your feet shoulder-width apart for balance.
- Place your hands behind your head on your neck.
- Bend your torso upward and twist to the right. Your left elbow should almost touch your right thigh.
- Come back to the starting position, making sure your abdomen is still tight. Do not extend back the whole way as that would release the tension in your abdomen.
- Repeat this to the left.

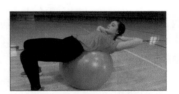
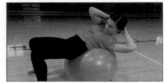

Side crunches

BACK EXTENSIONS

muscle focus: erector spinae (iliocostales, longissimi, and spinales)

- Place the fitness ball on the floor.
- Place your abdomen on the ball. Your legs should be extended behind you and about shoulder-width apart for balance.
- Place your hands behind your head on your neck (like when doing a crunch).
- Lift your upper body so that you are hyperextending your back.
- Come back down to the starting position.

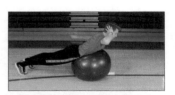
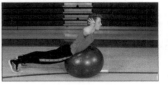

Back extensions

Have a trusted adult or friend evaluate you for correct form for the previous exercises. Did you respond positively to the feedback?

Reciprocate and evaluate your friend. Were you able to provide feedback in a positive manner?

The following is a suggested use of the fitness ball in a strength-building workout. Exercise to your level of fitness.

- Warm up and cool down.
- Perform each exercise 2 to 3 days per week.
- Begin with 1 set of 10 repetitions. Increase sets and the number of repetitions when the current number is too easy.
- Your goal should be to reach 3 sets of 10 to 15 repetitions.

PREDICT IF USING A FITNESS BALL IS AN EXERCISE THAT YOU WILL PURSUE IN COLLEGE OR A CAREER SETTING

| 1 | I will not consider the fitness ball as an exercise option in college or a career setting. |
| 2 | I will consider the fitness ball as an exercise option in college or a career setting. |

💻 RESEARCH INTEGRATION

Research how to improve flexibility with a fitness ball.

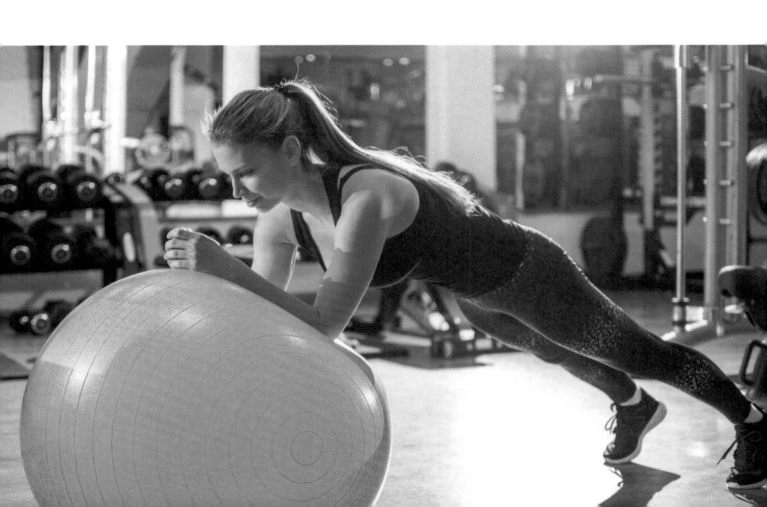

PUSH-UP HANDLES

Push-up exercises improve muscular strength and muscular endurance. In addition to strengthening your arms, these exercises help strengthen your core, particularly your chest and abdominal muscles.

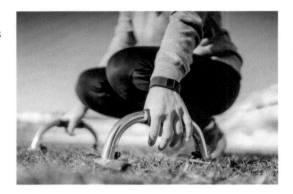

You can strength train with push-up handles almost anywhere. Push-up handles are portable and do not require a lot of space to use. They make a push-up harder by increasing the range of motion of the push-up. Begin exercising at your level of fitness and increase accordingly. Knee push-ups are an option if you are having difficulty with a standard push-up.

The purpose of this lesson is to include push-up handles in strength training.

 CAUTION: Place the push-up handles on a hard, flat, non-slippery surface.

PUSH-UP HANDLES STRENGTH-BUILDING EXERCISES

TIPS FOR USING PUSH-UP HANDLES

- Hold a handle in each hand.
- Keep your shoulders, elbows, and wrists in line.
- Keep your back straight.
- Lock your wrists; do not flex them.
- Exercise slowly and at your ability level. You may have to do knee push-ups until your strength level increases.

Practice each of the following exercises. Concentrate on proper form prior to engaging in a workout.

PUSH-UPS

muscle focus: pectoralis majors, biceps, triceps, and abdominal muscles

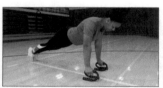
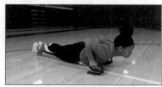
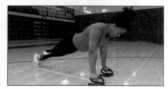

- Lie prone on the ground with the handles shoulder-width apart in front of you.
- Place your hands on the handles and get into a push-up position. Your body should be off the ground. Put your feet together and your toes on the ground.
- Hold the handles and lower your body toward the ground, but do not touch the ground. Keep your back straight.
- Come back to the starting position.
- Focus on different muscles by moving the handles closer together or farther apart. Move them closer together to do a close push-up. Move them just outside your shoulders to do a wide push-up.

Push-ups

IN-AND-OUT PUSH-UPS

muscle focus: pectoralis majors, biceps, triceps, deltoids, abdominal muscles, and hip abductors and adductors

- Lie prone on the ground with the handles shoulder-width apart in front of you.

- Place your hands on the handles and get into a push-up position. Your body should be off the ground. Put your feet together with your toes on the ground.

- Keep your back straight as you lower your body toward the ground. Do not touch the ground.

- Come back to the starting position.

- Spread your legs hip-width apart and lower your body again toward the ground.

- Come back to the starting position and put your feet together.

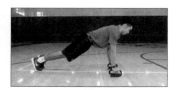
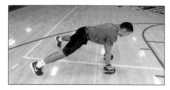
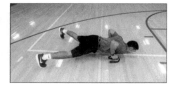

In-and-out push-ups

LEGS-UP PUSH-UPS

muscle focus: pectoralis majors, biceps, triceps, deltoids, abdominal muscles, gastrocnemii, and solei

- Get a stepper and place it behind you.

- Lie prone on the ground with the handles shoulder-width apart in front of you.

- Place your feet on the stepper.

- Place your hands on the handles and get into a push-up position. Your body should be off the ground.

- Keep your back straight as you lower your body toward the ground. Do not touch the ground.

- Come back to the starting position.

- Focus on different muscles by moving the handles closer together or farther apart. Move them closer together to do a close push-up. Move them just outside your shoulders to do a wide push-up.

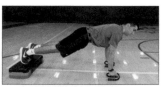
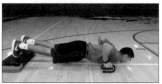
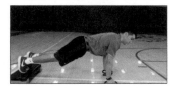

Legs-up push-ups

DIPS

muscle focus: triceps and abdominal muscles

- Place the handles behind you shoulder-width apart.

- Sit on the ground so that your legs are straight out in front of you.

- Place your hands on the handles and lift your buttocks off the ground.

- Bend your elbows and lower your buttocks toward the ground. Try not to touch the ground.

- Come back to the starting position.

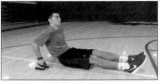
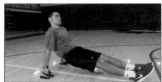

Dips

The following is a suggested use of the push-up handles in a strength-building workout. Exercise to your level of fitness.

- Warm up before your workout. Cool down after your workout.

- Perform each push-up exercise 2 to 3 days per week. Do not exercise the same muscle group on consecutive days.

- Begin with 1 set of 10 repetitions. Increase sets and the number of repetitions when the current number is too easy.

- Your goal should be to reach 3 sets of 10 to 15 repetitions.

PREDICT IF USING THE PUSH-UP HANDLES IS AN EXERCISE THAT YOU WILL PURSUE IN COLLEGE OR A CAREER SETTING

1	I will not consider using push-up handles as an exercise option in college or a career setting.
2	I will consider using push-up handles as an exercise option in college or a career setting.

RESEARCH INTEGRATION

Research anaerobic exercise and its relation to push-ups.

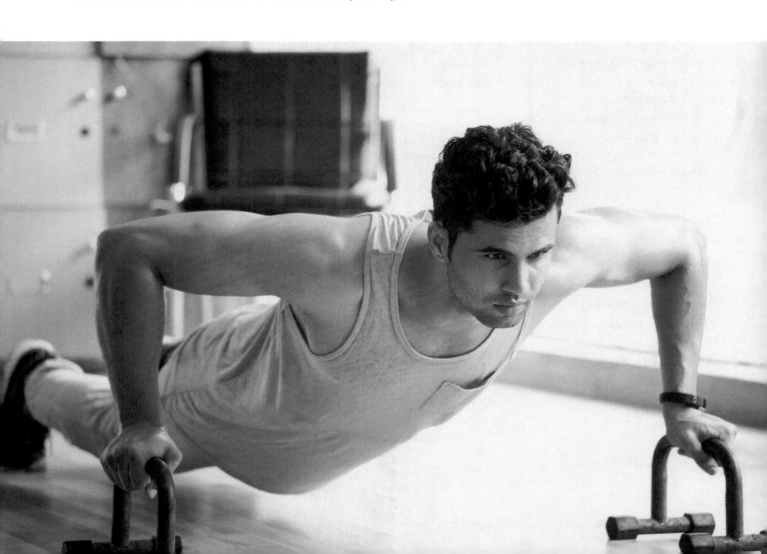

RESISTANCE BANDS

Many people make a lifetime commitment to strength training with resistance bands. Working with resistance bands applies less force on the joints than traditional weightlifting, which decreases the risk of injury. Physical therapists use resistance band exercises for rehabilitation purposes.

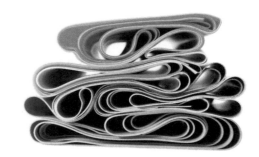

There are different types of resistance bands: handles, loops, tubes, flat, and so on. All of the bands are easy to carry with you and the exercises do not require a lot of space. Regular use of resistance bands helps to improve muscular strength, muscular endurance, and flexibility. When using resistance bands, start with the lightest resistance and gradually increase to a higher resistance as you get stronger.

The purpose of this lesson is to increase muscular strength and endurance using resistance bands.

FITNESS TIP: When using resistance bands, you should make sure that the band is secured in a way that the length is appropriate to give resistance for the entire exercise. Wrap the band around your hands if you need an increased resistance level.

CAUTION: Check the resistance bands for damage or wear before exercising. When exercising, secure the band before adding any resistance.

RESISTANCE BANDS STRENGTH-BUILDING EXERCISES

BENEFITS OF STRENGTH TRAINING WITH RESISTANCE BANDS

- is an effective overall strength workout that does not require weights
- offers a variety of resistance adjustments for beginner through advanced levels
- requires inexpensive pieces of equipment
- requires equipment that is easy to carry with you when you are traveling

Practice each of the following exercises. Concentrate on proper form prior to engaging in a workout.

TRICEPS EXTENSIONS

muscle focus: triceps and biceps

- Sit on the exercise ball with the middle of the band under you. You should be sitting on the band.
- Hold the right handle in your right hand and the left handle in your left hand.
- Place both hands over your head with your elbows bent.
- Extend both hands above your head, straightening your elbows.

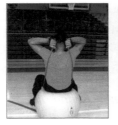
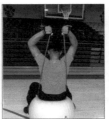
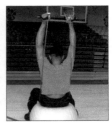

Triceps extensions

BICEPS HAMMER CURLS

muscle focus: biceps and triceps

- Stand on the middle of the exercise band with your feet shoulder-width apart.
- Hold both ends of the resistance band with your palms facing in toward your body.
- Bend at your elbows, and slowly bring each hand toward the respective shoulder while keeping your elbows by your sides and your palms toward your body.
- Return your arms slowly back to the starting position without fully straightening your elbows.

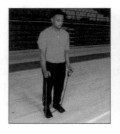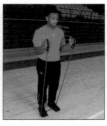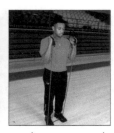

Biceps hammer curls

LATERAL RAISES

muscle focus: deltoids

- Place an end of the resistance band under your right foot and hold the other end in your right hand.
- Keep your arm straight at your side and make sure that the tension of the resistance band is at a good level. If the resistance is not enough, wrap the band around your hand until the resistance is comfortable.
- Keep your arm straight and raise it out to your side so that it is parallel with the floor.
- Bring your arm slowly back down to your side. Make sure you are keeping your arm straight during the entire exercise.

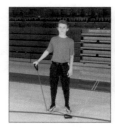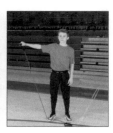

Lateral raises

BENT-OVER FLIES

muscle focus: trapezii, rhomboids, deltoids, and biceps

- Stand in the middle of the resistance band with your feet shoulder-width apart.
- Grab the left handle of the band with your right hand and the right handle of the band with your left hand. The band should now be crisscrossed.
- Bend your knees slightly and bend at the waist.
- Begin with your arms slightly bent.
- Lift both arms up and out to your sides.
- Bend your arms slowly down to the starting position.

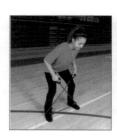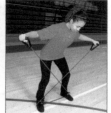

Bent-over files

BENT-OVER ROWS

muscle focus: trapezii, rhomboids, deltoids, and biceps

- Stand in the middle of the resistance band with your feet shoulder-width apart.
- Grab the left end of the band with your right hand and the right end of the band with your left hand. The band should now be crisscrossed, and your arms should start off straight.
- Bend your knees slightly. Bend at your waist and stick out your buttocks.
- Bend your elbows and bring them up toward the ceiling. Pinch your shoulder blades together.
- Straighten your arms slowly back to the starting position.

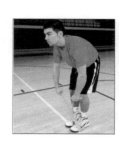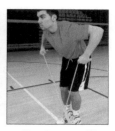

Bent-over files

CHEST PRESSES

muscle focus: pectoralis majors, anterior deltoids, and triceps

- Sit on the exercise ball and place the band behind your back.
- Place your hands in front of your shoulders in the loops of the band. You may need to hold closer to the middle of the band if it is too long for you.
- Push your arms straight out in front of you while holding onto the loops of the resistance band.
- Lower your arms slowly back toward your body, but do not go so far that your arms return to a resting position.

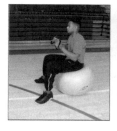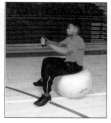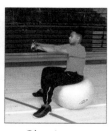

Chest presses

RESISTANCE PUSH-UPS

muscle focus: pectoralis majors, pectoralis minors, deltoids, triceps, and abdominal muscles

- Tie the resistance band around your chest, making sure that you have 2 even ends.
- Place a handle in each hand. You may need to wrap the band around your hands to get the proper tension.
- Get into a push-up position. Lie face down on the floor or yoga mat with your palms flat on the floor and shoulder-width apart. Bend your elbows and straighten your legs out behind you with your toes on the floor.
- Straighten your elbows as you push your body up off the floor. Keep your back straight and look straight ahead.
- Lower yourself slowly back to the starting position.

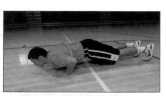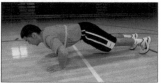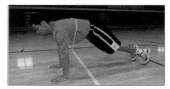

Resistance Push-ups

SEATED ROWS

muscle focus: erector spinae, trapezii, rhomboids, and latissimi dorsi

- Sit on the ground. Your feet and legs should be straight out in front of you.
- Place the middle of the band around the bottom of both feet. The resistance band should be across the instep of both feet. Hold an end in each hand.
- Start with your arms straight out in front of you. Make sure there is good tension with the resistance band.
- Make sure your forearms and wrists are rotated so that your thumbs are on top of the grip. Your palms should be facing each other.
- Keep your back upright. In a single motion, bend your elbows back and pinch your shoulder blades together. Do not bring your elbows so far back that they are almost touching; bring them back so that they are slightly behind you.
- Bring your arms slowly straight in front of you, back to the starting position.

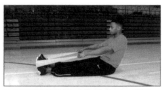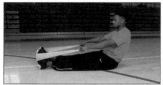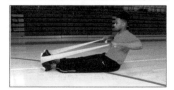

Seated rows

MONSTER WALK

muscle focus: hip abductors and glutes

- Stand with your feet shoulder-width apart.
- Tie the resistance band around both ankles.
- Bend your knees and waist into a squatting position.
- Hold your arms at your sides with your elbows bent.
- Take a step to the right with your right foot. Bring your left foot to meet your right foot. Make sure that your knees are aligned over top of your feet.
- Repeat to the left after completing the repetitions to the right.

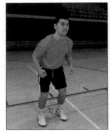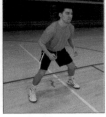

Monster walk

SQUATS

muscle focus: quadriceps, hamstrings, and glutes

- Stand on the middle of the band with your feet shoulder-width apart.
- Hold an end of the band in each hand with your elbows bent and your hands by your ears.
- Hold onto the band and bend as if you were sitting down in a chair.
- Bend until your knees are at 90-degree angles while still holding onto the resistance band with your elbows bent and your hands by your ears. Make sure your knees do not go past your toes.
- Stand back up to your starting position, but do not lock your knees.

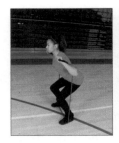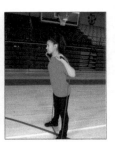

Squats

BAND EXPLOSIONS

muscle focus: glutes, hamstrings, quadriceps, gastrocnemii, solei, triceps, and deltoids

- Stand with your feet shoulder-width apart.
- Place a handle of the resistance band under your right foot and hold the other handle with your right hand.
- Bend your elbow so that your fist is at shoulder level. Your palm should be facing forward.
- Bend your knees, making sure they do not go past your toes. Bend at the waist into a squatting position.
- Straighten your elbow and lift the band as you stand back up, bringing your upper arm to touch your ear.

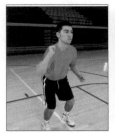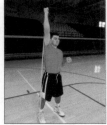

Band explosions

LEG EXTENSIONS

muscle focus: quadriceps, hamstrings, and glutes

- Lie with your back flat on the ground and your right knee bent to your chest.
- Wrap the band around the bottom of your right foot, holding an end in each hand.
- Keep your left leg flat on the ground.
- Hold the band firmly in your hands and push your right leg straight out without fully straightening your knee.
- Bring your leg slowly back to the starting position.
- Switch to your left leg after completing the set.

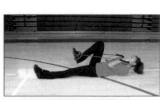
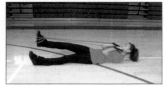

Leg extensions

CALF RAISES

muscle focus: gastrocnemii and solei

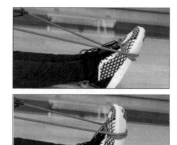

- Sit on the ground. Your feet and legs should be straight out in front of you.
- Place the middle of the resistance band around the bottom of both feet. The band should be across the balls of your feet (closer to the toes, but not on the toes). Hold an end in each hand.
- Flex your feet and point your toes away from your leg.
- Bring your toes slowly up toward your leg.

Calf raises

The following is a suggested use of resistance bands in a strength-building workout. Exercise to your level of fitness.

- Warm up before your workout. Cool down after your workout.
- Perform each resistance band exercise 2 to 3 days per week. Do not exercise the same muscle group on consecutive days.
- Begin with 1 set of 10 repetitions for each exercise. Increase sets and the number of repetitions when the current number is too easy.
- Your goal should be to reach 3 sets of 10 to 15 repetitions.
- Wrap the band to increase resistance as necessary.

PREDICT IF USING RESISTANCE BANDS IS AN EXERCISE THAT YOU WILL PURSUE IN COLLEGE OR A CAREER SETTING

1	I will not consider using resistance bands as an exercise option in college or a career setting.
2	I will consider using resistance bands as an exercise option in college or a career setting.

⌨ RESEARCH INTEGRATION

Research resistance band flexibility exercises.

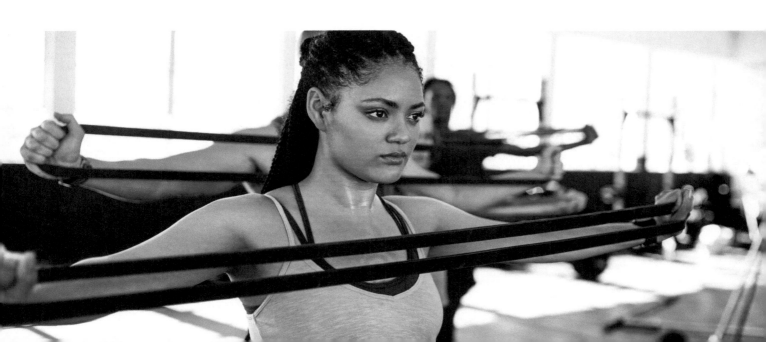

WEIGHTED BALL

There are many ways to increase muscular strength and endurance. Exercising with a weighted ball is a convenient way to improve strength. Experiencing a variety of exercise options may help you commit to strength training. If you are bored or feel stagnant doing 1 type of strength training, you can try another type. It is important to continue some form of strength training for a lifetime of fitness.

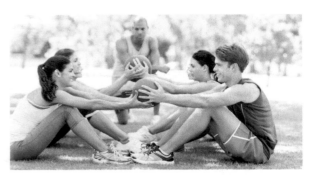

The purpose of this lesson is to increase muscular strength and endurance using a weighted ball.

FITNESS TIP: Have a certified trainer plan for you and supervise you when you are working with any type of weights.

CAUTION: Make sure that nobody is close to you before using the weighted ball. Do not walk into the path of another person who is using a weighted ball. Make sure to hold the ball and maneuver it without dropping it. Have a good grip on the ball before exercising. Keep the weighted ball movements controlled to avoid injury.

BENEFITS OF STRENGTH TRAINING WITH A WEIGHTED BALL

- requires only 1 piece of equipment
- can be done almost anywhere
- boosts metabolism and burns fat even after the exercise is over

WEIGHTED BALL STRENGTH-BUILDING EXERCISES

Practice each of the following exercises. Concentrate on proper form prior to engaging in a workout.

LUNGES WITH TWISTS

muscle focus: oblique abdominal muscles, quadriceps, hamstrings, and glutes

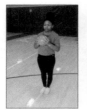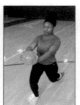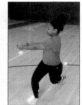

Lunges with twists

- Place your feet shoulder-width apart and relax your shoulders.
- Hold the weighted ball a few inches in front of your chest with both hands.
- Step forward into a lunge with your right leg. Make sure that your knee does not go past your toes.
- Make sure that your right thigh is parallel to the floor once you are in the lunge position. Then, extend your arms in front of you with the ball in both hands.
- Rotate your torso to the right, moving the ball in the same direction at the same time.
- Hold this for 2 seconds and then come back to the starting position.
- Do the same with the left leg.

FIGURE-8S

muscle focus: erector spinae, trapezii, deltoids, hamstrings, quadriceps, and abdominal muscles

- Stand with your feet shoulder-width apart.
- Hold the weighted ball out in front of you with your right hand on top of it and your left hand under it. Extend your arms at chest level.
- Step out into a side lunge with your left leg.
- Bring the ball down to the outside of your left thigh in a smooth motion.
- Come back to the standing position and quickly move into a side lunge to the right.
- Make a figure-8 with the ball, moving the ball to the outside of your right thigh. This is 1 repetition.
- Continue to make a figure-8 with the ball as you lunge from side to side.

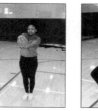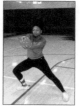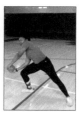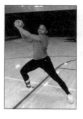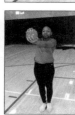

Figure-8s

CHEST PRESSES

muscle focus: pectoralis majors, pectoralis minors, deltoids, triceps, and abdominal muscles

- Lie flat on your back on a bench or the floor.
- Hold the weighted ball with both hands at your chest.
- Lift the ball toward the ceiling with both hands.
- Bring the ball back down to the starting position.

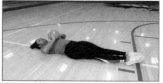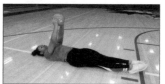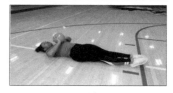

Chest presses

SHOULDER PRESSES

muscle focus: deltoids, triceps, and biceps

- Sit in a chair with your back straight or stand with your feet shoulder-width apart.
- Hold the weighted ball in front of your chest with both hands.
- Extend your arms toward the ceiling with the ball in your hands.
- Lower the ball slowly back to the starting position.

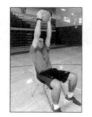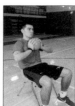

Shoulder presses

SQUATTING SHOULDER PRESSES

muscle focus: quadriceps, hamstrings, deltoids, and triceps

- Hold the weighted ball with both hands—1 on either side of the ball—in the middle of your chest.
- Stand with your feet shoulder-width apart.
- Bend your knees and lower your buttocks toward the ground to get into a squatting position. Do not let your knees go past your toes.
- Straighten your knees and hips while lifting the ball straight up in the air in a single motion.
- Return to the squatting position while bringing the ball back to your chest.

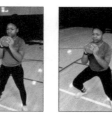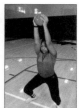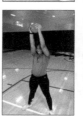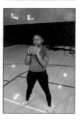

Squatting shoulder presses

TRICEPS EXTENSIONS

muscle focus: triceps

- Stand with your feet shoulder-width apart.
- Holding the weighted ball with both hands, extend your arms above your head. Your inner arms should almost be touching your ears.
- Bend your elbows and lower the ball behind your head. Your arms should be at 45-degree angles.
- Straighten your arms and bring the ball back up to the starting position.

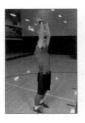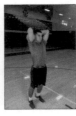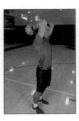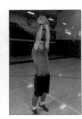

Triceps extensions

BICEPS CURLS

muscle focus: biceps

- Stand with your feet shoulder-width apart.
- Hold the weighted ball with both hands and extend your arms down toward the ground.
- Bring the ball slowly up to your chest.
- Lower the ball down to the starting position. Do not lock your elbows when you are doing this.

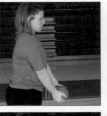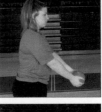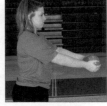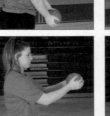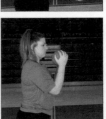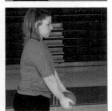

Biceps curls

LUNGES WITH PASSES

muscle focus: quadriceps, hamstrings, gastrocnemii, solei, glutes, biceps, and triceps

- Stand with your feet together.
- Hold the weighted ball close to your chest with both hands.
- Step forward with your right foot. Bend your right knee so that it is over your toes, not past them. Bend your left knee so that it is almost touching the ground; lift your heel.
- Pass the ball from your left hand to your right hand under your right leg.
- Grab the ball with both hands and come back to the starting position.

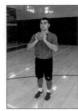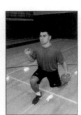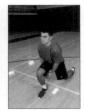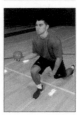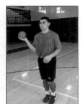

Lunges with passes

BACK EXTENSIONS WITH ROLLS

muscle focus: erector spinae, deltoids, and triceps

- Lie face down on the ground with the weighted ball in front of you.
- Extend your arms and legs. Your arms should be shoulder-width apart, and your legs should be hip-width apart.
- Place your right hand on the ball.
- Extend your spine and lift your chest and thighs off the ground. As you do this, roll the ball from your right hand to your left hand.
- Continue rolling the ball back and forth while keeping your chest and thighs off the ground.

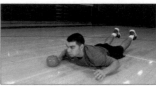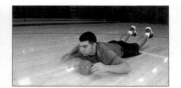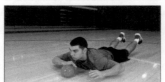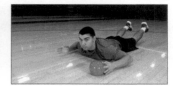

Back extensions with rolls

The following is a suggested use of a weighted ball in strength-building workouts. Exercise to your level of fitness.

- Warm up before your workout. Cool down after your workout.

- Perform each exercise 2 to 3 days per week. Do not exercise the same muscle group on consecutive days.

- Begin with 1 set of 10 repetitions. Increase sets and the number of repetitions when the current number is too easy.

- Your goal should be to reach 3 sets of 10 to 15 repetitions.

RESEARCH INTEGRATION

Research weighted ball (medicine ball) exercises for building core strength.

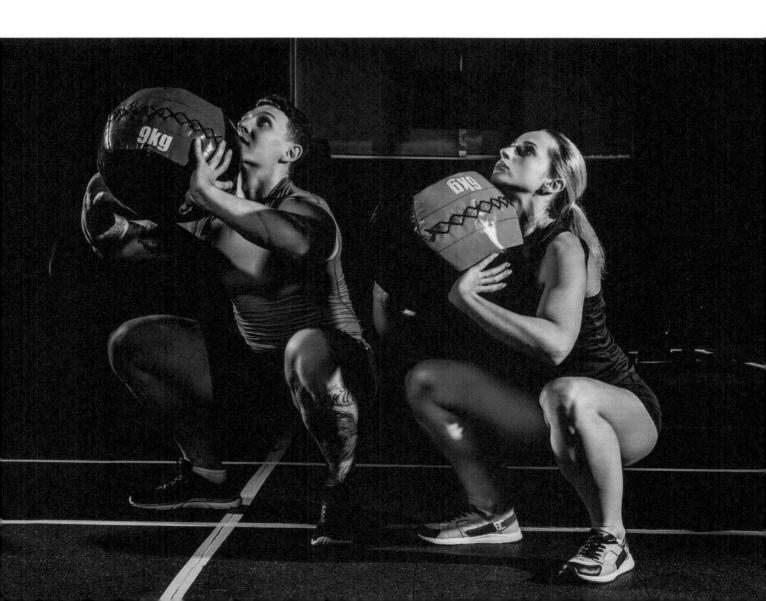

STRENGTH-TRAINING PROGRAM: USING WHAT YOU HAVE LEARNED

Strength training, also known as resistance training, tones and defines your muscles. You can choose to exercise to build muscle bulk or to refine lean muscle. Lifting heavier weights with fewer repetitions builds bulk (for example, 3 sets of 8 repetitions), while using lighter resistance with more repetitions tones muscles (for example, 3 sets of 15 repetitions). Strength training is important as you age. It improves balance, posture, and metabolism while strengthening bones and contributing to overall health.

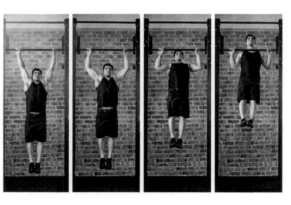

Using body weight, a fitness ball, push-up handles, resistance bands, a weighted ball, or other portable strength-training equipment provides you with exercise opportunities in dorm rooms, at home, or in limited spaces. Access to equipment in a convenient location will help you commit to your strength-training routine.

Fibers that make up your skeletal muscles break down during the exercise phase. After your strength workout, when your muscles are resting, the fibers repair and strengthen. It is recommended that you allow 24 hours between training the same muscle group to allow the muscle fibers to repair and strengthen.

The purpose of this lesson is to encourage you to design your personal strength-training program and perform exercises 2 to 3 days per week to obtain health benefits. A certified trainer should help you set up a balanced, effective strength program.

 CAUTION: Have a certified trainer plan for you and supervise you when you are working with weights.

STRENGTH-TRAINING PROGRAM

There are a variety of exercises from which to choose. Do strength exercises for the muscles of your upper body, lower body, and core. Opposing muscles (antagonistic muscles), such as biceps and triceps, should be equally trained because they work together. Choose the intensity of the exercise to fit your fitness level. For example, if you are struggling doing a right-angle push-up, switch to a knee push-up. Limit excuses and make a commitment to exercise!

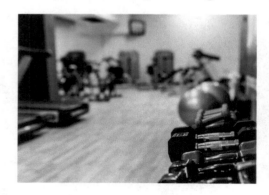

STRENGTH-TRAINING EXERCISE IDEAS

Weightlifting machines: You can use large stationary machines like those typically found in gyms.

Free weights: You can use free-weight equipment such as dumbbells, barbells, medicine balls, kettlebells, resistance bands, and weighted ropes to perform strength-training exercises.

Pilates or yoga: Pilates and yoga sessions are excellent workouts for muscle lengthening and muscle strengthening.

Personal workouts: You can use your own body weight as a source of resistance and create your own strength-training workouts. Create a personal workout by blending basic strength-building exercises such as sit-ups, push-ups, pull-ups, planks, and so on, and design the intensity and duration of each exercise according to your level of fitness. Include upper-body, lower-body, and core exercises in your workout. Perform your personal routine for some or all your strength-training workouts.

MUSCULAR STRENGTH AND MUSCULAR ENDURANCE SAMPLE WORKOUT

The following workout regimen is strictly an example of how to use the FITT principle to increase muscular strength and muscular endurance. The exercises are described in the Flexibility section, Muscular Endurance section, and PE Equipment Kit section of your PE Manual.

In the following chart, you will find a block plan for a weekly schedule based on increasing your muscular strength and muscular endurance. The charts include the days of the week, muscle groups, exercises, sets and repetitions (for example, 3 · 10 = 3 sets of 10 repetitions), and the type of equipment used.

There is a column on the chart for you to design your personal workout. You can use fitness equipment or your own body weight. The plan you design should be for your fitness level. Personalized exercise plans work for all fitness levels and body types.

- Have a certified trainer plan for you and supervise you when you are working with any type of weights.
- Before working out, warm up properly to prepare your body. The warm-up should increase your heart rate, breathing rate, and body temperature.
- Never begin vigorous exercise with cold muscles.
- Cool down after working out to allow your body to return to its baseline.

Warm-up: Complete 3 sets of this warm-up before exercising.

Exercise	Duration
• basic jump rope	• 1 minute
• high knees	• 30 seconds
• forward arm circles	• 30 seconds
• backward arm circles	• 30 seconds
• rear kicks	• 30 seconds

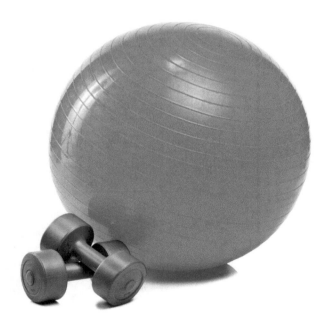

Day	Muscle Group	Exercise Sample	Sets/ Reps	Equipment	Personal Workout for Each Muscle Group
Mon. Wed.	chest shoulder	chest presses with weighted ball	3 · 15	weighted ball	
		bent-over flies	3 · 15	resistance band	
		bent-over rows	3 · 15	resistance band	
		squatting shoulder presses	3 · 15	weighted ball	
		shoulder presses	3 · 15	weighted ball	
		legs-up push-ups	3 · 15	push-up handles	
		wide-arm push-ups	3 · 15	body weight	
Mon. Wed.	biceps triceps	triceps extensions	3 · 15	resistance band	
		biceps hammer curls	3 · 15	resistance band	
		biceps curls	3 · 15	weighted ball	
		triceps extensions	3 · 15	weighted ball	
		dips	3 · 15	push-up handles	
		triceps push-ups (narrow push-ups)	3 · 10	body weight	
Tue. Thur.	legs hips	single-leg squats	3 · 15	fitness ball	
		squats with twists	3 · 15	fitness ball	
		leg extensions	3 · 15	resistance band	
		calf raises	3 · 15	resistance band	
		monster walk	3 · 15	resistance band	
		lunges with passes	3 · 15	weighted ball	
		figure-8s	3 · 15	weighted ball	
		in-and-out push-ups	3 · 15	push-up handles	
Tue. Thur.	back	back extensions	3 · 15	fitness ball	
		side crunches	3 · 15	fitness ball	
		seated rows	3 · 15	resistance band	
		back extensions with rolls	3 · 15	weighted ball	
		pull-ups	3 · 10	body weight	
Mon. Wed. Fri.	core	crunches	3 · 15	fitness ball	
		plank rollouts	3 · 15	fitness ball	
		resistance push-ups	3 · 15	resistance band	
		lunges with twists	3 · 15	weighted ball	
		planks	3 · 30 seconds	body weight	

Cool-down: Complete this cool-down after exercising.

Exercise	Duration
• hamstring stretch	• 30 seconds
• quadriceps stretch	• 30 seconds
• shoulder/triceps stretch	• 30 seconds
• side stretch	• 30 seconds
• lower back/hip stretch	• 30 seconds
• groin stretch	• 30 seconds

💻 RESEARCH INTEGRATION

Research how strength training is beneficial to your health and daily living.

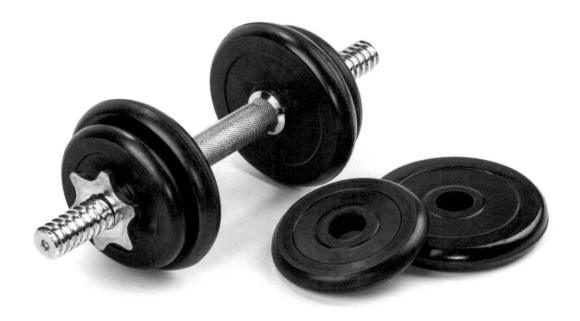

CROSS-TRAINING CARDIOVASCULAR AND STRENGTH CIRCUIT: USING WHAT YOU HAVE LEARNED

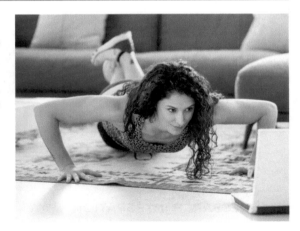

Time, cost, and facilities are 3 obstacles that keep some people from exercising regularly. A cross-training circuit can help you to overcome those obstacles. The following cross-training circuit alternates strength exercises with aerobic movements. Cross-training saves time by giving you a single workout that has both strength and aerobic benefits. This type of workout can be done in a small place such as at home or in a college dorm room. The equipment used in the following workout is not costly. It is also possible to create a workout using only body-weight exercises.

Workouts can be divided into 10- to 15-minute intervals and can be done 2 to 3 times per day to get in the recommended amount of exercise time. For example, you can exercise 15 minutes in the morning and 15 minutes in the evening to reach your 30-minute goal.

Keep in mind that skills you take for granted, such as balance and coordination, just like fitness levels, diminish with age if you do not use them. It is important to plan around obstacles, set your own goals based on your ability level, and determine your intensity and duration based on your individual target heart rate zone.

The purpose of this lesson is to encourage you to create and implement a cross-training circuit workout. The workout would be included in the recommended 60 minutes of daily physical activity and would count as both an aerobic and a strength workout. **The Cardiovascular Endurance section of this manual includes the target heart rate zone formula and the Borg Rating of Perceived Exertion Scale to help you to determine if you are exercising for heart health.** You can also use available technology to monitor your pulse rate and intensity.

CROSS-TRAINING CIRCUIT WORKOUT: CARDIOVASCULAR AND STRENGTH

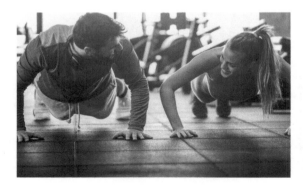

Review the following example and use the information to establish a workout regimen that fits into your schedule. Adhere to the FITT principle (frequency, intensity, time, and type of exercise). This workout requires a jump rope, fitness ball, push-up handles, resistance bands, stepper, and weighted ball. You should have a mat or cushioned surface for sit-ups and push-ups. You should have a hard, flat surface for the stepper and push-up handles.

SAMPLE CROSS-TRAINING CIRCUIT WORKOUT

Build cardiovascular endurance, strength, and flexibility in a cross-training circuit workout using exercises from the appropriate sections of your manual: Cardiovascular Endurance, Muscle Strength, Muscle Endurance, and Flexibility. Review the Aerobic Exercise and Proper Nutrition, Jump Rope, Fitness Ball, Resistance Bands, and Weighted Ball sections to practice correct forms for the skills.

Warm-up: Perform 5 to 10 minutes of light cardio to increase your heart rate, breathing rate, and body temperature. Do some dynamic stretches to increase flexibility.

Perform each exercise for 30 seconds. Rest and hydrate when necessary. Set the workout to music.

1. jumping jacks
2. sit-ups
3. high knees
4. weighted ball lunges with passes
5. jump rope
6. resistance band monster walk
7. stepper side step-ups
8. fitness ball side crunches
9. jog in place
10. push-ups with push-up handles
11. jump rope
12. fitness ball leg extensions
13. stepper squat jumps
14. weighted ball chest passes with sit-ups
15. stepper quick step-ups
16. resistance band explosions
17. jump rope
18. fitness ball plank rollouts
19. burpees
20. in-and-out push-ups with push-up handles

Repeat for a 20-minute workout.

Cool-down: Walk slowly until your heart rate, breathing rate, and body temperature have returned to baseline. Do some static stretches to increase flexibility.

DISCUSS WITH A FRIEND OR AN ADULT BARRIERS TO EXERCISE AND CREATE A PERSONAL CIRCUIT WORKOUT WITHOUT EQUIPMENT

Objective: to overcome exercise barriers you may face now and in the future

Use the cross-training information to create a personal circuit workout without equipment. Design your own personal aerobic/strength workout that can be done almost anywhere to eliminate several barriers to exercise: insufficient time, lack of access to a gym, expense, and lack of enjoyment.

 ### RESEARCH INTEGRATION

Research how much time you need to devote to exercise weekly to obtain health benefits.

 ### HEALTH INTEGRATION

Use available technology to monitor your pulse rate and intensity. Apply the results to your overall fitness plan.

TRAINING FOR A 5K RACE

Have you ever wanted to run a 5K or some other sort of race? A 5K is 3.107 miles. There are ways you can train to accomplish such goals and prevent injury. You should train properly before entering a race.

This section explains the proper preparation and training that are needed to run in a 5K race. If you are not interested in a race, you can use these training methods to improve your personal running workouts.

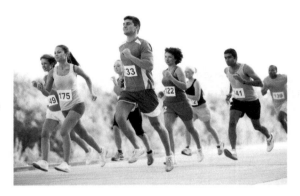

TRAINING FOR A 5K RACE

TIPS FOR RUNNING

- Keep yourself hydrated before, during, and after jogs, runs, and races.

- Invest in a good pair of running shoes.

- Watch for a side ache. This can be related to weak conditioning, weak abdominal muscles, shallow breathing, a large meal before exercise, or dehydration. This is common with beginner runners. You can relieve the pain by holding your arm over your head and stretching your aching side while taking deep breaths.

- Be sure to pace yourself. Pacing is the ability to run at a steady speed (continuous running, not running and then walking) for a given length of time. Do not start off too fast; you want to be able to sustain a run for a given length of time.

INTERVAL TRAINING

- Start training with interval training. Interval training involves moving from 1 intensity of exercise to another intensity of exercise in different set time frames.

- Build up your cardiovascular endurance as well as your muscular endurance in your legs.

- Start off slowly. This will also help you build up to where you can sustain a good pace when running.

EXAMPLE WORKOUT

- Do a 5-minute warm-up walk. Then, alternate between jogging for 60 seconds and walking for 90 seconds for a total of 20 minutes. Finally, do a 5-minute cool-down consisting of walking and stretching. The total workout time is 30 minutes. Do this 3 to 4 days a week (not back-to-back days).

- Increase your jogging and walking time when you feel comfortable. For example, jog for 90 seconds and then walk for 2 minutes for a total of 20 minutes. Remember to warm up for at least 5 minutes and cool down for at least 5 minutes.

- Continue this cycle until you can jog for a longer period of time with shorter walks in between. Gradually, you will be able to jog for a longer period of time.

- Increase your jogging time to a full 20 to 30 minutes. It may take a long time to get to this point, and that is okay.

INCREASING YOUR SPEED

Once you can jog continuously for 20 to 30 minutes, you should be able to run a 5K race. Now, focus on trying to decrease your time by building up your cardiovascular and muscular endurance. To do this, increase the pace at which you run. There are steps that you can take to increase your speed without running a longer distance.

- Vary your intensities. Start by running a short distance but at a high intensity. Another day, run a longer distance but at a medium intensity. Perform the high intensity runs 3 days a week, separated by slower, easier runs.

- Be consistent in your training. Continue to run year-round. Taking a little time off is good, but avoid taking long periods of time off. Continue to run even when you are not training for a specific event.

- Run hills. Adding hills to your runs will challenge you more and give you greater fitness gains. Running uphill develops aerobic endurance and leg strength.

- Include sprinting in your training. This will help increase your stride power and running endurance.

- Strengthen your core. This will help reduce the amount of energy your body loses while running.

- Follow these steps to help you perform better and decrease your time when running a 5K race.

PREDICT IF RUNNING IS AN EXERCISE OPTION THAT YOU WILL PURSUE IN COLLEGE OR A CAREER SETTING

1	I will not consider running as an exercise option in college or a career setting.
2	I will consider running as an exercise option in college or a career setting.

♥ HEALTH INTEGRATION

Use available technology to monitor your pulse rate and intensity. Apply the results to your overall fitness plan.

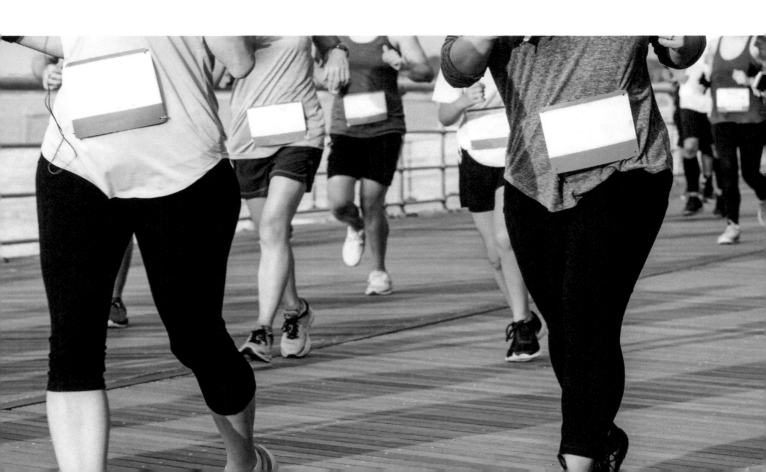

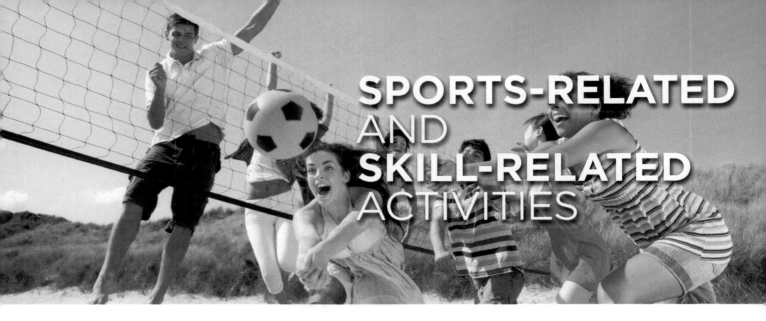

SPORTS-RELATED
AND
SKILL-RELATED
ACTIVITIES

FITNESS TIP: Prior to beginning your physical education activities, read the following safety information that applies to every lesson, review the timeline, and review the assessment rubric.

SAFETY ALERT: Before you exercise, make sure that you are properly warmed up and have enough room to perform each activity. Wear proper equipment and follow activity-specific safety rules. Stay hydrated and take breaks as needed. Exercise only if you are healthy, and always exercise at your own pace. If an exercise starts to hurt, if you feel dizzy, or if you feel light-headed, stop the exercise completely and get help. Upon completion of any workout, cool down and stretch.

TIMELINE

Review all of the activity information before beginning. Use the scoring rubrics as assessment tools. You may ask a trusted adult or friend to observe your performance and provide feedback. Progress according to your skill level. The time that it takes you to complete a module will depend on your personal progress.

Practice and assess the first skill until competent.

Apply skills in a game situation.

Continue to progress until you have practiced and assessed each skill until competent.

ASSESSMENT RUBRIC

You will find a rubric assessment tool following some of the basic skills. Use this tool to evaluate and score your progress in learning the elements of a new skill.

SKILL	PROGRESSING	COMPETENT	PROFICIENT
skill 1	1 or 2 of the elements	3 or 4 out of 5 elements	all elements met

CAN JAM

If you are more likely to commit to exercise by playing in games with others, can jam may be a good choice for you. Can jam is played by 2 opposing teams, each made up of 2 players. Points are scored by throwing a flying disc into a can (goal). The rules are easy to follow, but the game is challenging and competitive. Can jam is a fun, social game that provides exercise, improves coordination, and is easy to set up.

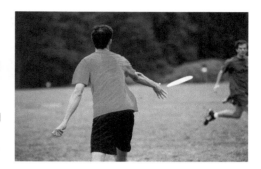

The purpose of this lesson is for you to practice disc-throwing skills and to encourage participation in games for physical activity.

CAM JAM SKILLS

BACKHAND GRIP

- Hold the disc in your dominant hand.

- Hold the disc parallel to the ground with your thumb on top.

- Rest your index finger on the edge of the disc, and curl your remaining fingers under the disc.

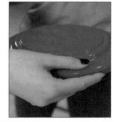

SKILL	PROGRESSING	COMPETENT	PROFICIENT
grip	1 of the elements	2 out of 3 elements	all elements met

BACKHAND THROW

- Hold the disc in your dominant hand.

- Bend your elbow and keep the disc close to your body so it is touching your forearm. The back of your hand should be facing the target.

- Step toward the target with your dominant foot.

- Snap your wrist and release the disc while extending your arm.

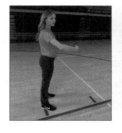 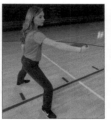 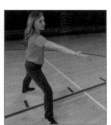

SKILL	PROGRESSING	COMPETENT	PROFICIENT
throw	1 or 2 of the elements	3 out of 4 elements	all elements met

DEFLECTING

- Use your hands to move the disc to the target without catching, carrying, or double hitting the disc.

- Make quick contact and release the disc with your hands.

- Tap or push it to the target.

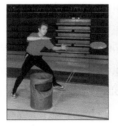 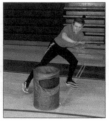 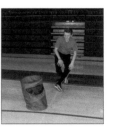

SKILL	PROGRESSING	COMPETENT	PROFICIENT
deflecting	1 of the elements	2 out of 3 elements	all elements met

PRACTICE THE SKILLS

- Using the backhand grip, practice throwing toward the target.
- Increase your distance as you improve.
- Pass and deflect with a partner.

PLAYING THE GAME

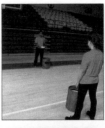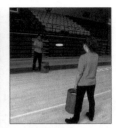
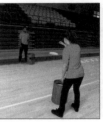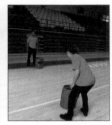

- The game requires 4 players (2 per team).
- Set the goals 50 feet apart.
- Mark a throw line with cones set 25 feet from each goal.
- For each team, 1 player (the deflector) stands near the goal and the other player (the thrower) stands at the throw line.
- Each team gets 1 disc.
- The thrower throws the disc toward the goal.
- The deflector redirects the disc toward the goal or into the goal.
- Switch roles with your teammate.
- After both players from the starting team throw and deflect, it is the other team's turn.
- Continue to alternate throws until a team reaches 21 points.

SCORING

dinger	1 point	redirected hit	Deflector redirects the thrown disk to hit any side of the goal.
deuce	2 points	direct hit	Thrower hits the side of the goal, unassisted by partner.
bucket	3 points	slam dunk	Deflector redirects the thrown disk and it lands inside the goal.
instant win	game over	direct entry	Thrower lands the disk inside the goal, unassisted by partner. The disk can enter through the slot opening on the side or through the top of the goal. When an instant win occurs, the throwing team is declared the winner and the opposing team does not receive a "last toss" option.

RULES

1. Players must remain behind the line when throwing. No points are awarded if the player crosses the line.
2. No points are awarded when a throw hits the ground before hitting the goal.
3. Deflectors can move anywhere within the playing area to redirect the disc.
4. No points are awarded if a deflector double hits, catches, or carries the disc.
5. If an opponent interferes with a play or defends the goal, 3 points are awarded. If the score is 19 or 20, 1 or 2 points are awarded respectively.
6. A team must reach an exact score of 21 points to win. If a play places a team's score above 21 points, the points from that play are deducted from the team's current score, and play continues. For example, if a team has 20 points and scores a bucket (3 points), that team's score is reduced to 17.
7. Teams must complete an equal number of turns before the game is over. Unless an instant win is thrown, the team with the hammer (last toss) will always get to throw last.
8. If the game is tied, the winner is decided in a tiebreaker method of overtime. Each team completes 1 round of throws, and the team to score first wins. Overtime rounds continue until the tie is broken.

DEMONSTRATE POSITIVE GAME BEHAVIOR

- Follow the rules.
- Make no physical contact with an opposing player.
- Be supportive and encouraging to your teammate.
- Treat your opponents with respect.

SKILL	PROGRESSING	COMPETENT	PROFICIENT
game behavior	1 or 2 of the elements	3 out of 4 elements	all elements met

EXTENSION: Set up a can jam tournament with friends.

 HEALTH INTEGRATION

Count and analyze your pulse during and after playing can jam to determine if you are exercising in your personal target heart rate zone. Apply the results to your overall fitness plan. Many people choose to get their aerobic workouts by playing in casual games with friends.

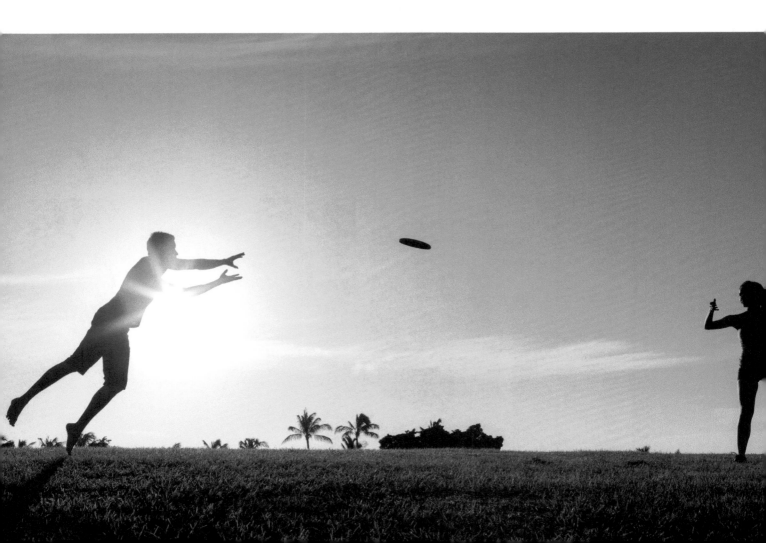

PICKLEBALL

Pickleball is a lifetime sport enjoyed by players of all ages. If you enjoy racket sports, pickleball may be a good choice for you. Pickleball is a paddle sport that combines elements of badminton, tennis, and table tennis. It is played with a paddle, a pickleball ball, and a low net on a court with a hard-surface. This striking activity helps you develop concentration, hand-eye coordination, footwork, and fitness.

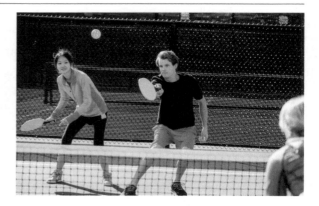

The purpose of this lesson is for you to practice skills and participate in a game of pickleball.

⚠️ **CAUTION: Make sure that nobody is close to you before you swing the paddle. Do not walk into the path of another person who is swinging a paddle.**

PICKLEBALL STROKES

READY POSITION

Wait for the ball and keep your paddle in the middle of your chest. This way, you are ready to return the ball from wherever it comes.

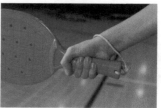

- Bend your knees and stand with your feet shoulder-width apart.
- Keep your head up and your weight on the balls of your feet.
- Hold the paddle in your dominant hand.

HANDSHAKE GRIP

- Hold the paddle in your dominant hand away from your body and at waist height.
- Place the head of the paddle vertical to the ground and point the handle toward your belly button.

UNDERHAND STROKE

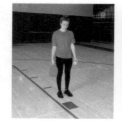 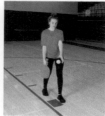 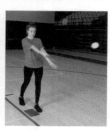

- Hold the paddle so that the head is facing the ground and positioned under the ball.
- Flick your wrist to hit the ball with the center of the paddle.
- Rotate your forearm so that it faces upward on contact.
- Follow through to your target.

SKILL	PROGRESSING	COMPETENT	PROFICIENT
underhand stroke	1 or 2 of the elements	3 out of 4 elements	all elements met

OVERHAND STROKE

- Bend your elbow slightly and position the paddle under the ball.
- Flick your wrist to hit the ball with the center of the paddle.
- Extend your arm as you make contact.
- Follow through to your target.

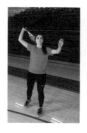 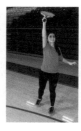 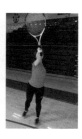

SKILL	PROGRESSING	COMPETENT	PROFICIENT
overhand stroke	1 or 2 of the elements	3 out of 4 elements	all elements met

FOREHAND STROKE

- Hold the paddle on the same side of your body as your dominant hand.
- Face the palm of your hand forward.
- Extend your arm and flick your wrist to hit the ball.
- Point the face of the paddle up to get the ball over the net.
- Follow through to your target.

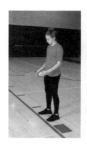 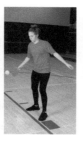 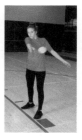 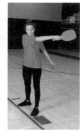

SKILL	PROGRESSING	COMPETENT	PROFICIENT
forehand stroke	1 or 2 of the elements	3 or 4 out of 5 elements	all elements met

BACKHAND STROKE

- Rotate the paddle and extend it across your body.
- Rotate your feet and shoulders in the same direction as the paddle.
- Face the back of your hand (the side that your knuckles are on) forward.
- Flick your wrist as you hit the ball with the center of the paddle.
- Follow through to your target.

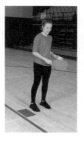 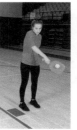 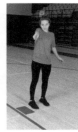

SKILL	PROGRESSING	COMPETENT	PROFICIENT
backhand stroke	1 or 2 of the elements	3 or 4 out of 5 elements	all elements met

OPTION: 2-HANDED BACKHAND STROKE

- Place your non-dominant hand below your dominant hand.
- Rotate the paddle.
- Rotate your feet and shoulders in the same direction as the paddle.
- Flick your wrists as you hit the ball with the center of the paddle.
- Follow through to target

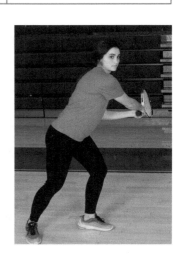

UNDERHAND SERVE

- Hold the paddle in your dominant hand. Hold the ball in your non-dominant hand.
- Hold the head of the paddle down toward the ground.
- Step forward with your non-dominant foot.
- Drop the ball slightly below your waist.
- Hit the ball with the center of the paddle. Flick your wrist as you make contact.
- Follow through to your target.
- Serve successfully 70 percent of the time.

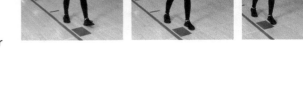

SKILL	PROGRESSING	COMPETENT	PROFICIENT
underhand serve	1, 2, 3, or 4 of the elements	5 or 6 out of 7 elements	all elements met

PRACTICE THE STROKES

- Practice each stroke by hitting the ball against a wall with the paddle.
- Allow the ball to bounce before striking it.
- Volley the ball against the wall. This means that you should not allow the ball to bounce off the ground.
- Strike the ball toward the wall using various levels of force.
- Aim and strike the ball to the left of the target.
- Aim and strike the ball to the right of the target.
- Hit the ball back and forth with a partner. How many times can you hit it back and forth?

SHOTS

DINK SHOT

The most effective short-hand shots, or dinks, are those that bounce in front of the no-volley line (the area 7 feet from the net, where volleying is not allowed). Dinks should be short and low.

LOB

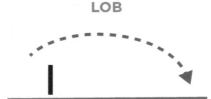

A lob is high and pushes your opponent to the rear of the court. This slows down the game to give you a chance to get ready for your opponent's shot.

DRIVE

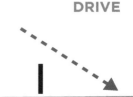

A drive is a hard, fast hit that is difficult to return.

PRACTICE THE SHOTS

Practice the shots independently by bouncing or tossing the ball at the appropriate height for each shot. Practice with a net set up.

- Practice the dink shot forward and crosscourt.
- Practice the lob shot.
- Practice the drive shot.
- Describe a shot and then execute it. Do this for the 3 shots.
- Have a partner toss the ball for you. Practice each shot and then switch roles. Be supportive and encouraging to your partner.

PLAYING A GAME

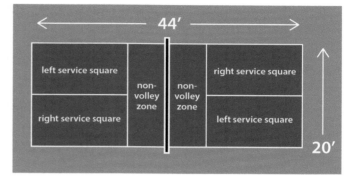

- Pickleball is a singles game with 2 players or a doubles game with 4 players.

- Start by serving the ball underhand from the right side of the court. Serve diagonally to your opponent on the left. Stand behind the serving line when you start your serve.

  - If a point is scored, the server then serves from the left side of the court. Continue this side-to-side pattern until the serve is lost. In a doubles game, the other teammate then serves. Once the second teammate loses the serve, the opposing team serves.

- The ball must land in the service box.

- Your opponent must let the ball bounce once before returning the serve.

- After each team hits the ball once, you may either let the ball bounce once or hit it. This starts the game.

- Points are only scored when a player is serving.

- Games are played to 11 points. A team must win by 2 points.

- Faults include the following.

  - hitting the ball out of bounds

  - serving faults

  - allowing the ball to bounce more than once

  - hitting the ball on the fly in the non-volley zone

  - hitting the ball to the wrong service court

PICKLEBALL OPTIONS

- Play at picnics and group outings.

- Make a net by tying jump ropes together and then tying the jump ropes to the tops of chairs. If there are 2 trees in your playing area, tie the jump ropes to the trees. You may also go to a park with a tennis court and set smaller boundaries on the tennis court.

DEMONSTRATE POSITIVE GAME BEHAVIOR

- Follow the rules.

- Call for a shot, when appropriate, to identify that you are going to hit it. This is for safety and game efficiency.

- Be supportive and encouraging to your teammate.

- Treat your opponents with respect.

SKILL	PROGRESSING	COMPETENT	PROFICIENT
game behavior	1 or 2 of the elements	3 out of 4 elements	all elements met

PREDICT IF PLAYING PICKLEBALL IS AN EXERCISE THAT YOU WILL PURSUE IN COLLEGE OR A CAREER SETTING

1	I will not consider playing pickleball as an exercise option in college or a career setting.
2	I will consider playing pickleball as an exercise option in college or a career setting.

🖥 RESEARCH INTEGRATION

Research the locations of pickleball courts near your home.

♥ HEALTH INTEGRATION

Count your pulse during and after playing pickleball to determine if you are exercising in your personal target heart rate zone. Many people choose to get their aerobic workouts by playing in casual games with friends.

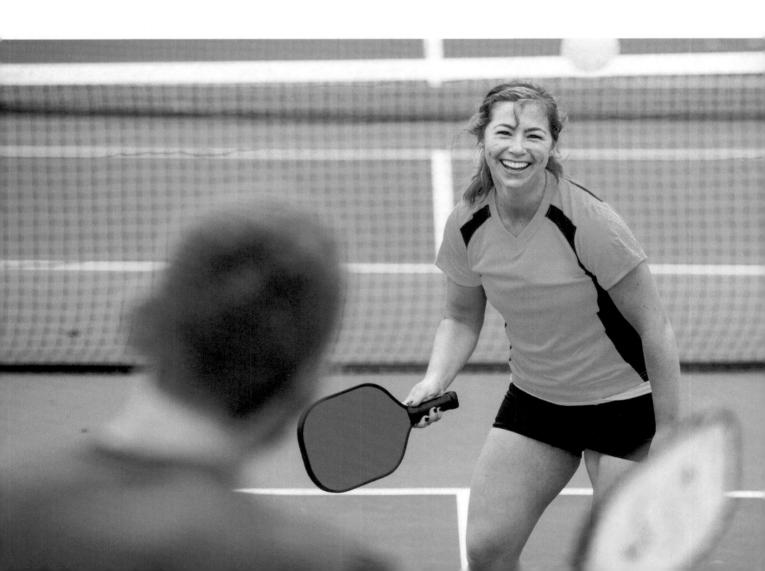

VOLLEYBALL

If you are more likely to commit to exercise by playing in games with others, volleyball may be a good choice for you. The official game of volleyball is played by 2 teams of 6 players on an indoor volleyball court. Another popular version of volleyball is beach volleyball, which is played by 2 teams of 2 to 6 players on a sand surface. The object of the game is to strike a ball over a net and onto the ground so that the opposing team cannot return it.

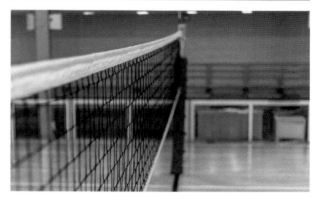

You may play volleyball as a competitive sport or as an opportunity for social play. Casual games of volleyball can be played by as few as 2 players and set up in a yard, park, beach, or gym.

The purpose of this lesson is for you to participate in aerobic exercise and in skill-building activities. When you play volleyball, be sure to follow the rules, communicate with teammates in a positive and effective manner, and exhibit appropriate behavior with your team and the opposing team.

 CAUTION: Do not overinflate the ball.

VOLLEYBALL SKILLS

READY POSITION

The ready position will enable you to react quickly.

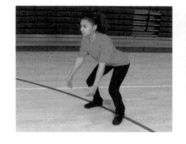 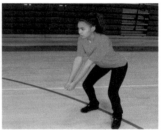

- Stand with your legs shoulder-width apart.
- Balance on the balls of your feet.
- Bend your knees slightly.
- Hold your shoulders rounded and slightly forward.
- Hold your arms in front of you and ready to react.

SKILL	PROGRESSING	COMPETENT	PROFICIENT
ready position	1 or 2 of the elements	3 or 4 out of 5 elements	all elements met

FOREARM GRIP

Try both of the following grips to decide which works better for you.

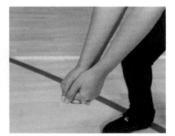

- Right-handed players: Make a fist with your left hand, wrap the fingers of your right hand around your left hand, and line up your thumbs side by side on top.
- Left-handed players: Make a fist with your right hand, wrap the fingers of your left hand around your right hand, and line up your thumbs side by side on top.
- Place 1 hand out flat with your palm up. Place the other hand underneath with the palm up. Curl your thumbs until they are next to each other, centered, and pointing down.

FOREARM PASS (BUMP)

- Stand in the ready position.
- Use the correct grip.
- Contact the ball with your forearm platform.
- Follow through toward your target.

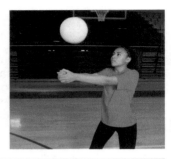

SKILL	PROGRESSING	COMPETENT	PROFICIENT
forearm pass	1 or 2 of the elements	3 out of 4 elements	all elements met

FOREARM PASS (BUMP) PRACTICE

- Forearm pass and catch: Toss the ball to yourself to begin. Pass it back up with your forearm platform, reaching toward your target and catching it. Do not allow your swing to be out of control.
- Forearm pass: Toss the ball to yourself to begin, then continue to pass it. How many times can you pass in a row?
- Wall forearm passes: Toss the ball to yourself to begin, then pass it against a wall. How many times can you pass in a row?
- Partner wall forearm passes: Take turns passing against a wall with a partner.
- Partner toss, forearm pass, and catch: Toss the ball to your partner. Your partner passes it back to you. You catch it. Switch roles.
- Partner forearm passes: How many times can you pass back and forth with a partner?

OVERHAND PASS (SET)

- Stand in the ready position.
- Hold your hands level with your forehead with your elbows bent. Form the size and shape of the ball with your fingers and thumbs.
- Contact the ball with your finger pads, not tips.
- Use a soft touch near your forehead and extend your elbows to push the ball up into the air.

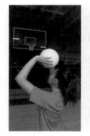 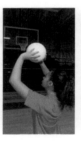 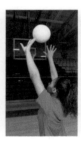 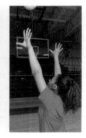

SKILL	PROGRESSING	COMPETENT	PROFICIENT
overhand pass	1 or 2 of the elements	3 out of 4 elements	all elements met

OVERHAND PASS (SET) PRACTICE

- Set and catch: Toss the ball to yourself to begin, set it back up with your finger pads, and catch it.
- Set: Toss the ball to yourself to begin, then continue to set it. How many times can you set in a row?
- Wall sets: Toss the ball to yourself to begin, then set it against a wall. How many times can you set in a row?
- Partner wall sets: Take turns setting against a wall with a partner.
- Partner toss, set and catch: Toss the ball to your partner. Your partner sets it back to you. You catch it. Switch roles.
- Partner sets: How many times can you set back and forth with a partner?

UNDERHAND SERVE

Put your non-dominant foot forward.

Hold the ball on the palm of your non-dominant hand. Position that arm across your body at waist height.

Make a fist with your striking hand.

Bring your striking arm back and then forward, striking the ball with the heel of your hand.

Shift your weight to your front foot.

Serve successfully 70 percent of the time.

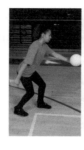 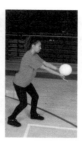 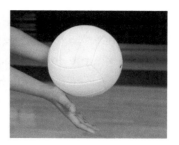

SKILL	PROGRESSING	COMPETENT	PROFICIENT
underhand serve	1 or 2 of the elements	4 or 5 out of 6 elements	all elements met

UNDERHAND SERVE PRACTICE

- Wall serves: Practice serving toward a wall.
- Partner serves: Serve to a partner and volley back and forth using the set and bump skills.

CHALLENGING VOLLEYBALL SKILLS

The following advanced skills are for students who have mastered the basic skills. The challenge level is recommended if you want to further explore the volleyball activity.

OVERHAND SERVE

- Put your non-dominant foot forward.
- Turn the non-dominant side of your body slightly toward the net or target.
- Hold the ball in your non-dominant hand.
- Bend your striking arm with your hand cupped near your ear.
- Contact: Toss the ball 2 to 3 feet in the air, placing your weight on your back foot. Shift your weight to your front foot as you strike the ball approximately 12 inches above your head.
- Follow through in the direction of the ball.

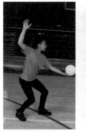 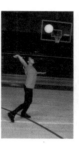 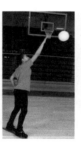 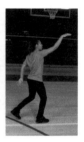

SKILL	PROGRESSING	COMPETENT	PROFICIENT
overhand serve	1 or 2 of the elements	3, 4, or 5 out of 6 elements	all elements met

OVERHAND SERVE PRACTICE

- Wall serves: Practice serving toward a wall.
- Partner serves: Serve to a partner and volley back and forth using the set and bump skills.

ANALYZE AND IMPROVE THE OVERHAND SERVE

- Practice several times a week to improve skills and game play.
- Concentrate on body position.
- Concentrate on cupping your striking hand and keeping your elbow bent.
- Practice the toss.
- Use various amounts of force and speed to improve the placing of the serve.
- Practice the overhand serve technique without a ball.
- Practice and refine the overhand serve with a ball.

OVERHAND HITTING (SPIKE)

1 player: Follow the overhand serve techniques.

2 players: Spike after your teammate hits the ball up high near the net.

- As a hitter, approach from behind using a 4-step approach.
- Place your dominant foot forward.
- Step forward with your non-dominant foot, then quick step with your dominant then non-dominant foot. For example, if you are right-handed, you would start with your right foot forward, step left, then right, then left.
- Begin with your arms at waist height in front of your body. Swing them backward then forward until both of your arms are reaching high with your dominant arm slightly forward.
- Strike the ball with the fleshy part of your dominant hand.
- Follow through, facing the direction in which you want the ball to go.

SKILL	PROGRESSING	COMPETENT	PROFICIENT
overhand hit (spike)	1 or 2 of the elements	3, 4, or 5 out of 6 elements	all elements met

EXTENSION

If you have an available outdoor wall or garage door and permission from your parent or guardian, you can place a horizontal line of tape or chalk mark 7 feet 4½ inches from the ground to represent the height of a net. Begin approximately 10 feet back and practice the underhand and overhand serves. When you are successful, move back farther. Continue this until you are able to serve from 30 feet back, which is the official serving distance.

VOLLEYBALL GAMES

REGULATION VOLLEYBALL GAME

- There are 6 people on a team: 3 front row players and 3 back row players.
- Players rotate in order to reach the serving position.
- The players from the same team all rotate 1 position clockwise when it is their team's turn to serve.
- The serving position is behind the end line. Most players will serve from the right end line; however, for left-handed servers, you may serve from anywhere behind the end line.
- The objective is to serve the ball across the net into the opponent's court within the boundaries. The ball can hit the net on the way over and still be playable.
- Each team is allowed 3 hits, but no player can hit the ball twice in a row.
- A player may not make contact with any part of the net.
- A ball contacting the net is considered playable.

SCORING

- The serve starts the game.
- When the serving team wins the rally, a point is scored.
- If the rally is won by the non-serving team, that team gets a point and a chance to serve.
- The first team to score 25 points and be ahead by at least 2 points wins the game.
- A match consists of either winning 2 out of 3 games or 3 out of 5 games.

OPTIONAL VOLLEYBALL GAMES

2-ON-2 GAME

You have 2 players on each side. You will want about 4 teams to play. Start by tossing the ball over the net. Each team can only hit the ball twice: a pass and a set. The team that wins the rally stays on the court and wins a point. The team that lost the rally leaves the court, and a new team steps on.

RULER OF THE COURT GAME

This game is played with 2 to 4 players on each side. You will need about 4 teams to play. The first team serves the ball. The teams rally back and forth, and the team that wins the rally stays on the court and gets a point. The team that loses the rally quickly gets off the court and another team quickly runs on to rally with the team that won. The first team to get 10 points—or however many points you decide on at the beginning of the game—wins.

DEMONSTRATE POSITIVE GAME BEHAVIOR

- Follow the rules.
- Call out when you are attempting to strike the ball to avoid collisions.
- Be supportive and encouraging to your teammates.
- Treat your opponents with respect.

SKILL	PROGRESSING	COMPETENT	PROFICIENT
game behavior	1 or 2 of the elements	3 out of 4 elements	all elements met

PREDICT IF PLAYING VOLLEYBALL IS AN EXERCISE THAT YOU WILL PURSUE IN COLLEGE OR A CAREER SETTING

1	I will not consider playing volleyball as an exercise option in college or a career setting.
2	I will consider playing volleyball as an exercise option in college or a career setting.

RESEARCH INTEGRATION

Research the types of volleyball that are played in the Olympics.

HEALTH INTEGRATION

Count your pulse to determine if you are exercising in your personal target heart rate zone. Count your pulse after practicing skills and after playing in a game. Apply the results to your overall fitness plan.

ANATOMY **SECTION**

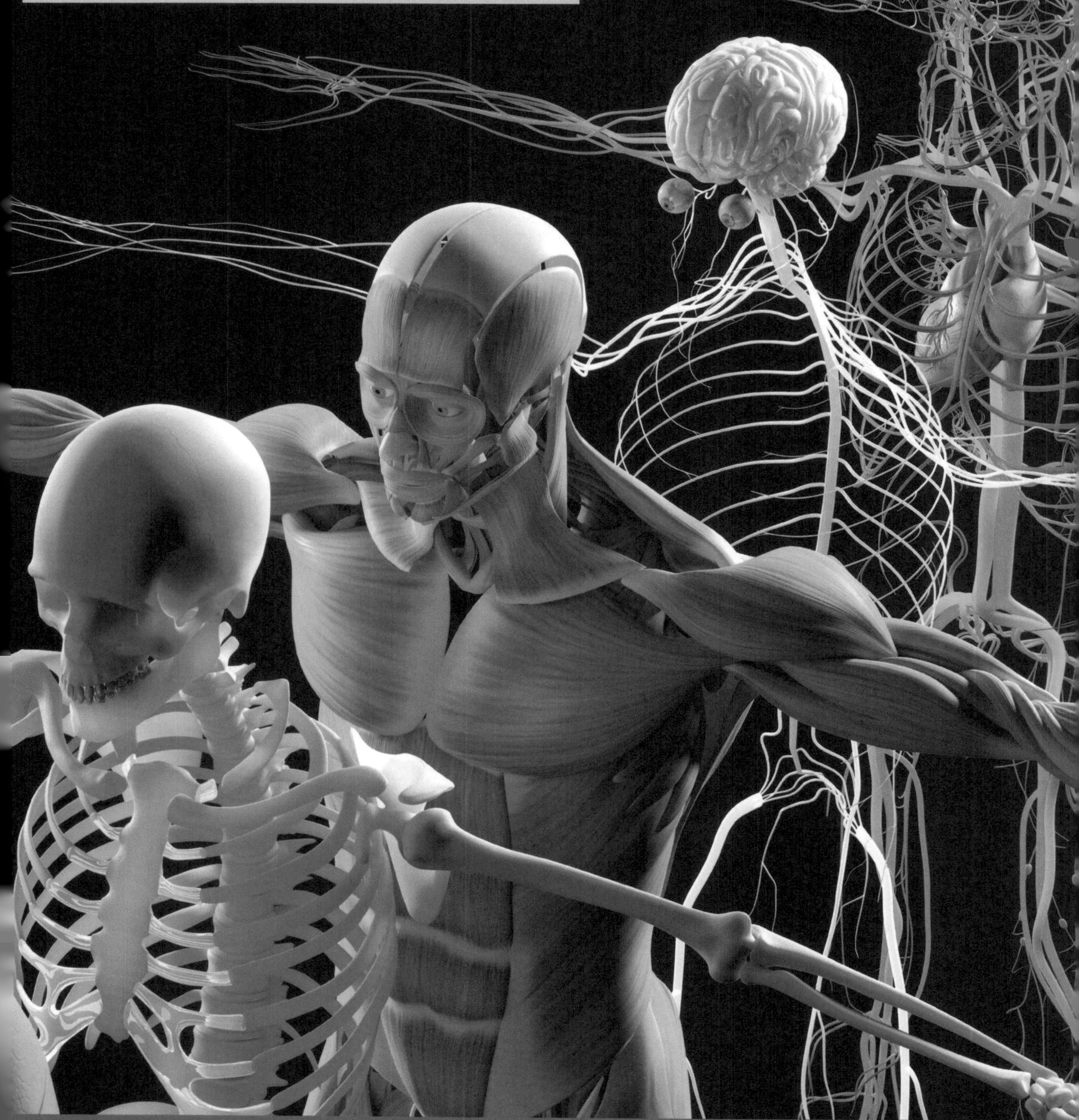

ANATOMY

The study of Anatomy is an excellent way to learn important things about your body. It is important to learn proper terminology of the body parts. Use this section as a reference when learning the muscles that are used during the exercises shown in this physical education workbook.

SKELETAL SYSTEM

The skeletal system consists of 206 bones. They are connected by tendons, ligaments and cartilage. The skeletal system supports the body, aids in movement, and protects internal organs.

Impact exercises and eating healthfully—especially foods high in calcium—help to keep your bones strong.

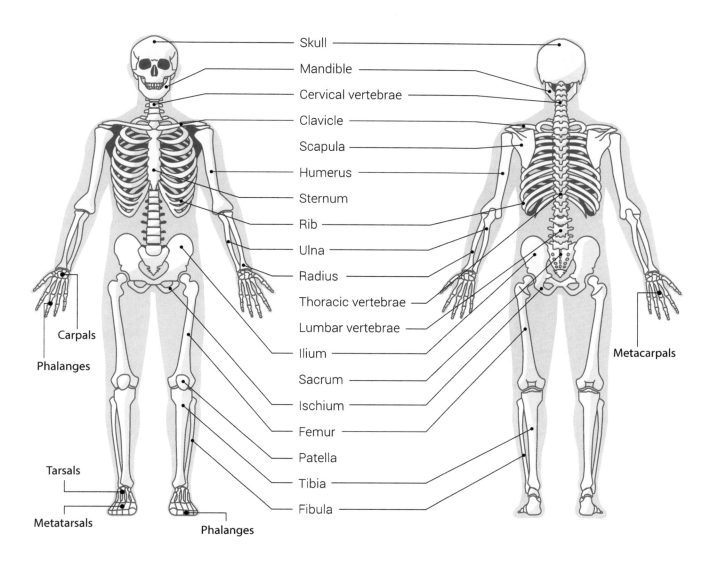

MUSCULAR SYSTEM

The **muscular system** is made up of over 600 muscles. Inside this system are thousands of thin, long cells called muscle fibers. These fibers allow our muscles to relax and contract in order for us to move around. The muscles in our body are all shapes and sizes and help us have strength, balance, posture, movement, and heat.

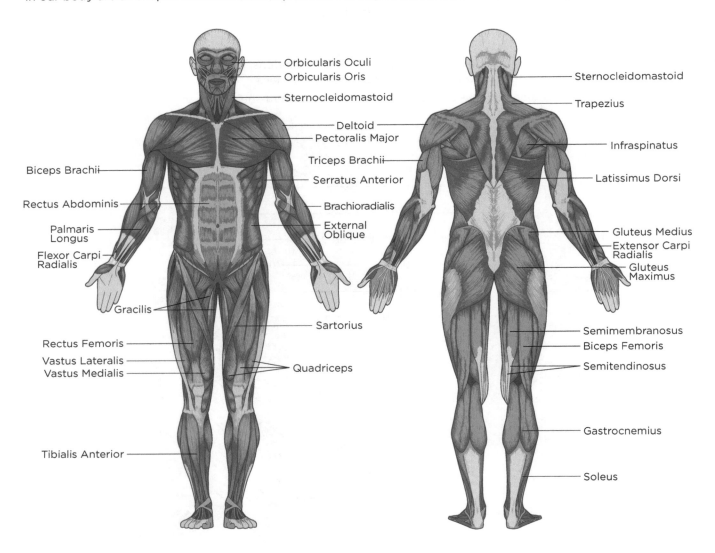

Types of Muscles

- Skeletal Muscles - these are the muscles we use to move around. They cover our skeleton and move our bones. These muscles are voluntary because we control them directly with signals from our brain. Sometimes they are called striped muscles because they come in long, dark bands of fiber and look striped. Opposing muscles, or antagonistic muscles, work in pairs to pull on bones to create movements and should be equally trained (for example, triceps and biceps or quadriceps and hamstrings are antagonistic muscles).

- Smooth Muscles - these are special muscles that don't connect to bones, but control organs in our body. These organs include the esophagus, stomach, intestines, bladder, blood vessels, respiratory system, and uterus (female). Smooth muscles are involuntary and are controlled by the nervous system, so you do not have to think about controlling them.

- Cardiac Muscle - this is a special muscle that pumps our heart and blood through our body. It can stretch like a smooth muscle and contract like a skeletal muscle. Like the smooth muscle, cardiac muscle is involuntary.

CIRCULATORY SYSTEM

The **circulatory system** allows blood to circulate throughout the body and transport nutrients, oxygen, carbon dioxide, hormones, and blood cells. Arteries carry oxygen rich blood from the heart to the rest of the body. Veins carry deoxygenated blood back to the heart.

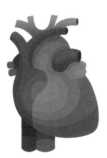

Your heart is a muscle that is about the size of your fist. It pumps blood throughout your body by way of your blood vessels. A child's heart pumps blood through approximately 60 thousand miles of blood vessels (2 ½ times around Earth). Your heart is a part of your circulatory system, which also includes blood, blood vessels, and lungs.

Your blood contains important nutrients and oxygen for your body's cells. Your body is made up of cells that require nutrients and oxygen. Cardiovascular exercise, also referred to as aerobic exercise, helps to keep your heart muscle pumping strong. Exercise almost every day to keep your heart strong.

Your heart is made up of four chambers: the right atrium, right ventricle, left atrium, and left ventricle. The **right atrium** and **right ventricle** receive "waste" blood by way of your veins. This blood collects a waste called carbon dioxide gas, which needs to be sent to your lungs so you can breathe it out. The blood then picks up oxygen and enters the **left atrium** and **left ventricle**. Your blood is now filled with fresh oxygen and nutrients and is ready to be pumped to your body's cells.

Circulatory System

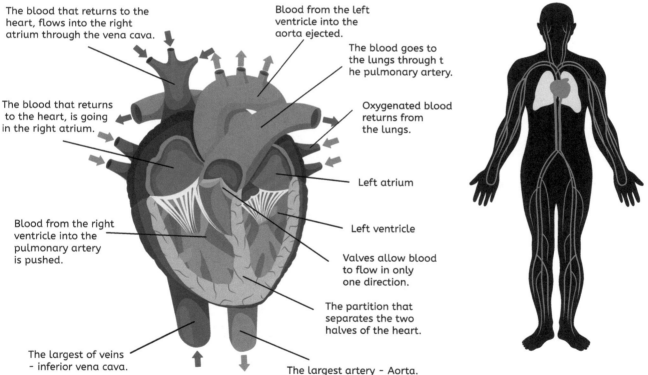

The blood that returns to the heart, flows into the right atrium through the vena cava.

The blood that returns to the heart, is going in the right atrium.

Blood from the right ventricle into the pulmonary artery is pushed.

The largest of veins - inferior vena cava.

Blood from the left ventricle into the aorta ejected.

The blood goes to the lungs through the pulmonary artery.

Oxygenated blood returns from the lungs.

Left atrium

Left ventricle

Valves allow blood to flow in only one direction.

The partition that separates the two halves of the heart.

The largest artery - Aorta.

RESPIRATORY SYSTEM

Your lungs are part of your **respiratory system**, which also includes your nose, mouth, trachea (windpipe), and diaphragm (muscle). An exchange of gases occurs when you breathe. You breathe in oxygen and breathe out carbon dioxide, which is a waste gas.

Regular exercise is important for clear, healthy lungs. Exercise makes you breathe in more air than usual, helping to clear out carbon dioxide.

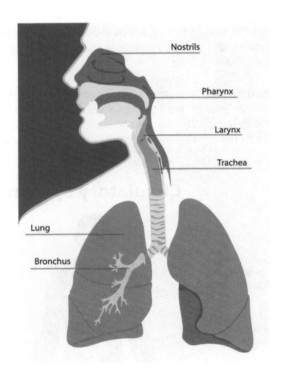

NERVOUS SYSTEM

Your brain is part of your **nervous system**, which also includes your nerves and spinal cord. Messages travel between your nerves and brain. Your brain controls just about everything you think, do, and feel. It coordinates and controls body systems that involve movement, personality, thinking, heartbeat, breathing, and more.

Research has connected exercise to a healthy brain. Compared to the rest of your body, your brain is small; however, it uses a quarter of the oxygen you breathe in. The increased blood flow from exercise brings important oxygen and nutrients to your brain. Regular exercise is associated with improved learning.

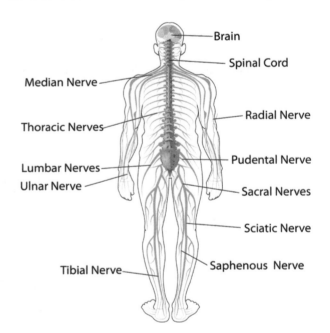

DIGESTIVE SYSTEM

Your stomach is part of your **digestive system**, which also includes your mouth, esophagus, and intestines. When food enters your mouth, the digestive process begins with your saliva and the chewing of the food. Your tongue pushes the chewed food into your esophagus, which is attached to your stomach.

Healthful eating is very important to a healthy body. Your body needs the nutrients and vitamins from healthful foods to work at its best. Proper nutrition and regular exercise should be lifelong commitments.

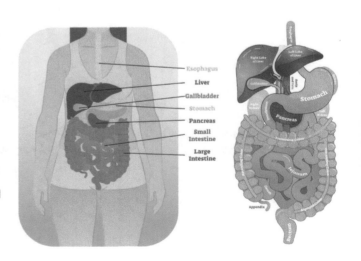

ANATOMICAL TERMINOLOGY

Abduction - movement of an appendage away from the midline.

Adductor Brevis - posterior muscle located in the upper thigh.

Adductor Longus - posterior muscle located in the upper thigh.

Adductor Magnus - posterior muscle located in the upper thigh.

Anterior - front of the body.

Appendage - an external body part that projects from the body.

Biceps Brachii - anterior muscle of the upper arm.

Biceps Femoris - posterior, upper leg muscle.

Brachioradialis - anterior muscle located in the lower arm.

Circumduction - movement of an appendage in a circle around a joint.

Deltoid - thick, triangular muscle located at the top of the shoulder.

Distal - away from or farthest from the trunk or point of origin.

Dorsiflexion - moving the ankle joint to stand on your heel.

Eversion - turning the sole of the foot away from the midline.

External Oblique - torso muscle that extends around the sides of the body.

Extension - a movement that increases the angle between two bones.

Extensor Carpi Radialis - a pair of muscles that are located in the lower arm.

Flexion - a movement that decreases the angle between two bones.

Flexor Carpi Radialis - a pair of muscles that are located in the lower arm.

Flexor Carpi Ulnaris - a pair of muscles that are located in the lower arm.

Gastrocnemius - calf muscle in the posterior, lower leg.

Gluteus Maximus - large muscle in the buttocks.

Gluteus Medius - medium muscle in the buttocks.

Gracilis - a pair of muscles that are located in the anterior, upper leg.

Hamstrings - group of muscles located in the posterior side of the upper leg. Muscles include Biceps Femoris, semimembranosus, semitendinosis.

Inferior - away from the head; lower.

Infraspinatus - posterior muscle located below the scapula (shoulder blade).

Internal Oblique - torso muscle that is located at the sides of the body.

Inversion - turning the sole of the foot toward the midline.

Joint - where two bones come together. Types of joints include: hinge, ball and socket, pivot, gliding, saddle, and immovable.

Lateral - away from the midline of the body; located toward the sides of the body.

Latissimus Dorsi - posterior lower back muscles.

Medial - toward the midline of the body.

Midline - an imaginary line that divides the body into right and left halves.

Orbicularis Oculi - circular muscle around the eye.

Orbicularis Oris - circular muscle around the mouth.

Pectoralis Major - anterior chest muscle.

Pectoralis Minor - anterior chest muscle under the pectoralis major.

Plantarflexion - moving the ankle joint to point your toe.

Posterior - back.

Pronation - turning the palm posterior.

Proximal - toward or nearest the trunk or point of origin of a part.

Quadricep - the four major muscles in the anterior, upper leg. Muscles; rectus femoris, vastus lateralis, vastus intermedius, vastus mediais.

Rectus Abdominis - anterior stomach muscle.

Rectus Femoris - anterior muscles located in the upper leg. One of the four muscles in the quadriceps.

Rotation - movement of a bone around an axis.

Sartorius - anterior muscles that are located in the upper leg. It is the longest muscle in the body.

Semimembranosus - posterior, upper leg.

Semitendinosis - posterior, upper leg.

Serratus Anterior - anterior muscle that is connected to the first 8 ribs and wraps around the side of the chest, ending below the scapula (shoulder blade).

Soleus - anterior muscle located in the lower leg.

Supination - turning the palm anterior.

Sternocleidomastoid - muscles located in the sides of your neck.

Superior - toward the head of the body; upper.

Temporalis - a facial muscle that is located on either side of the head.

Teres Major - posterior muscle that is located in the upper back.

Trapezius - posterior muscles in the upper back.

Triceps Brachii - three posterior muscles in the upper arm.

Vastus Intermedius, Lateralis & Medialis - anterior muscles in the upper leg. These muscles and the rectus femoris make up the quadriceps.

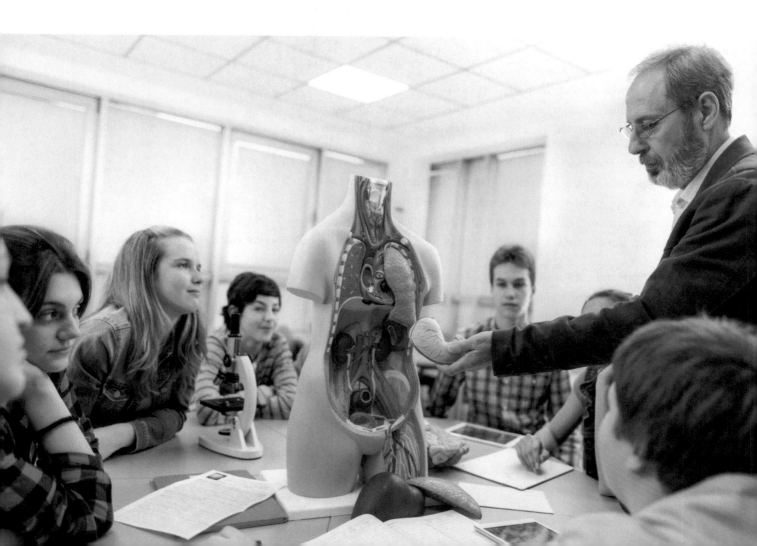

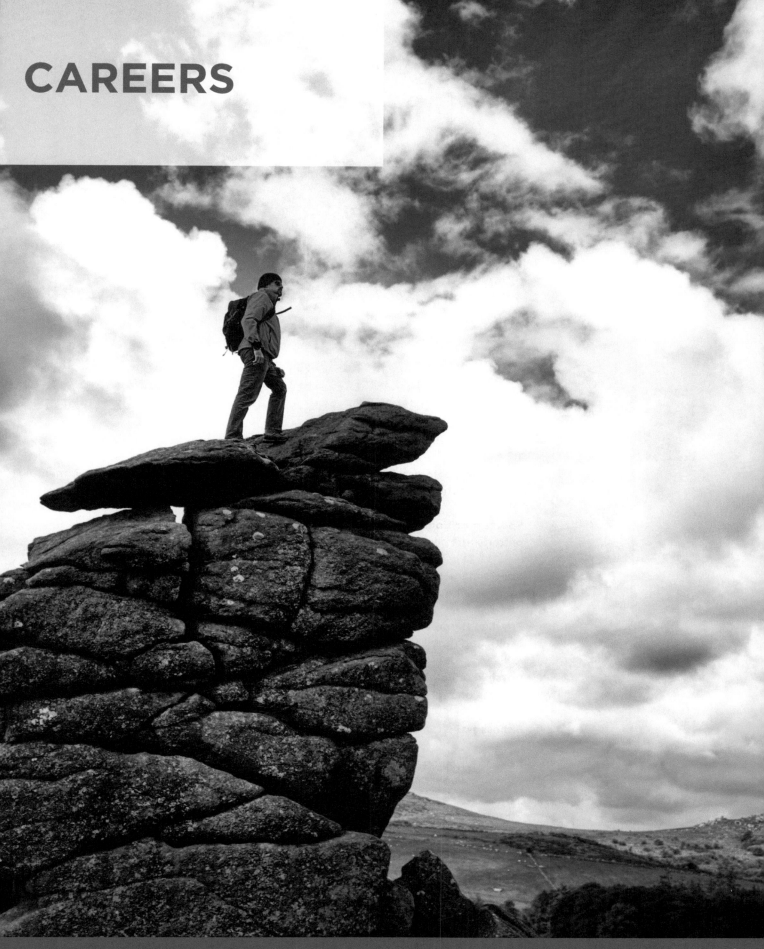

CAREERS

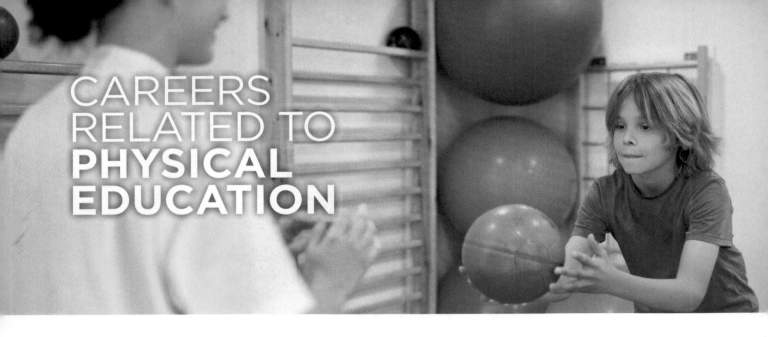

CAREERS RELATED TO PHYSICAL EDUCATION

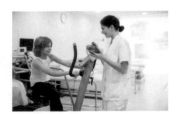

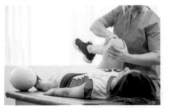

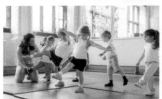

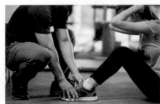

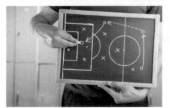

ARE YOU INTERESTED IN PHYSICAL ACTIVITY AND HOW IT RELATES TO HEALTH AND SPORTS? IF SO, YOU MAY BE INTERESTED IN THE FOLLOWING CAREER OPPORTUNITIES:

Sports medicine: a doctor who helps to treat and prevent sport injuries

Sports psychologist: a trained professional who helps athletes improve their mental skills for better sport performance

Sports nutritionist: a dietician who educates athletes about proper nutrition for better sport performance

Sports manager: a trained professional who organizes and budgets sports and sport activities

Physical therapist: a trained professional who works with patients to improve their health and mobility

Physical education teacher: a trained professional who teaches students about exercise and its connection to health

Fitness trainer: a certified trainer who helps people improve their fitness levels

Coach: a person with a sport background who leads players in a sport at the high school, college, or professional level

Chiropractor: a health care professional who treats back, joint, and muscle problems

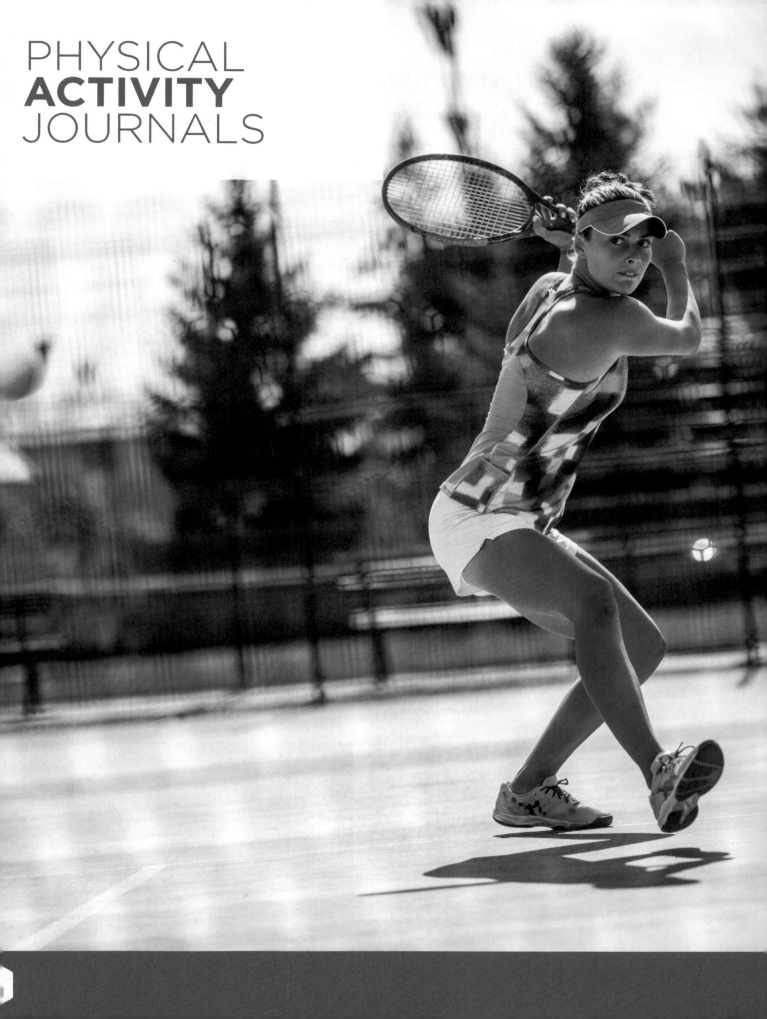

PHYSICAL
ACTIVITY
JOURNALS

PHYSICAL ACTIVITY JOURNALS

Activity journals are a wonderful way to express fitness progress and ideas. Keeping a journal can help you record the progression of your fitness goals and achievements. In addition, these journals help to promote proper writing, spelling, and math skills. Parents are encouraged to check the Physical Activity Journals as a way of monitoring the development of these skills. **** *Please note that these journals are for personal use only and are not required to be submitted for course credit.* ****

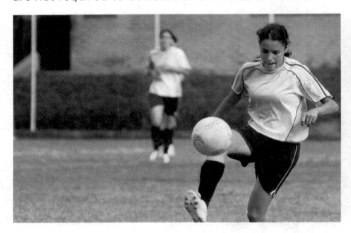 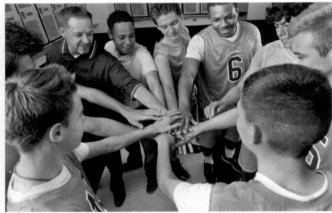

FITNESS WORKOUT JOURNAL

The fitness workout journal is used to record progress in your cardiovascular fitness. The electronic movement band is a great tool to help with record this progress. This journal can be helpful if you want to walk or run in a 5K race or any race of significant distance. As you progress, you can see the changes in your time and distance by utilizing the fitness workout journal. *Please note that this journal is for personal use only and is not required to be submitted for credit.*

STRENGTH-TRAINING JOURNAL

The strength-training journal should be used to help record your progression in muscular strength and muscular endurance. When lifting weights, it is important to document the amount of weight with which you are training in order to gain muscular strength and endurance. *Please note that this journal is for personal use only and is not required to be submitted for credit.*

PHYSICAL EDUCATION JOURNAL

The Physical Education journal is a tool that you can use weekly to record each day that you are active. Using the journal, record the date, nature of activity, and amount of time used to complete the activity. At the end of each week, you can can total the minutes of activity completed and covert the time (minutes) into hours. *Please note that this journal is for personal use only and is not required to be submitted for credit.*

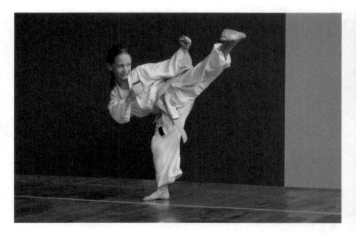 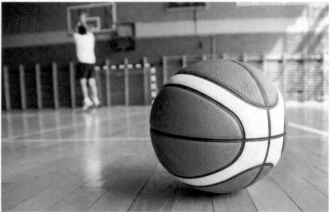

FITNESS WORKOUT JOURNAL

The Fitness Workout Journal is used to record progress in your cardiovascular fitness. The electronic movement band is a great tool to help with recording this progress. This journal can be helpful if you want to walk or run in a 5K race or any race of significant distance. As you progress, you can see the changes in your time and distance by utilizing the Fitness Workout Journal. *Please note that this journal is for personal use only and is not required to be submitted for credit.*

Date	Activity	Distances/Strides	Time	Heart Rate
09-01	Walking	1,000 Steps	1.5 hours	90 bpm

STRENGTH-TRAINING JOURNAL

The Strength-Training Journal should be used to help record your progression in muscular strength and muscular endurance. When lifting weights, it is important to document the amount of weight with which you are training in order to gain muscular strength and endurance. *Please note that this journal is for personal use only and is not required to be submitted for credit.*

Date	repetitions/ sets weight	repetitions/ sets weight	repetitions/ sets weight	repetitions/ sets weight	repetitions/ sets weight	repetitions/ sets weight	repetitions/ sets weight	repetitions/ sets weight	repetitions/ sets weight
Chest Press									
Pecs									
Upper Back									
Vertical Traction									
Shoulder Press									
Arm Extension									
Arm Curl									
Lower Back									
Ab Crunch									
Leg Curl									
Multi-Hip									
Glutes									
Leg Extension									
Leg Press									
Pull-Ups									
Incline Sit-Ups									

PHYSICAL EDUCATION JOURNAL

GRADES 7 THROUGH 12 ~ 72 HOURS

WEEK _____

	Cardiovascular	Strength	Flexibility	Sport or Other Physical Activity
Monday	Activity Time:	Activity Time:	Activity Time:	Activity Time:
Tuesday	Activity Time:	Activity Time:	Activity Time:	Activity Time:
Wednesday	Activity Time:	Activity Time:	Activity Time:	Activity Time:
Thursday	Activity Time:	Activity Time:	Activity Time:	Activity Time:
Friday	Activity Time:	Activity Time:	Activity Time:	Activity Time:
Sat./Sun.	Activity Time:	Activity Time:	Activity Time:	Activity Time:

Total Weekly Time:

Personal Fitness Inventory
Students should check BMI, height, and weight at the beginning of the year.

BMI_____%
Height_____in.
Weight_____lb.

Check weight weekly if overweight and high percent BMI.

Strength Training
3x weekly

Push-Ups_____1 min.

Sit-Ups_____1 min.

Cardiovascular Training
3x weekly

Resting Heart Rate_____min.

Target Heart Rate_____min.

Make copies of this page as needed to complete your physical education course and for future workouts. Please note that this journal is for personal use only. You must submit the electronic form for grading

GLOSSARY
OF TERMS

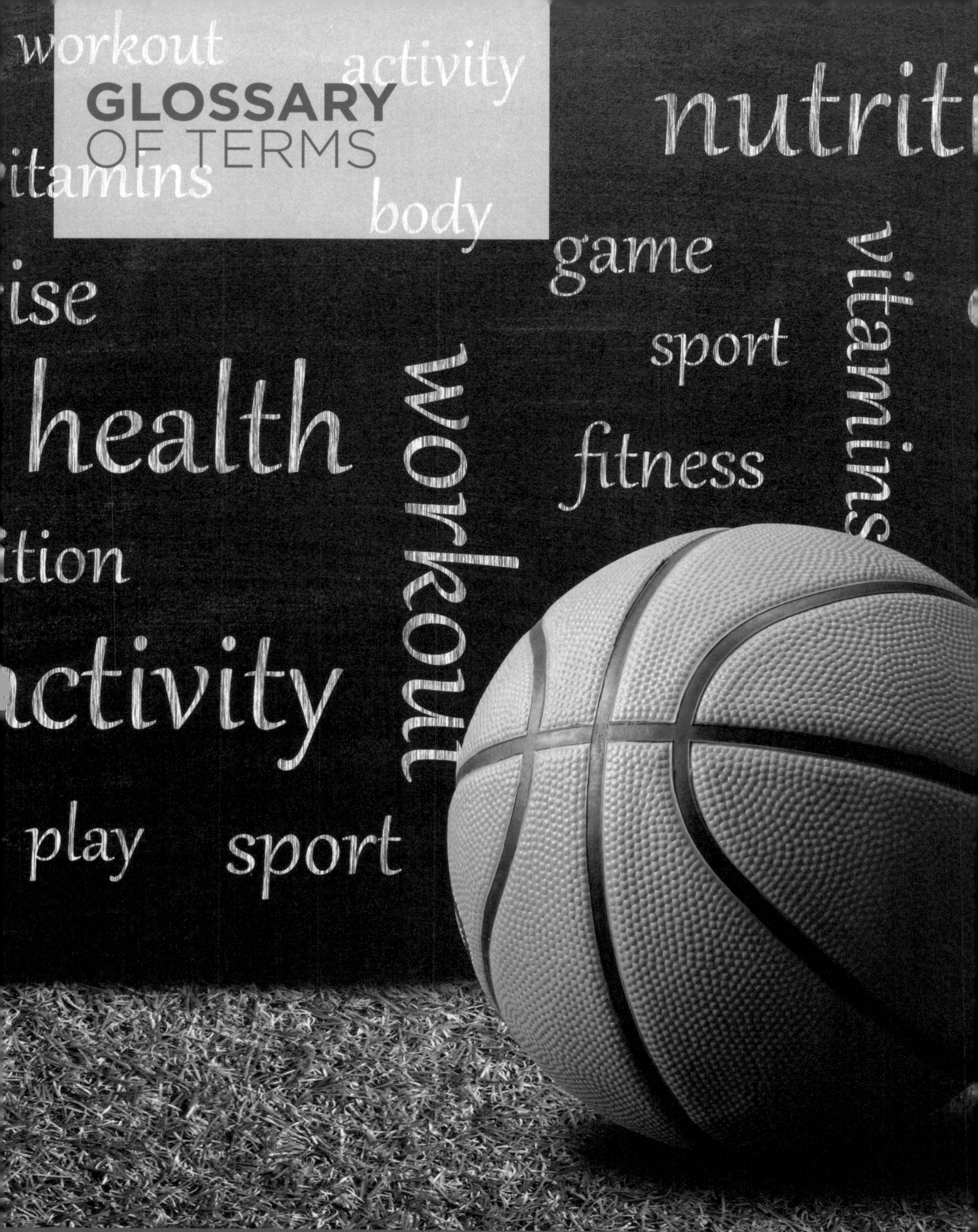

workout
activity
vitamins
body
nutriti
ise
game
sport
health
workout
vitamins
fitness
ition
activity
play
sport

PHYSICAL EDUCATION GLOSSARY OF TERMS

Abductors - muscles that pull the arm or leg away from the midline of the body.

Adductors - muscles that pull the arm or leg toward the midline of the body.

Aerobic - physical activity or exercise done at a steady pace for an extended period of time so that the heart can supply as much oxygen as the body needs (e.g., walking, running, swimming, cycling).

Agility - a component of physical fitness that relates to the ability to rapidly change the position of the body in space with speed and accuracy.

Anaerobic - physical activity or exercise done in short, fast bursts that cause the heart to not be able to supply oxygen as fast as the body needs (e.g., sprinting, weightlifting).

Anterior - front side of the body.

Artery - a blood vessel that carries blood away from the heart.

Balance - a skill related component of physical fitness that relates to the maintenance of equilibrium while stationary or moving.

Blood Pressure - the force of circulating blood on the walls of the arteries.

Body Mass Index (BMI) - the measurement of body fat based on height and weight.

Body Alignment - body control using such skills as balance, coordination, spatial judgments, and postural efficiency.

Body Composition - a health-related component of physical fitness that relates to the percent of fat tissue and lean tissue in the body.

Body Systems - anatomically or functionally related to parts of the body (e.g., skeletal, muscular, circulatory).

Calorie - the unit of measuring the energy produced by food when oxidized in the body.

Cardiorespiratory - relating to both the heart and respiratory system.

Cardiorespiratory Fitness - a health related component of physical fitness relating to the ability of the circulatory and respiratory systems to supply oxygen during sustained physical activity.

Cardiovascular Endurance - the body's ability to use oxygen to meet energy demands of muscles through aerobic exercise.

Carotid Artery - main artery located in the neck.

Circuit Training - exercise program, similar to an obstacle course, in which the person goes from one place to another doing a different exercise at each place.

Circulatory System - the heart and system of blood vessels in the body, including arteries, capillaries, and veins.

Conditioning - engaging in regular physical activity or exercise that results in an improved state of physical fitness.

Continuous - two or more repetitions of the same skill such as dribbling in basketball or soccer.

Contract - muscle shortens.

Cool-down - brief, mild exercise done after vigorous exercise to help the body safely return to a resting state.

Coordination - a skill related component of physical fitness that relates to the ability to use the senses together with body parts in performing motor tasks smoothly and accurately.

Dehydration - excess fluid loss from the body.

Directions - forward, backward, left, right, up, down.

Dynamic Balance - equilibrium used when in motion, starting, and stopping.

Dynamic Flexibility - is the ability to move quickly or at normal speed into a stretched position.

Effort - this concept defines how the body moves. It consists of three components: *time* (faster or slower), *force* (harder or softer), and *flow* (bound or free).

Equilibrium - state at which there is no change in the motion of the body.

Exercise - physical activity that is planned, structured, repetitive, and results in the improvement or maintenance of personal fitness.

Extend - muscle lengthens or becomes longer.

External Oblique - muscles located on the anterior side of the abdomen or stomach area.

Fitness - capability of the body of distributing inhaled oxygen to muscle tissue during increased physical activity.

FITT - is an acronym for Frequency, Intensity, Time, and Type, which are four key ways that activity can be manipulated to create a desired fitness outcome.

Flex - muscle shortens.

Flexibility - the elasticity of muscles and connective tissues, which determines the range of motion of the joints.

Frequency - the amount of time you repeat an exercise.

Goal - something that you want to achieve in your physical activities. A predetermined plan of action.

Health-Related Fitness - components of physical fitness that have a relationship with good health. Components are cardiorespiratory endurance, muscular strength, muscular endurance, flexibility, and body composition.

Heart - muscle that pumps blood throughout the body.

Heart Rate - the number of heartbeats occurring within a specified length of time.

Individual Sport - a sport with one participant, such as archery, cycling, golf, running, swimming, tennis.

Individuality - the training principle that takes into account that each person begins at a different level of fitness. Each person has personal goals and objectives for physical activity and fitness.

Intensity - the level of effort exerted during a workout, measured with target heart rate.

Interval Training - an anaerobic exercise program that consists of runs of short distance followed by rest.

Journal - written record of activities or events.

Kinesthetic - the sense perception of movement, the muscular sense.

Kinetic - energy that an object possesses because it is moving, such as a pitched baseball or person running.

Learning Stages - Three Stages:
   Cognitive Stage - the first stage of motor learning when the participant requires intense concentration with no distraction.
   Associative Stage - the second and intermediate stage. Skill is used in combination with other skills when the learner is improving the quality of performance.
   Automatic Stage - the final stage. Advanced, proficient and dynamic, skill is used in combination with other skills in an open environment.

Levels - positions of the body (e.g., high, medium, low).

Lifelong Activity - a non-impact physical activity that you can enjoy into adulthood. Walking, hiking, biking, golf, tennis, etc.

Linear Movement - movement which occurs in a straight path.

Locomotor Movement - movement producing physical displacement of the body by weight transfer of feet. Basic locomotor steps are walk, run, hop, skip, slide, gallop, and jump.

Manipulative Skills - a skillful movement done to or with objects such as throwing a ball, striking a soccer ball, catching a Frisbee, or juggling.

Maximum Heart Rate - the highest number of times the heart can beat in one minute. Generally calculated by subtracting a person's age from 220.

Moderate Physical Activity - sustained, repetitive, large muscle movements (e.g., walking, running, cycling) done at less than 60% of maximum heart rate for age.

Motor Skills - non-fitness abilities that improve with practice and relate to one's ability to perform specific sports and other motor tasks (e.g. tennis serve, shooting a basketball).

Muscular Endurance - a health related component of physical fitness that relates to the ability to contract your muscles repeatedly without excessive fatigue.

Muscular Strength - a health related component of physical fitness that relates to the maximal force that you can exert when you contract your muscles.

Muscular System - is an organ system consisting of skeletal, smooth, and cardiac muscles. It permits movement of the body, maintains posture, and circulates blood.

Non-locomotor - movement in the space that the body or its parts can reach without traveling away from starting point.

Non-manipulative Skills - skillful movements done with the body like turning, twisting, or rolling.

Nutrient - a basic component of food that nourishes the body. There are six nutrients: carbohydrates, lipids, proteins, vitamins, minerals, and water.

Obesity - a condition in which the body has excessive adipose (fat) tissue.

Pathways - patterns of travel while performing locomotor movements (e.g., straight, curved, zigzag).

Physical Activity - body movement that is produced by the contraction of skeletal muscles.

Physical Education - a planned, sequential, movement-based program of curricula and instruction that helps the students to develop knowledge, motor skills, and self-management skills needed to maintain a physically active life.

Physical Fitness - a level of physical ability to perform daily tasks effectively with enough energy for additional recreational activities and physical challenges.

Posterior - back side of the body.

Power - a skill-related component of physical fitness that relates to the ability to move your body parts swiftly while at the same time applying maximum force on your muscles.

Progression - a rate at which you change the frequency, intensity, and time of your exercise.

Psychomotor - physical activity relating to fitness and skill.

Pulse - the rhythmical throbbing of arteries produced by the regular contraction of the heart. Common areas to check pulse are the wrist and neck.

Radial Artery - main artery located on the anterior wrist.

Range of Motion (ROM) - varying degrees of motion around a joint.

Reaction Time - a skill related component of physical fitness that relates to the time elapsed between stimulation and the beginning of the response to it.

Recovery Time - time or rest between exercises.

Repetition - number of times a skill is repeated.

Resistance - opposition of some force to another.

Respiratory System - system in the body that takes in and distributes oxygen during the breathing process.

Rubric - a scoring tool that lists the criteria for a fitness test.

Self-space - all the space that the body or its parts can reach without traveling from a starting position.

Serial - two or more different skills performed with each other, such as fielding a ball and throwing it to a target, or dribbling a basketball and shooting it.

Set - a group of several repetitions.

Skeletal System - internal framework of bones; helps provide the body with shape and support, protects vital organs, and produces blood cells.

Skilled-related Fitness - consists of components of physical fitness that have a relationship with performance in sports and motor skills. The components are agility, balance, power, reaction time, and speed.

Speed - a skill related component of physical fitness that relates to the ability to perform a movement or cover a distance in a short period of time.

Static Balance - maintaining equilibrium while holding a pose or remaining motionless.

Strength - the quality of being strong, such as body or muscle power.

Strength Training - the use of resistance to muscular contraction to build the strength, anaerobic endurance, and size of skeletal muscles.

Target Heart Rate - a figure used to represent the number of heart beats per minute required to reach during exercise in order to achieve desired positive results.

Team Sports - includes any sport which involves players working together to win the contest. (e.g., basketball, volleyball, football, soccer, lacrosse, etc.).

Torque - a turning, or rotary force.

Warm-up - a variety of low intensity activities designed to prepare your body for more vigorous activities.

Vigorous Physical Activity - sustained, repetitive, large muscle movements (e.g., running, swimming, soccer) done at 60% or more of maximum heart rate for age. Activity makes person sweat and breathe hard.

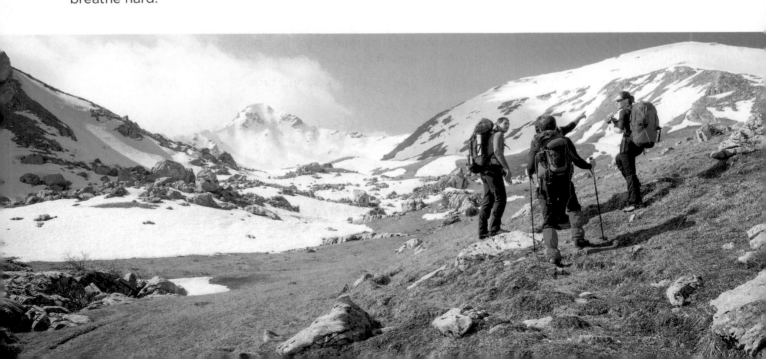

SHAPE AMERICA NATIONAL STANDARDS FOR PHYSICAL EDUCATION

Standard 1: *Demonstrates competency in a variety of motor skills and movement patterns.*
Standard 2: *The physically literate individual applies knowledge of concepts, principles, strategies and tactics related to movement and performance.*
Standard 3: *The physically literate individual demonstrates the knowledge and skills to achieve and maintain a health-enhancing level of physical activity and fitness.*
Standard 4: *The physically literate individual exhibits responsible personal and social behavior that respects self and others.*
Standard 5: *The physically literate individual recognizes the value of physical activity for health, enjoyment, challenge, self-expression and/or social interaction.*

NATIONAL STANDARD OUTCOMES FOR PHYSICAL EDUCATION

Each outcome is fully defined in the online program.

Primary Outcomes
Embedded Outcomes (Secondary Outcomes)

STANDARD OUTCOMES FOR THE FRONT INFORMATIONAL SECTIONS

Section: Physical Education Requirements
S3.M8.7
S3.M8.8
S3.H4.L1
S4.M7.7
S4.M2.8
S4.M7.8
S4.H1.L1

Section: PE Log
S3.M16.7
S3.M16.8
S3.H11.L2

Section: Organized or Team Sports Verification Log
S4.M2.7
S4.M2.8
S3.H6.L1

Section: Essentials of Fitness
S3.M7.7
S3.M7.8

S3.M1.8
S3.H12.L2
S5.M1.7
S5.M1.8
S5.M2.7
S5.M4.7
S5.M2.8
S5.M4.8
S5.H1.L1

Section: Principles of Fitness
S3.M11.7
S3.M11.8
S3.M15.7
S3.M15.8
S3.H3.L2

Section: Planning and Preparing: Warm-Up and Cool-Down
S3.M9.7
S3.M9.8
S3.M10.8
S3.M12.7
S3.M12.8)

S3.M18.7
S3.H9.L1

Section: Planning and Preparing: Weather Precautions
S3.H3.L1

Section: Measuring Fitness
S3.M15.7
S3.M15.8
S3.M16.8
S3.H11.L1
S5.M3.8
S5.M6.8
S5.H1.L1

Section: Health-Related Fitness Components: Body Composition
S3.M10.7
S3.H8.L1
S3.H1.L2
S3.H13.L1
S4.H1.L2

Section: Health-Related Fitness Components: Cardiovascular Endurance
S3.M10.7
S3.M13.7
S3.M13.8
S3.M8.7
S3.M18.7
S3.H3.L2
S3.H8.L2
S3.H10.L1
S3.H10.L2
S3.H14.L1
S4.M7.7
S4.M7.8
S4.M2.7
S4.H5.L1
S5.M1.7
S5.M2.7
S5.M1.8
S5.H1.L1

Section: Health-Related Fitness Components: Flexibility
S3.M9.7

S3.M9.8
S3.M10.8
S3.H9.L1

Section: Health-Related Fitness Components: Muscular Strength
S3.M3.7
S3.M4.7
S3.M6.7
S3.M6.8
S3.H7.L1
S4.M7.7
S4.M7.8
S4.H5.L1

Section: Muscular Endurance
S3.M3.7
S3.M4.7
S3.M6.7
S3.M6.8
S3.H7.L1
S4.M7.7
S4.M7.8
S4.H5.L1

STANDARDS AND STANDARD OUTCOMES FOR GRADES 7–PE EQUIPMENT KIT SECTION

WARM-UP AND COOL-DOWN GRADES 7–12

Module: Warm-Up
S3.M9.7
S3.M12.7
S3.M9.8

S3.M10.8
S3.M12.8
S5.M1.7
S5.M1.8

Module: Cool-Down
S3.M9.7
S3.M12.7
S3.M17.7

S3.M9.8
S3.M10.8
S3.M12.8
S5.M1.8

SEVENTH GRADE PE EQUIPMENT KIT

Module: Aerobic Exercise
S1.M1.7
S1.M1.8
S2.M12.7
S3.M1.7
S3.M2.7
S3.M6.7
S3.M8.7
S3.M10.7
S3.M12.7
S3.M18.7
S3.M2.8

S3.M3.8
S3.M5.8
S3.M8.8
S3.M12.8
S3.M13.8
S3.M14.8
S3.M16.8
S4.M2.7
S4.M7.
S4.M1.8
S4.M2.8
S4.M7.8
S5.M2.7
S5.M4.7

S5.M5.7
S5.M2.8
S5.M4.8
S5.M5.8

Module: Dance
S1.M1.7
S2.M12.7
S3.M2.7
S3.M6.7
S4.M2.7
S4.M6.7
S5.M1.7

S5.M4.7
S5.M5.7
S5.M6.7

Module: Jump Rope
S1.M24.7
S3.M2.7
S3.M5.7
S3.M6.7
S3.M7.7
S4.M1.7
S4.M2.7
S4.M3.7

S4.M7.7
S5.M1.7
S5.M3.7
S4.M5.7
S5.M6.7

Module: Strength Training
S3.M1.7
S3.M2.7
S3.M3.7
S3.M4.7
S3.M6.7

S3.M8.7
S3.M10.7
S3.M12.7
S3.M14.7
S4.M7.7
S5.M1.7
S5.M2.7
S5.M4.7
S5.M5.7

Module: Resistance Bands

S3.M2.7
S3.M3.7
S3.M4.7
S3.M6.7
S3.M8.7
S3.M10.7
S4.M3.7
S4.M7.7
S5.M1.7

Module: Badminton

S1.M11.7
S1.M12.7
S1.M13.7
S1.M14.7
S2.M1.7
S2.M6.7
S2.M7.7
S2.M8.7
S2.M9.7
S2.M10.7
S2.M12.7
S2.M13.7
S3.M5.7
S4.M1.7
S4.M2.7
S4.M3.7
S4.M4.7
S4.M6.7
S4.M7.7
S5.M4.7
S5.M5.7

Module: Basketball

S1.M2.7
S1.M5.7
S1.M6.7
S1.M7.7
S1.M8.7
S1.M9.7
S1.M10.7
S1.M24.7
S2.M1.7
S2.M2.7
S2.M3.7
S2.M4.7
S2.M5.7
S2.M6.7
S2.M9.7
S2.M13.7
S3.M1.7
S3.M2.7
S4.M1.7
S4.M2.7
S4.M3.7
S4.M4.7
S4.M5.7
S4.M6.7
S4.M7.7
S5.M1.7
S5.M4.7
S5.M5.7
S5.M6.7

Module: Golf

S1.M19.7
S1.M22.7
S1.M24.7
S2.M8.7
S2.M9.7
S2.M10.7
S2.M13.7
S3.M5.7
S4.M2.7
S4.M6.7
S4.M7.7
S5.M1.7
S5.M4.7
S5.M5.7

Module: 4 Square (Playground Ball Games)

S1.M11.7
S1.M12.7
S1.M13.7
S1.M15.7
S1.M16.7
S1.M22.7
S2.M1.7
S2.M2.7
S2.M8.
S2.M9.7
S2.M10.7
S2.M13.7
S4.M1.7
S4.M2.7
S4.M3.7
S4.M4.7
S4.M5.7
S4.M6.7
S4.M7.7
S5.M3.7
S5.M4.7
S5.M5.7
S5.M6.7

Module: Team Handball (Playground Ball Games)

S1.M2.7
S1.M3.7
S1.M5.7
S1.M6.7
S1.M7.7
S1.M10.7
S1.M11.7
S1.M21.7
S1.M22.7
S2.M1.7
S2.M2.7
S2.M3.7
S2.M4.7
S2.M5.7
S2.M6.7
S2.M13.7

S3.M2.7
S3.M5.7
S4.M1.7
S4.M2.7
S4.M3.7
S4.M4.7
S4.M5.7
S4.M6.7
S4.M7.7
S5.M3.7
S5.M4.7
S5.M5.7
S5.M6.7

Module: Soccer

S1.M2.7
S1.M4.7
S1.M6.7
S1.M7.7
S1.M10.7
S1.M11.7
S1.M22.7
S2.M1.7
S2.M2.7
S2.M3.7
S2.M4.7
S2.M6.7
S2.M10.7
S2.M13.7
S3.M1.7
S3.M2.7
S3.M5.7
S4.M1.7
S4.M2.7
S4.M3.7
S4.M4.7
S4.M5.7
S4.M6.7
S4.M7.7
S5.M4.7
S5.M5.7
S5.M6.7

Module: Short-Handled Racket Tennis

S1.M13.7

S1.M15.7
S1.M16.7
S1.M17.7
S2.M1.7
S2.M6.7
S2.M8.7
S2.M9.7
S2.M10.7
S2.M12.7
S2.M13.7
S3.M5.7
S4.M1.7
S4.M2.7
S4.M3.7
S4.M4.7
S4.M6.7
S4.M7.7
S5.M4.7
S5.M5.7
S5.M6.7

Module: Wiffle Ball

S1.M2.7
S1.M3.7
S1.M6.7
S1.M18.7
S1.M19.7
S1.M20.7
S1.M21.7
S1.M22.7
S2.M8.7
S2.M9.7
S2.M10.7
S2.M11.7
S2.M13.7
S3.M5.7
S3.M14.7
S4.M1.7
S4.M2.7
S4.M4.7
S4.M6.7
S4.M7.7
S5.M4.7
S5.M5.7
S5.M6.7

EIGHTH GRADE PE EQUIPMENT KIT

Module: Aerobic Exercise

S1.M1.8
S3.M2.8
S3.M3.8
S3.M5.8
S3.M8.8
S3.M12.8
S3.M13.8
S3.M14.8
S3.M16.8
S4.M1.8
S4.M2.8
S4.M7.8
S5.M2.8
S5.M4.8
S5.M5.8

Module: Hip-Hop Dance

S1.M1.8
S2.M12.8
S3.M2.8
S3.M3.8
S3.M5.8
S4.M1.8
S4.M2.8
S4.M5.8
S4.M6.8
S5.M2.8
S5.M4.8
S5.M5.8
S5.M6.8

Module: Jump Rope

S1.M1.8
S1.M24.8
S2.M12.8
S2.M13.8
S3.M2.8
S3.M7.8
S3.M16.8
S4.M1.8
S4.M3.8
S4.M7.8
S5.M2.8
S5.M4.8
S5.M5.8
S5.M6.8

Module: Strength Training

S3.M1.8
S3.M2.8
S3.M9.8
S3.M11.8
S3.M12.8
S3.M18.8
S4.M1.8
S4.M2.8
S4.M7.8
S5.M5.8
S5.M6.8

Module: Fitness Ball

S3.M2.8
S4.M1.8

S4.M2.8
S4.M7.8
S5.M6.8

Module: Cross-Training Circuit

S1.M1.8
S3.M1.8
S3.M2.8
S3.M4.8
S3.M6.8
S3.M8.8
S3.M9.8
S3.M11.8
S3.M12.8
S3.M13.8
S3.M16.8
S4.M1.8
S4.M7.8
S5.M4.8
S5.M5.8

Module: Floor Hockey

S1.M4.8
S1.M6.8
S1.M7.8
S1.M9.8
S1.M10.8
S1.M15.8
S1.M19.8
S2.M1.8
S2.M3.8

S2.M4.8
S2.M5.8
S2.M6.8
S2.M7.8
S2.M8.8
S2.M9.8
S2.M10.8
S2.M11.8
S3.M5.8
S4.M2.8
S4.M4.8
S4.M5.8
S4.M6.8
S4.M7.8
S5.M4.8
S5.M5.8
S5.M6.8

Module: Juggling

S1.M24.8
S3.M2.8
S3.M18.8
S4.M1.8
S4.M7.8
S5.M4.8
S5.M5.8

Module: Pickleball

S1.M12.8
S1.M13.8
S1.M14.8
S1.M16.8
S1.M17.8

S2.M1.8
S2.M6.8
S2.M7.8
S2.M8.8
S2.M9.8
S2.M11.8
S2.M12.8
S2.M13.8
S3.M5.8
S4.M2.8
S4.M3.8
S4.M6.8
S4.M7.8
S5.M4.8
S5.M5.8
S5.M6.8

Module: Speed Ball: Basketball Version

S1.M2.8
S1.M5.8
S1.M6.8
S1.M7.8
S1.M8.8
S1.M9.8
S1.M11.8
S1.M18.8
S1.M21.8
S2.M1.8)
S2.M2.8
S2.M3.8
S2.M4.8
S2.M5.8
S2.M6.8

S2.M9.8
S2.M10.8
S2.M11.8
S3.M2.8
S3.M5.8
S4.M1.8
S4.M2.8
S4.M3.8
S4.M4.8
S4.M5.8
S4.M6.8
S4.M7.8

S5.M4.8
S5.M5.8

Module: Tennis
S1.M13.8
S1.M14.8
S1.M15.8
S1.M17.8
S1.M19.8
S1.M20.8
S1.M22.8

S2.M1.8
S2.M6.8
S2.M7.8
S2.M8.8
S2.M9.8
S2.M13.8
S3.M2.8
S3.M5.8
S4.M1.8
S4.M2.8
S4.M3.8
S4.M4.8

S4.M7.8
S5.M4.8
S5.M5.8
S5.M6.8

Module: Volleyball
S1.M12.8
S1.M13.8
S1.M17.8
S2.M7.8
S2.M8.8

S2.M9.8
S3.M2.8
S3.M5.8
S4.M1.8
S4.M2.8
S4.M3.8
S4.M5.8
S4.M6.8
S4.M7.8
S5.M4.8
S5.M5.8
S5.M6.8

HIGH SCHOOL 9–12 PE EQUIPMENT KIT

Module: Warm-Up and Cool-Down
S3.H9.L
S4.H5.L1

CARDIOVASCULAR EXERCISE TRAINING

Module: Aerobic Exercise and Proper Nutrition
S1.H2.L2
S1.H3.L1
S3.H1.L
S3.H2.L1
S3.H2.L2
S3.H5.L1
S3.H5.L2
S3.H6.L1
S3.H6.L2
S3.H8.L1
S3.H8.L2

S3.H10.L1
S3.H10.L2
S3.H11.L2
S3.H12.L1
S3.H13.L1
S3.H13.L2
S3.H14.L1
S3.H14.L2
S4.H1.L1
S4.H4.L2
S4.H5.L1
S5.H1.L1
S5.H2.L2
S5.H3.L1

Module: Jump Rope
S1.H1.L1
S2.H2.L1
S2.H3.L1)
S3.H5.L2
S3.H8.L2
S3.H10.L1
S3.H10.L2
S4.H1.L1
S4.H5.L1)
S5.H1.L1
S5.H2.L2

Module: Stepper
S1.H1.L1
S2.H2.L1
S2.H3.L1
S3.H5.L2
S3.H8.L2
S3.H10.L1
S3.H10.L2
S3.H11.L1
S3.H14.L2
S4.H1.L1
S4.H5.L1
S5.H1.L1
S5.H2.L2

Module: Training for a 5K
S1.H3.L1
S2.H3.L1
S3.H6.L2
S3.H8.L2
S3.H10.L1
S3.H10.L2
S4.H1.L1
S4.H5.L1
S5.H2.L2
S5.H3.L1

DANCE

Module: Social Dance
S1.H2.L1
S1.H2.L2
S2.H1.L2
S2.H4.L2
S3.H6.L2
S4.H2.L1
S4.H5.L1

S5.H3.L2
S5.H3.L2
S5.H4.L1
S5.H4.L2

Module: Creative Dance
S1.H2.L1

S1.H2.L2
S2.H1.L2
S2.H4.L2
S4.H2.L1
S4.H5.L)
S5.H3.L1
S5.H3.L2
S5.H4.L1

S5.H4.L2

Module: Hip-Hop Dance
S1.H2.L1
S1.H2.L2
S3.H11.L1
S2.H1.L2

S2.H4.L2
S4.H2.L1
S4.H5.L1
S5.H3.L1
S5.H3.L2
S5.H4.L1
S5.H4.L2

STRENGTH BUILDING

Module: Fitness Ball
S3.H7.L1
S4.H5.L1

Module: Push-Up Handles
S3.H7.L1
S3.H8.L2
S3.H11.L1
S4.H5.L1

S5.H2.L2

Module: Resistance Bands
S3.H7.L1
S4.H5.L1
S5.H2.L2

Module: Kettlells

S1.H3.L1
S2.H2.L1
S3.H7.L1
S4.H5.L1
S5.H2.L2

Module: Weighted Ball
S1.H3.L1
S2.H2.L1
S3.H7.L1

S4.H5.L1
S5.H2.L2

Module: Double Grip Medicine Ball
S1.H3.L1
S2.H2.L1
S3.H7.L1
S4.H5.L1
S5.H2.L2

Module: Slider
S1.H3.L1
S2.H2.L1
S3.H9.L1
S3.H11.L1
S4.H5.L1
S5.H2.L2

STRENGTH AND CIRCUIT TRAINING

Module: Strength-Training Program
S1.H3.L2
S2.H2.L1
S3.H7.L2
S3.H9.L1
S3.H9.L2
S3.H11.L2

S4.H1.L1
S4.H5.L1
S5.H1.L1
S5.H2.L
S5.H3.L2

Module: Cross-Training Circuit

S1.H3.L2
S3.H1.L1
S3.H2.L2
S3.H5.L2
S3.H6.L1
S3.H7.L1
S3.H7.L2
S3.H8.L2

S3.H10.L1
S3.H10.L2
S3.H12.L1
S4.H1.L1
S4.H2.L1
S4.H3.L1
S4.H3.L2
S4.H4.L1

S4.H4.L2
S4.H5.L1
S5.H1.L1
S5.H2.L2
S5.H3.L1

SPORT RELATED OUTCOMES GRADES 9–12

RACKET SPORTS

Module: Badminton
S1.H1.L1
S1.H1.L2

S2.H1.L1
S2.H1.L2
S2.H2.L1

S2.H2.L2
S2.H3.L1
S2.H3.L2

S2.H5.L1
S2.H5.L2
S3.H4.L1

S3.H6.L1
S3.H10.L2
S4.H2.L1

S4.H4.L1
S4.H3.L1
S4.H5.L1
S5.H1.L1
S5.H2.L2

Module: Pickleball
S1.H1.L1
S1.H1.L2)
S2.H1.L1

S2.H2.L1
S2.H2.L2
S2.H3.L1
S2.H3.L2
S2.H5.L1
S2.H5.L2
S3.H4.L1
S3.H6.L1
S3.H10.L1
S3.H10.L2

S4.H2.L1
S4.H3.L1
S4.H4.L1
S4.H5.L1
S5.H1.L1
S5.H2.L2

Module: Tennis
S1.H1.L1
S1.H1.L2

S2.H1.L1
S2.H2.L1
S2.H2.L2
S2.H3.L1
S2.H5.L1
S2.H5.L2
S3.H4.L1
S3.H6.L1
S3.H10.L1
S3.H10.L2

S4.H2.L1
S4.H3.L1
S4.H4.L1
S4.H5.L1
S5.H1.L1
S5.H2.L2

TEAM SPORTS

Module: Basketball
S1.H3.L2
S2.H2.L1
S2.H3.L1
S2.H3.L2
S2.H5.L1
S2.H5.L2
S3.H1.L1
S3.H3.L2
S3.H4.L1
S3.H5.L1
S3.H5.L2
S3.H10.L1
S4.H1.L1

S4.H2.L1
S4.H2.L2
S4.H3.L1
S4.H3.L2
S4.H4.L1
S4.H5.L1
S5.H1.L1
S5.H2.L2
S5.H4.L2

Module: Soccer
S1.H1.L2
S1.H3.L2

S2.H2.L1
S2.H3.L1
S2.H3.L1
S2.H5.L1
S2.H5.L2
S3.H1.L1
S3.H4.L1
S3.H5.L2
S3.H10.L1
S4.H1.L
S4.H2.L1
S4.H2.L2
S4.H3.L1
S4.H3.L2

S4.H4.L1
S4.H5.L1
S5.H1.L1
S5.H2.L2
S5.H4.L1

Module: Volleyball
S1.H1.L1
S1.H1.L2
S2.H1.L1
S2.H2.L1
S2.H2.L2
S2.H3.L1

S2.H5.L1
S2.H5.L2
S3.H4.L1
S3.H6.L1
S3.H10.L1
S3.H10.L2
S4.H2.L1
S4.H3.L1
S4.H4.L1
S4.H5.L1
S5.H1.L1
S5.H2.L2

THROWING ACTIVITIES

Module: Can Jam
S1.H1.L2
S2.H1.L1
S2.H1.L2
S2.H2.L1
S2.H3.L1
S2.H5.L1
S2.H5.L2
S3.H6.L1
S3.H10.L1

S4.H2.L1
S4.H3.L1
S4.H4.L1
S4.H5.L1
S5.H1.L1
S5.H2.L2

Module: Football
S2.H2.L1
S2.H5.L1

S2.H3.L1
S2.H5.L2
S3.H10.L1
S4.H1.L1
S4.H2.L1
S4.H3.L1
S4.H3.L2
S4.H4.L
S4.H5.L1
S5.H1.L1

S5.H2.L2
S5.H4.L1

Module: Velcro Catch Set
S1.H1.L1
S1.H1.L2
S2.H1.L2
S2.H2.L1
S2.H2.L2

S2.H5.L1
S2.H5.L2
S3.H10.L1
S4.H2.L1
S4.H3.L1
S4.H5.L1
S5.H1.L1
S5.H2.L2
S5.H4.L1
S5.H4.L1

STANDARD OUTCOMES FOR THE ANATOMY, JOURNALS, AND GLOSSARY SECTIONS

Section: Careers
S3.H5.L2
S4.H3.L2

Section: Anatomy
S3.M14.7

S3.M14.8
S3.H9.L2

Section: Journals
S3.M16.7
S3.M16.8

S4.M2.7
S4.M2.8
S3.H6.L1
S3.H11.L2

Section: Glossary

S2.H1.L1

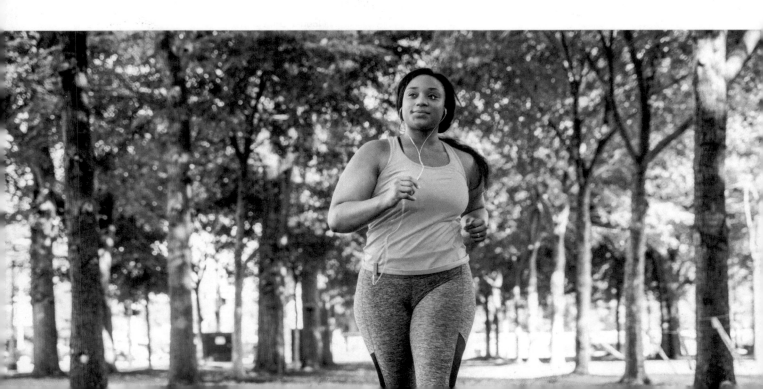